PEDIATRIC THERAPY

· An Interprofessional Framework for Practice ·

T0198155

PEDIATRIC THERAPY
• An Interprofessional Framework for Practice •

Editor

Catherine Rush Thompson, PT, PhD, MS
Professor of Physical Therapy
Physical Therapy Education
Rockhurst University
Kansas City, Missouri

Associate Editors

Ketti Johnson Coffelt, OTD, MS, OTR/L
Assistant Professor of Occupational Therapy
Rockhurst University
Kansas City, Missouri

Pamela Hart, PhD, CCC-SLP
Associate Professor of Communication Sciences and Disorders
Rockhurst University
Kansas City, Missouri

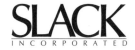

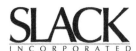

SLACK Incorporated
6900 Grove Road
Thorofare, NJ 08086 USA
856-848-1000   Fax: 856-848-6091
www.Healio.com/books
© 2018 by SLACK Incorporated

Senior Vice President: Stephanie Portnoy
Vice President, Editorial: Jennifer Kilpatrick
Vice President, Marketing: Michelle Gatt
Acquisitions Editor: Tony Schiavo
Managing Editor: Allegra Tiver
Creative Director: Thomas Cavallaro
Cover Artist: Christine Seabo
Project Editor: Joseph Lowery

All contributing authors to this book have no financial interests in any resources shared in this book. All therapists are clinicians and/or academicians who hope to add to the body of knowledge in pediatric therapy.

All rights reserved. No part of this book may be reproduced, stored in a retrieval system or transmitted in any form or by any means, electronic, mechanical, photocopying, recording or otherwise, without written permission from the publisher, except for brief quotations embodied in critical articles and reviews.

The procedures and practices described in this publication should be implemented in a manner consistent with the professional standards set for the circumstances that apply in each specific situation. Every effort has been made to confirm the accuracy of the information presented and to correctly relate generally accepted practices. The authors, editors, and publisher cannot accept responsibility for errors or exclusions or for the outcome of the material presented herein. There is no expressed or implied warranty of this book or information imparted by it. Care has been taken to ensure that drug selection and dosages are in accordance with currently accepted/recommended practice. Off-label uses of drugs may be discussed. Due to continuing research, changes in government policy and regulations, and various effects of drug reactions and interactions, it is recommended that the reader carefully review all materials and literature provided for each drug, especially those that are new or not frequently used. Some drugs or devices in this publication have clearance for use in a restricted research setting by the Food and Drug and Administration or FDA. Each professional should determine the FDA status of any drug or device prior to use in their practice.

Any review or mention of specific companies or products is not intended as an endorsement by the author or publisher.

SLACK Incorporated uses a review process to evaluate submitted material. Prior to publication, educators or clinicians provide important feedback on the content that we publish. We welcome feedback on this work.

Library of Congress Cataloging-in-Publication Data

Names: Thompson, Catherine Rush, 1954- editor. | Coffelt, Ketti Johnson,
    editor. | Hart, Pamela (Associate professor of communication sciences and
    disorders), editor.
Title: Pediatric therapy : an interprofessional framework for practice /
    editor, Catherine Rush Thompson ; associate editors, Ketti Johnson
    Coffelt, Pamela Hart.
Other titles: Pediatric therapy (Thompson)
Description: Thorofare, NJ : SLACK Incorporated, [2018] | Includes
    bibliographical references and index.
Identifiers: LCCN 2018000340 (print) | LCCN 2018000721 (ebook) | ISBN
    9781630911782 (Epub) | ISBN 9781630911690 (Web) | ISBN 9781630911775
    (paperback : alk. paper)
Subjects: | MESH: Pediatrics--methods | Interprofessional Relations |
    Intersectoral Collaboration | Cooperative Behavior | Clinical Competence |
    Child | Adolescent | Infant
Classification: LCC RJ499.3 (ebook) | LCC RJ499.3 (print) | NLM WS 366 | DDC
    618.92/89--dc23
LC record available at https://lccn.loc.gov/2018000340

For permission to reprint material in another publication, contact SLACK Incorporated. Authorization to photocopy items for internal, personal, or academic use is granted by SLACK Incorporated provided that the appropriate fee is paid directly to Copyright Clearance Center. Prior to photocopying items, please contact the Copyright Clearance Center at 222 Rosewood Drive, Danvers, MA 01923 USA; phone: 978-750-8400; website: www.copyright.com; email: info@copyright.com

Printed in the United States of America.

Last digit is print number: 10   9   8   7   6   5   4   3   2   1

DEDICATION

*"I wanted a perfect ending. Now I've learned, the hard way, that
some poems don't rhyme, and some stories don't have a clear beginning,
middle, and end. Life is about not knowing, having to change,
taking the movement and making the best of it,
without knowing what's going to happen next.
Delicious Ambiguity."*
—Gilda Radner

We dedicate this book to our own families who have provided support in our professional and personal lives, to our students who have asked the challenging questions that explore ambiguity and inspire critical thinking, to our colleagues who have shared their professional expertise, and, *most importantly*, to those families who have inspired us and trusted us with their children's care. It has been a privilege to learn and to grow together.

CONTENTS

ACKNOWLEDGMENTS

"Alone we can do so little; together we can do so much."
—Helen Keller

We would personally like to thank our professional colleagues who have supported this effort and provided valuable insight regarding the importance of interprofessionalism for pediatric therapists. More specifically, we would like to thank those who contributed their time and effort to this book through authoring and reviewing the book's contents for accuracy and relevance. We are also indebted to family members, friends, students, and families who provided an incentive for developing a manual promoting interprofessional care for children and their families.

ABOUT THE PRIMARY EDITOR

Catherine Rush Thompson, PT, PhD, MS is a professor in the Department of Physical Therapy Education at Rockhurst University in Kansas City, Missouri, and a consultant for Community Living Opportunities—helping individuals with developmental disabilities achieve fulfilling lives in the community. Her pediatric therapy experience spans over 40 years, including owning a private practice and working alongside pediatric professionals serving pediatric populations and their families. Catherine has practiced in early intervention, home-based therapy, and educational, medical, and community-based settings, offering screenings and child- and family-centered care to infants, children, adolescents, adults, and older adults with and without developmental disabilities and other health care needs. With research and teaching experience in health promotion, pediatrics, motor imagery, neurorehabilitation, professional development, and clinical decision making, as well as interprofessional service in Ecuador, Guatemala, Haiti, and Kyrgyzstan, she brings a deep appreciation of interprofessional collaboration and cultural competency for providing high-quality care to all communities. Her most recent publication, *Prevention Practice and Health Promotion: A Health Care Professional's Guide to Health, Fitness, and Wellness, Second Edition*, addresses health care issues across the lifespan and emphasizes holistic care. She hopes that *Pediatric Therapy: An Interprofessional Framework for Practice* will provide a foundation for engaging students and clinicians in interprofessional discussions and activities that will enhance the quality of care in pediatrics.

ABOUT THE ASSOCIATE EDITORS

Ketti Johnson Coffelt, OTD, MS, OTR/L is a professor in the Department of Occupational Therapy Education at Rockhurst University and an occupational therapist for the Olathe School District, providing consultative services with students receiving extensive homebound services due to medically related variables. She has over 28 years of experience as an occupational therapist, working primarily in pediatrics and school systems. She has served on many school teams as a team member and as a facilitator, developing and implementing student Individualized Education Programs (IEPs), mentoring team members, and participating in collaborative consultation with other educational professionals. She saw firsthand the value of forming effective preschool- and school-age early intervention teams with other professionals and families to facilitate a shared partnership and commitment to meeting each child's ever-changing learning needs. Her collaborative teaming experiences bring a depth of understanding of the opportunities and challenges of the interprofessional team collaborative process used to support children and youth learning. Her research endeavors include a peer-reviewed publication, *Continuing Competence Trends of Occupational Therapy Practitioner*, and critical appraisal of the effectiveness of visual task sequencing in the establishment of skills and routines of children with disabilities. She has presented at regional and national professional occupational therapy conferences, with research focused on the use of video modeling with tasks in the home environment for children and adults with disabilities and on exploring the sensory-adaptive approach of pressure undergarments for children with attention deficit/hyperactivity disorder.

Pamela Hart, PhD, CCC-SLP is an associate professor in the Department of Communication Sciences and Disorders at Rockhurst University. She teaches and conducts research in the areas of augmentative and alternative communication, autism spectrum disorders, research methods, and child language disorders. Of specific interest to Dr. Hart is the qualitative study of the ways that rehabilitation and educational teams work together to provide interdisciplinary services to clients with complex communication needs to support language and literacy development. She has numerous national and regional presentations and publications related to this topic. Clinically, Dr. Hart provides speech-language pathology services as part of an interdisciplinary team that evaluates and implements treatments for individuals who are nonverbal and require augmentative and alternative communication strategies. She has many years of experience working alongside occupational therapists, physical therapists, educators, and others with the goal of helping individuals with complex needs to meet their highest potential. The combination of Dr. Hart's research interests and clinical experiences provide a strong basis for the concepts presented in this book. Her publications and presentations include, but are not limited to, effective teaming, facilitation of language with clients using augmentative and alternative communication, play and technology in early childhood, assistive technology for literacy interventions, interventions for children with complex communication needs and physical impairments, educational placement decisions for children with complex communication needs, and improving graduate students' skills and confidence through structured lab experiences. She brings a wealth of clinical and educational experience to her writing.

CONTRIBUTING AUTHORS

Joan Delahunt, OTD, MS, OTR/L (Sections 9 & 10)
Assistant Professor of Occupational Therapy
Rockhurst University
Kansas City, Missouri

Brandi Dorton, DPT (Section 10)
Physical Therapist
Physical and Occupational Therapy
Children's Mercy Hospital
Kansas City, Missouri

Lynn Drazinski, MA, CCC-SLP (Section 10)
Professional Faculty
Communication Sciences and Disorders
Augustana College
Rock Island, Illinois

Carol Koch, EdD, CCC-SLP (Section 6)
Associate Professor of Communication Sciences and
Disorders
Samford University
Birmingham, Alabama

Lauren Little, PhD, OTR/L (Section 7)
Assistant Professor
Department of Occupation Therapy
Rush University
Chicago, Illinois

Grace McConnell, PhD, CCC-SLP (Section 5)
Assistant Professor of
Communication Sciences and Disorders
Rockhurst University
Kansas City, Missouri

Mildred Oligbo, PT, DPT (Section 9)
Clinical Assistant Professor of Physical Therapy
University of Kansas Medical Center
Kansas City, Kansas

Stephanie Orr, PT, DPT, PCS (Section 10)
Physical Therapist
Pediatric Certified Specialist
Physical and Occupational Therapy
Children's Mercy Hospital
Kansas City, Missouri

PREFACE

"Interprofessional education is a collaborative approach to develop healthcare students as future interprofessional team members and a recommendation suggested by the Institute of Medicine. Complex medical issues can be best addressed by interprofessional teams. Training future healthcare providers to work in such teams will help facilitate this model resulting in improved healthcare outcomes for patients."[1]

This book is designed to engage clinicians and students in interprofessional learning experiences that cultivate collaborative practice and optimize the outcomes of those served. According to the American Speech-Language-Hearing Association, "There is a growing emphasis on interprofessional education in health care as a result of research demonstrating the benefits of interprofessional collaborations in health care that require continuous interaction, coordinated efforts, and knowledge sharing among healthcare professionals."[2] These ongoing interprofessional interactions are especially important for pediatric therapists serving families whose children are dynamically growing and developing new skills.

Pediatric therapies typically include physical therapy, occupational therapy, and speech-language pathology. Other valuable team members include family members, medical and nursing staff, special educators, case workers, and others engaged in a child's care and education.

When working with families and other professionals and paraprofessionals, all team members benefit from competency in key pediatric skills, whether services are provided in the classroom, clinic, school, or community. Common foundational knowledge across all disciplines includes[2-7]:

- Recognizing philosophies and frameworks underlying pediatric care (eg, child- and family-centered care)
- Screening for typical growth and development
- Assessing the abilities of infants, children, youth, and adolescents in various situations
- Performing standardized and criterion-referenced tests and measures of infants, children, youth, and adolescents
- Recognizing legal and ethical issues impacting pediatric care
- Addressing unique issues related to specific practice settings
- Using the clinical reasoning process for designing and modifying interventions
- Implementing evidence-based practice

This manual will provide learners across disciplines with learning experiences emphasizing foundational knowledge and essential skills for effective interprofessional collaboration in pediatric settings. These skills include[3-9]:

- Recognizing typical and atypical development of children from birth to adulthood
- Realizing the importance of holistic care
- Respecting the roles, frames of reference, and approaches favored by each discipline
- Providing services within the scope of practice determined by professional and legal standards
- Developing essential skills for interprofessional care to improve health care and educational outcomes for children and their families

Each section of this manual offers learning objectives, key concepts, and case-based learning activities requiring integration of information and critical reasoning. The appendices offer additional opportunities for interprofessional engagement. Common pediatric conditions discussed in this manual include autism spectrum disorder, cerebral palsy, developmental delay (including children "at risk" for developmental delay), Down syndrome, and other common health impairments. Although this manual does not outline specific pediatric pathologies and their discipline-specific management, it encourages learners to explore current evidence-based literature to understand the most recent developments related to pediatric pathologies and their management. Using interprofessional skills, professionals can embrace their distinctive roles in pediatric care while sharing theoretical frameworks and therapeutic approaches across practice settings. The ultimate goal is to improve the child's and family's quality of life.

Upon completion of this manual, learners should be able to demonstrate the following interprofessional skills:

- Discuss the roles and responsibilities of professionals providing pediatric care
- Describe family-centered, routine-based care and its importance in healthy growth and development
- Differentiate pediatric care provided in the home, schools, and medical settings
- Select valid and reliable tests and measures of growth and development of infants, toddlers, youth, and adolescents
- Collaborate with others in the development of goals and evidence-based pediatric interventions
- Select and design appropriate interprofessional interventions for children with special needs and their caregivers
- Educate others about preventive care for healthy growth and development
- Discuss current, evidence-based resources for children, their families, and others
- Engage in interprofessional clinical reasoning to address common problems faced in dynamic pediatric practice

Overall, this manual is designed to offer learners a guide for developing interprofessional competencies needed in pediatric therapeutic practice settings.

REFERENCES

1. Bridges DR, Davidson RA, Odegard PS, Maki IV, Tomkowiak J. Interprofessional collaboration: three best practice models of interprofessional education. *Med Educ Online*. 2011;16(10). http://www.tandfonline.com/doi/full/10.3402/meo.v16i0.6035. Accessed February 2, 2017.
2. Interprofessional education and its impact on the education of audiologists and speech-language pathologists. American Speech-Language-Hearing Association Web site. http://www.asha.org/Articles/Interprofessional-Education-and-its-Impact-on-the-Education-of-Audiologists-and-Speech-Language-Pathologists/. Published June 2008. Accessed May 2, 2017.
3. Interprofessional Education Collaborative. Core competencies for interprofessional collaborative practice: Report of an expert panel. American Association of Colleges of Nursing Web site. http://www.aacn.nche.edu/education-resources/ipecreport.pdf. Published 2011. Accessed May 2, 2017.
4. Interprofessional Education and Collaborative Practice Resources. American Physical Therapy Association Web site. http://www.apta.org/Educators/Curriculum/Interprofessional/. Published March 31, 2017. Accessed May 2, 2017.
5. Goldberg LR. The importance of interprofessional education for students in communication sciences and disorders. *Commun Disord Q*. 2014;35:3-4.
6. Rapport MJ, Furze J, Martin K, et al. Essential competencies in entry-level pediatric physical therapy education. *Pediatr Phys Ther*. 2014;26(1):7-18.
7. American Occupational Therapy Association. Importance of interprofessional education in occupational therapy curricula. *Am J Occup Ther*. 2015;69:1-14.
8. Pecukonis E, Doyle O, Bliss DL. Reducing barriers to interprofessional training: promoting interprofessional cultural competence. *J Interprof Care*. 2008;22:417-428.
9. Poulton BC, West MA. The determinants of effectiveness in primary health care teams. *J Interprof Care*. 1999;13:7-18.

Section 1

Interprofessional Approaches to Pediatric Practice

Catherine Rush Thompson, PT, PhD, MS and Pamela Hart, PhD, CCC-SLP

OVERVIEW

This first section sets the tone for the entire book by describing and delineating *interprofessional competencies* for pediatric therapists and those unique to each profession, referred to as *complementary competencies*. Given the importance of understanding other professionals' roles and responsibilities, this section further provides an outline of the various professionals typically encountered in pediatric care. It then describes the importance of role clarification, collaborative leadership, and team functioning as key interprofessional competencies needed for effective teamwork, emphasizing the importance of appreciating the complementary competencies that define the roles and responsibilities of other team members. Finally, it describes the various team approaches used in pediatric care, including intradisciplinary, multidisciplinary, interdisciplinary, transdisciplinary, and collaborative team approaches.

INTERPROFESSIONAL COMPETENCIES

Interprofessional skills go beyond those practiced exclusively by those providing individualized care for children. This skill set recognizes key competencies for collaboration with other professionals when making decisions that impact all those providing care and those receiving care. These skills are referred to as *interprofessional competencies*.

What are these interprofessional competencies and how were they determined? Recognizing that effective teamwork is essential to family-centered care, experts in public health and health care began determining interprofessional competencies by exploring competencies expected of all health professionals, or *common competencies*.[1] These interprofessional competencies were compared with those that were deemed unique or defining of each profession, or *complementary competencies*. Finally, the common competencies that were considered essential for effective collaboration were identified as interprofessional competencies, as illustrated in Figure 1-1. Interprofessional competencies are those common competencies that should be developed to ensure effective teamwork when providing care.

In *Core Competencies for Interprofessional Collaborative Practice*, an expert panel from the Interprofessional Education Collaborative representing public health and health care fields distinguished the following 4 domains for what they determined to be core interprofessional competencies.[1] Each of these 4 domains is based upon a guiding principle that describes the domain and provides the basis of the competencies within that domain. The 4 domains are as follows:

Thompson CR. *Pediatric Therapy:
An Interprofessional Framework for Practice* (pp 1-13).
© 2018 SLACK Incorporated.

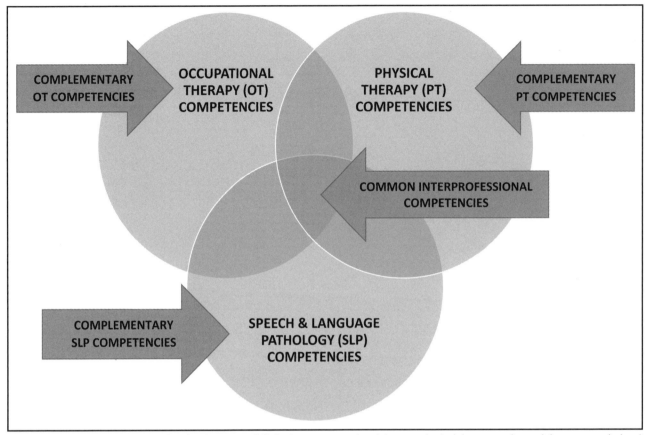

Figure 1-1. This diagram illustrates the complementary skills (unique to occupational therapy, physical therapy, and speech language pathology) and overlapping interprofessional skills that are shared across professions. These interprofessional competencies lay the foundation for effective teamwork.

1. *Competency Domain 1: Values/Ethics for Interprofessional Practice*[1]: The key principle for this domain is expressed in the following statement: *Work with individuals of other professions to maintain a climate of mutual respect and shared values.* In addition to abiding by professional values and standards, each professional is expected to share common values and ethics for interprofessional practice. This principle is supported by 10 interprofessional competencies, as outlined in Table 1-1.

2. *Competency Domain 2: Roles/Responsibilities*[1]: The second domain is based upon another key principle: *Use the knowledge of one's own role and those of other professions to appropriately assess and address the health care needs of the patients and populations served.* This guiding principle lays the foundation for its corresponding 8 competencies, as outlined in Table 1-2.

3. *Competency Domain 3: Interprofessional Communication*[1]: This competency focuses on the importance of communication with others, as outlined in the following statement: *Communicate with patients, families, communities, and other health*

professionals in a responsive and responsible manner that supports a team approach to the maintenance of health and the treatment of disease. This domain includes 8 competencies that address key communication skills, as outlined in Table 1-3.

4. *Competency Domain 4: Teams and Teamwork*[1]: The final domain emphasizes the importance of teamwork and is guided by the following statement: *Apply relationship-building values and the principles of team dynamics to perform effectively in different team roles to plan and deliver patient-/population-centered care that is safe, timely, efficient, effective, and equitable.* This domain incorporates 11 competencies that address key teamwork skills essential for interprofessional collaboration, as outlined in Table 1-4.

All of the competencies incorporate principles and values embraced by pediatric therapists. All therapists agree that care should be *patient centered* and community oriented. From the pediatric therapist's perspective, care should be *child centered, family centered,* and *context specific* to ensure success in all environments. In addition, care should focus on *relationship building,* so therapists must build trust with

	TABLE 1-1
	VALUES AND ETHICS COMPETENCIES
VE1	Place the interests of patients and populations at the center of interprofessional health care delivery.
VE2	Respect the dignity and privacy of patients while maintaining confidentiality in the delivery of team-based care.
VE3	Embrace the cultural diversity and individual differences that characterize patients, populations, and health care team.
VE4	Respect the unique cultures, values, roles/responsibilities, and expertise of other health professions.
VE5	Work in cooperation with those who receive care, those who provide care, and others who contribute to or support the delivery of prevention and health services.
VE6	Develop a trusting relationship with patients, families, and other team members.
VE7	Demonstrate high standards of ethical conduct and quality of care in one's contributions to team-based care.
VE8	Manage ethical dilemmas specific to interprofessional patient-/population-centered care situations.
VE9	Act with honesty and integrity in relationships with patients, families, and other team members.
VE10	Maintain competence in one's own profession appropriate to scope of practice.
	Adapted from Interprofessional Education Collaborative. Core Competencies for Interprofessional Collaborative Practice. American Association of Colleges of Nursing Web site. https://nexusipe-resource-exchange.s3-us-west-2.amazonaws.com/IPEC_CoreCompetencies_2011.pdf. Published 2016. Accessed May 2, 2017.

	TABLE 1-2
	ROLES AND RESPONSIBILITIES COMPETENCIES
RR1	Communicate one's roles and responsibilities clearly to patients, families, and other professionals.
RR2	Recognize one's limitations in skills, knowledge, and abilities.
RR3	Engage diverse health care professionals who complement one's own professional expertise, as well as associated resources, to develop strategies to meet specific patient care needs.
RR4	Explain the roles and responsibilities of other care providers and how the team works together to provide care.
RR5	Use the full scope of knowledge, skills, and abilities of available health professionals and health care workers to provide care that is safe, timely, efficient, effective, and equitable.
RR6	Communicate with team members to clarify each member's responsibility in executing components of a treatment plan or public health intervention.
RR7	Forge interdependent relationships with other professions to improve care and advance learning.
RR8	Engage in continuous professional and interprofessional development to enhance team performance.
	Adapted from Interprofessional Education Collaborative. Core Competencies for Interprofessional Collaborative Practice. American Association of Colleges of Nursing Web site. https://nexusipe-resource-exchange.s3-us-west-2.amazonaws.com/IPEC_CoreCompetencies_2011.pdf. Published 2016. Accessed May 2, 2017.

TABLE 1-3

INTERPROFESSIONAL COMMUNICATION COMPETENCIES

CC1	Choose effective communication tools and techniques, including information systems and communication technologies, to facilitate discussions and interactions that enhance team function.
CC2	Organize and communicate information with patients, families, and health care team members in a form that is understandable, avoiding discipline-specific terminology when possible.
CC3	Express one's knowledge and opinions to team members involved in patient care with confidence, clarity, and respect, working to ensure common understanding of information and treatment and care decisions.
CC4	Listen actively and encourage ideas and opinions of other team members.
CC5	Give timely, sensitive, instructive feedback to others about their performance on the team, responding respectfully as a team member to feedback from others.
CC6	Use respectful language appropriate for a given difficult situation, crucial conversation, or interprofessional conflict.
CC7	Recognize how one's own uniqueness, including experience level, expertise, culture, power, and hierarchy within the health care team, contributes to effective communication, conflict resolution, and positive interprofessional working relationships.
CC8	Consistently c ommunicate the importance of teamwork in patient-centered and community-focused care.

Adapted from Interprofessional Education Collaborative. Core Competencies for Interprofessional Collaborative Practice. American Association of Colleges of Nursing Web site. https://nexusipe-resource-exchange.s3-us-west-2.amazonaws.com/IPEC_CoreCompetencies_2011.pdf. Published 2016. Accessed May 2, 2017.

TABLE 1-4

TEAMS AND TEAMWORK INTERPROFESSIONAL COMPETENCIES

TT1	Describe the process of team development and the roles and practices of effective teams.
TT2	Develop consensus on the ethical principles to guide all aspects of patient care and teamwork.
TT3	Engage other health professionals—appropriate to the specific care situation—in shared patient-centered problem solving.
TT4	Integrate the knowledge and experience of other professions—appropriate to the specific care situation—to inform care decisions while respecting patient and community values and priorities/preferences for care.
TT5	Apply leadership practices that support collaborative practice and team effectiveness.
TT6	Engage self and others to constructively manage disagreements about values, roles, goals, and actions that arise among health care professionals and with patients and families.
TT7	Share accountability with other professions, patients, and communities for outcomes relevant to prevention and health care.
TT8	Reflect on individual and team performance for individual, as well as team, performance improvement.
TT9	Use process improvement strategies to increase the effectiveness of interprofessional teamwork and team-based care.
TT10	Use available evidence to inform effective teamwork and team-based practices.
TT11	Perform effectively on teams and in different team roles in a variety of settings.

Adapted from Interprofessional Education Collaborative. Core Competencies for Interprofessional Collaborative Practice. American Association of Colleges of Nursing Web site. https://nexusipe-resource-exchange.s3-us-west-2.amazonaws.com/IPEC_CoreCompetencies_2011.pdf. Published 2016. Accessed May 2, 2017.

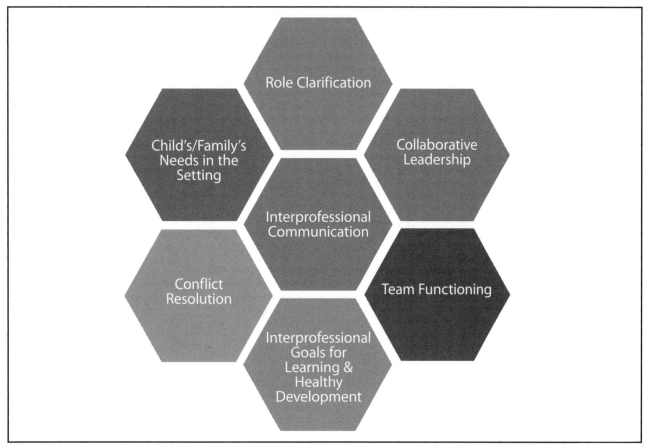

Figure 1-2. This diagram illustrates key interprofessional competencies essential to pediatric care.

children, their families, and others to ensure support and carryover between all settings, including the home, school, and community. Considerable evidence suggests that trust in clinicians is based upon (1) the clinician's technical competence, (2) respect for the family's/client's views, (3) sharing of relevant information, and (4) the client's own confidence in managing his or her illness.[2,3] Because parents play an essential role in their children's care, empowering children and their families to help manage health- and education-related issues through advocacy and self-advocacy are key elements of building trust in pediatrics.

As critical thinkers, pediatric therapists appreciate that interprofessional collaboration is *process oriented*. Shared decision making is an ongoing effort that requires continual assessment and critical input from all involved in care. Collaborative efforts ensure that children are engaged in *developmentally appropriate* learning activities and that therapists use educational strategies and behavioral assessments that guide their interactions with all involved. These efforts should be well integrated across the learning continuum and sensitive to differences in settings (eg, home, community, clinic, school).

To facilitate effective interprofessional collaboration, professionals need a common language and understanding of professional roles and responsibilities. Most importantly, team members must work toward common outcomes that address the goals of the child and family.

One framework, the National Interprofessional Competency (NIC) framework, describes competencies required for effective *interprofessional care*.[4] The NIC framework suggests key competencies foundational to collaborative decision making that honors the knowledge, skills, values, and experience of all involved. Figure 1-2 illustrates these key competencies deemed essential to interprofessional care.

This interprofessional framework offers key concepts that can be adapted to pediatric settings[4]:

1. *Role Clarification*: All team members must understand their own role, as well as the roles of others on their team. Respecting each other's roles and knowledge contributes to establishing and meeting appropriate goals.

2. *Child-/Family-/School-Centered Care*: Team members must value the input and engagement of each person, including the child, family members, community members, and others involved in the child's life.

3. *Interprofessional Communication*: All team members must clearly communicate with each other in a collaborative, responsive, respectful, and responsible manner. Professionals must be thoughtful in sharing and collecting information, allocating sufficient time to listen carefully to family members and other professionals working on the team.

4. *Conflict Resolution*: Team members must be able to deal with interprofessional conflict and problem solving that best meets the needs of children and their families. Factors that can reduce team conflict include (1) delineating a clear purpose or agenda for meetings, (2) determining a manageable team size and team composition, (3) having organizational support, (4) scheduling convenient team meetings, (5) developing clear goals and objectives, (6) reflecting on what is effective for reaching team goals and objectives, and (7) being open to needed changes.[5]

5. *Team Functioning*: All professional team members must appreciate the principles of team dynamics and group processes for effective interprofessional collaboration. Table 1-5 illustrates some characteristics of effective team dynamics and group processes, reinforcing the interprofessional competencies needed in pediatric care.

6. *Collaborative Leadership*: Decision making is not top-down or bottom-up; collaboration between team members should allow every voice to be equally heard and understood. All team members should work together to formulate a plan to meet the needs of each child and family, to implement the plan, and to evaluate the effectiveness of the plan. As needed, the plan can be modified to enhance the child's outcomes. The partnership between everyone on the team must be participatory, collaborative, and coordinated to ensure ongoing decision making that addresses the complex issues facing each child.

SCOPES OF PRACTICE FOR THERAPISTS AND OTHERS WORKING IN PEDIATRIC SETTINGS

All team members must understand and respect the knowledge of others. The scope of practice of therapists and paraprofessionals working in pediatric settings is supported by their respective professional organizations, such as the American Physical Therapy Association (APTA), the American Occupational Therapy Association (AOTA), and the American Speech-Language-Hearing Association (ASHA). The following are definitions of each professional with definitions of their practice expertise:

Physical therapists have advanced degrees (doctoral training), pass a national licensure examination, and are licensed by each state to work with individuals across their lifespan to manage pain and improve or restore mobility. Physical therapists are uniquely "movement experts" who examine all body systems and functions (musculoskeletal, neuromuscular, cardiopulmonary, integumentary, and other body systems) to determine how they contribute to postural control and mobility. Physical therapists evaluate growth, psychosocial and physical development, motor skills related to daily activities, and each individual's roles in life, as well as environmental, personal, and other factors that could impact any individual's ability to move and to participate fully and optimally in life, whether it be at home, school, work, or during leisure activities. Physical therapists provide professional care in a wide range of settings, including, but not limited to, hospitals, private practices, outpatient clinics, home health agencies, schools, sports and fitness facilities, work settings, and nursing homes. According to the Academy of Pediatric Physical Therapy:

> Pediatric physical therapists use their expertise in movement and apply clinical reasoning through the process of examination, evaluation, diagnosis, and intervention. As primary health care providers, physical therapists also promote health and wellness as they implement a wide variety of supports for children from infancy through adolescence in collaboration with their families and other medical, educational, developmental, and rehabilitation specialists. Pediatric physical therapy promotes independence, increases participation, facilitates motor development and function, improves strength and endurance, enhances learning opportunities, and eases challenges with daily caregiving.[6]

In many practice settings, *physical therapist assistants* assist in care. According to the APTA, physical therapist assistants "provide physical therapy services under the direction and supervision of a licensed physical therapist. Physical therapist assistants help people of all ages who have medical problems, or other health-related conditions that limit their ability to move and perform functional activities in their daily lives."[7] In the school setting, physical therapists provide consultation and support to staff to improve students' educational performance related to functional gross motor development, whereas physical therapist assistants help with therapeutic activities designed to support educational goals. In the hospital setting, physical therapist assistants provide health education and physical therapy interventions to improve their patients' health and wellness.

Another therapist commonly seen in pediatric settings is the *occupational therapist*. The AOTA describes the scope of practice of occupational therapy as "the therapeutic use of occupations, including everyday life activities, with

TABLE 1-5
DYNAMICS AND GROUP PROCESSES FOR PEDIATRIC INTERPROFESSIONAL TEAMS

CATEGORY	CHARACTERISTICS
Child/family focused	• Focuses care on the child and family • Recognizes need for holistic care for child and family • Values child's and family's needs and goals • Provides timely interventions to match needs
Culture	• Supports an interprofessional atmosphere, valuing contributions of all team members • Nurtures consensus, providing a safe environment for sharing ideas • Works toward common goals • Uses a proactive/health promotion approach • Facilitates an environment for team meetings (eg, adequate time for meeting preparation, discussion at meeting, and follow-up; convenient location for team meeting; good representation of those impacted by decision making; capacity of team members is clear; organization provides support; meetings are documented with decisions made)
Communication	• Holds regular case conferences to share information • Communicates both formally and informally • Shares information to ensure a holistic perspective • Possesses strong listening and clear communication skills • Avoids use of jargon
Learning	• Recognizes the need to learn with others • Supports a culture that enhances interprofessional learning and development of cultural competencies • Explores creative solutions to unique pediatric challenges
Roles and responsibilities	• Understands own and others' roles and responsibilities • Brings a high level of professional competency, knowledge, and skills • Provides a positive role model for the profession represented • Recognizes the need to practice professional autonomy, if needed • Incorporates resources for team building
Team members	• Recognizes the optimal size and structure for team needs • Appreciates contributions of all team members • Explores and accepts overlapping role(s) • Recognizes professional synergy through mutual support • Tolerates different opinions and perceptions • Recognizes the need for lateral leadership • Recognizes the level of learning of each team member
Adapted from Nancarrow S, Booth A, Ariss S, Smith T, Enderby P, Roots R. Ten principles of good interdisciplinary team work. *Hum Resour Health*. 2013;11:19.	

individuals, groups, populations, or organizations to support participation, performance, and function in roles and situations in home, school, workplace, community, and other settings."[8] As stated by Trombly, "Occupational therapists are experts in occupational functioning."[9] This role is evident across practice settings, similar to those of physical therapists, but also including mental health facilities. School-based occupational therapists use their knowledge of occupation areas (ie, activities of daily living, instrumental activities of daily living, rest and sleep, education, work, play, leisure and social participation) to assess and select interventions considering the limitations of the child and the activity demands within the school environment for optimal academic and nonacademic performance. In the school setting, occupational therapists provide services to students, supporting their educational and functional needs related to sensory responsiveness, motor performance, perceptual processing, and psychosocial and cognitive abilities.[10] Occupational therapists practicing in schools have strongly recognized the importance of providing support and collaborating with educational professionals, school staff, and the families of the children they serve.[11]

Similar to physical therapist assistants, *certified occupational therapy assistants* and *occupational therapy aides* are supervised by occupational therapists and perform activities that enhance occupational services in educational and medical practice settings.[12] In the school setting, certified occupational therapy assistants provide quality skilled occupational therapy services to children and consult with teachers and school staff under the direction of an occupational therapist. Certified occupational therapy assistants can contribute to all facets of school-based services with adherence to federal and state laws and AOTA documents.[12]

Speech-language pathologists play an important role in pediatric settings to help establish effective communication and safe feeding and swallowing strategies for young clients. According to ASHA:

> The speech-language pathologist is the professional who engages in clinical services, prevention, advocacy, education, administration, and research in the areas of communication and swallowing across the lifespan from infancy through geriatrics. Speech-language pathologists address typical and atypical impairments and disorders related to communication and swallowing in the areas of speech sound production, resonance, voice, fluency, language (comprehension and expression), cognition, and feeding and swallowing.[13]

In the school setting, speech-language pathologists provide assessment and intervention services for students with disorders in speech, language, cognition, swallowing/dysphagia, fluency, and/or voice. These disorders may be the result of developmental disabilities, hearing impairment, traumatic brain injury, cleft palate, or learning disabilities to name a few.

Speech-language pathology assistants are defined by ASHA as "support personnel who, following academic coursework, fieldwork, and on-the-job training, perform tasks prescribed, directed, and supervised by ASHA-certified speech-language pathologists."[14]

Physical therapists, occupational therapists, and speech-language pathologists are commonly seen working in both hospital and school settings. Similarly, nurses provide a valuable health care link in educational settings. *Nursing* involves "the protection, promotion, and optimization of health and abilities, prevention of illness and injury, facilitation of healing, alleviation of suffering through the diagnosis and treatment of human response, and advocacy in the care of individuals, families, groups, communities, and populations," according to the American Medical Association.[15] Although most nurses work in general medical and surgical hospitals, many work in elementary and secondary schools to provide health services on site.

A broad range of specialists work predominantly in medical vs educational settings. The following are some professionals who are most commonly encountered in these settings. For those not listed, therapists should consult professional websites and job descriptions for team members, as well as appreciate the experience that each individual contributes to interprofessional collaboration.

MEDICAL TEAMS

Medical care facilities are typically where specialists deal with acute and emergent medical conditions and recovery from illness. The emphasis in pediatric medical settings is on promoting a child's recovery to function and stabilizing a child's physiological and structural integrity. In addition to physical therapists, occupational therapists, speech-language pathologists, and nurses, children and their families engage with a wide range of health care professionals to manage acute and chronic conditions. Interprofessional teams in hospitals may include therapists, nurses, physicians, physician assistants, audiologists, recreation therapists, nutrition specialists, social workers, family members, and others. The following are team members commonly encountered in medical settings.

Physicians are medical experts who serve as the heads of medical teams in most health care settings. According to the American Medical Association (AMA), physician-led team-based health care is defined as "the consistent use by a physician of the leadership knowledge, skills, and expertise necessary to identify, engage, and elicit from each team member the unique set of training, experience, and qualifications needed to help patients achieve their goals, and to supervise the application of these skills."[15] In pediatrics, the specialists commonly seen by children include neonatologists, pediatricians, neurologists, cardiologists, urologists, orthopedists, physiatrists, and other experts who deal with childhood pathologies.

Physician assistants practice medicine on teams with physicians, surgeons, and other health care workers. They are licensed to diagnose and treat illness and disease and to prescribe medication for patients. They commonly work in physician's offices, hospitals, and clinics in collaboration with a licensed physician.[16]

Audiologists provide assessment and intervention services to individuals with disorders affecting auditory and/or balance function. Specific roles include prevention of hearing loss, assessment of hearing loss, fitting individuals with hearing aids and other assistive devices, as well as services to help individuals with cochlear implants achieve their highest level of function.[17]

Recreational therapists design therapeutic recreation, involving planning, directing, and coordinating recreation-based treatment programs for people with disabilities, injuries, or illnesses.[18] In the hospital setting, therapeutic recreation uses a range of leisure activities as interventions to engage children in problem solving. Activities can include games, sports, parties, and music.

A *nutrition specialist* holds a license to practice dietetics and nutrition services, whereas a *licensed dietitian* facilitates nutrition therapy. They are responsible for encouraging healthy food choices, assessing and coordinating nutritional menus, and working with families to encourage appropriate diets.[19] Nutrition specialists are typically employed at hospitals; however, they also provide consultation to schools and communities.

Social workers are highly trained and experienced professionals. According to the National Association of Social Workers, only those who have earned social work degrees at the bachelor's, master's, or doctoral level and have completed a minimum number of hours in supervised fieldwork are professional social workers.[20,21] Those working in pediatrics will most likely encounter social workers in schools, hospitals, mental health clinics, and numerous public and private agencies that serve individuals and families in need.[20,21]

Interprofessional team members and administrative staff in a hospital setting must collaborate efficiently and effectively to ensure that families transition into and out of medical care as easily as possible. This transition includes the provision of community resources and referrals to help children and their families optimally return to their daily lives.

TEAM MEMBERS IN THE SCHOOL SETTING

Team members in the school setting are committed to the education of all children and offer their expertise to help children achieve academic goals. Pediatric therapists will most likely encounter teachers (including special education teachers), counselors, school psychologists, resource specialists, and adaptive physical educators.

Teachers serve multiple roles in educational settings. Most importantly, school teachers educate our nation's children and adolescents about the world, teaching foundational knowledge and skills and engaging them in learning activities to develop their critical thinking skills. They develop lesson plans designed to teach their subjects, such as mathematics, reading, science, and social studies, and help students develop interpersonal communication skills. Teachers serve as role models for their students and encourage student development through exploration and discovery. In the school setting, teachers work diligently with support staff to help students meet educational goals and achieve academic success. Teachers evaluate the abilities and weaknesses of their students. They play a key role in identifying students who struggle with learning and making referrals to special education services.

Special education teachers are educators who are specially trained to work with students who have a wide range of learning, mental, emotional, and physical disabilities. As team leaders in the school setting, special education teachers provide direct and indirect instructional support and behavioral strategies to students' learning. Oftentimes, they must modify the general education curriculum for students with disabilities based upon a variety of instructional techniques and technologies and consult closely with pediatric therapists to optimize each student's outcomes.[22]

Counselors empower children and their families to accomplish mental health and wellness. The American Counseling Association notes that *professional counselors* are "graduate level (either master's or doctoral degree) mental health service providers, trained to work with individuals, families, and groups in treating mental, behavioral, and emotional problems and disorders."[23]

The *school psychologist* assists in the identification of the intellectual, social, and emotional needs of students. Their entry-level education for school psychology includes a specialist-level or master's degree in psychology and state licensure.[24] Given their specialized training, psychologists provide consultation and support to families and staff regarding behavior and conditions related to learning. They also plan behavioral programs to meet the special needs of children and often serve as facilitators during interprofessional team meetings to determine individualized programs for students.

Resource specialists are licensed or certified teachers who provide instructional planning and support and direct services to students whose needs have been identified in an Individualized Education Program (IEP).[23] Resource specialists are typically assigned to general education classrooms for the majority of their school day.

Adapted physical educators are trained to provide specially designed physical education programs for students who require special instruction in physical education. Physical education teachers need to meet all the qualifications for a teaching certification or licensure, and adapted physical educators may have additional certification through the Adapted Physical Education National Standards (APENS).[25] The APENS states that adapted physical education is "physical education which has been adapted or modified, so that it is as appropriate for the person with a disability as it is for a person without a disability."[25] These educators work with team members to ensure active engagement in physical activities in school settings and may serve on the team that helps to develop a child's IEP.

SERVICE DELIVERY

The provision of care in both medical and educational settings is based upon laws, regulations, and the funding available for each setting. In general, pediatric care that is provided in a medical setting is covered by insurance, public funding (for those qualified), and/or personal funds. Medical facilities range from outpatient clinics with limited health care options to hospital-based management that may feature more extensive care, ranging from neonatal and pediatric intensive care to inpatient and outpatient rehabilitation services. Depending upon the complexity, severity, and chronicity of illness, children may spend extended lengths of time in the hospital, receiving both medical and educational services, if needed. Payment for services in hospital-based care is generally covered by private insurance, Medicaid, and personal funds.

Educational settings are mandated by law to provide a free, appropriate public education (FAPE) in the least restrictive environment (LRE) with consideration given to any therapeutic, special education, or assistive technology necessary to help the child or adolescent meet goals listed in the student's IEP.[26] School districts are responsible for providing educational and therapeutic services to children with special needs 3 to 21 years.[26] Infants and toddlers may receive care through various state-funded, hospital-based, or private clinical facilities. To the greatest extent possible, infants and toddlers should be served in their natural environment, such as a home or day care setting.[26] Laws governing pediatric therapy will be discussed in greater detail in chapters related to therapy provided in educational settings.

Early intervention programs are typically offered to families in their home setting. These services are provided in hopes of empowering and educating families about how to help children with special needs learn about themselves and their environment and develop skills for interaction and engagement with other children, adults, and the community. As children grow older, they may receive additional therapeutic assistance to develop needed skills to function more independently in the adult world with others. Oftentimes, pediatric therapists help families with locating additional supports for their adolescents as they enter adulthood, aiding in the transition to independent living, group homes or returning home.

Another role of pediatric therapists is to encourage community involvement of children and their families. Therapists benefit their families by connecting them with local recreational settings, sports activities, community centers, sites supporting Special Olympics, adult day programs for older youth, and other local options that encourage participation and socialization.

REFERRAL PROCESS

Referrals to pediatric therapies are dependent upon multiple factors, including the practice environment, funding sources, and laws governing care provided in a chosen setting. For example, very premature newborns are commonly identified as needing pediatric therapy services while they are in the neonatal intensive care unit. Generally, these infants are monitored for their growth and development over time to determine whether they are physiologically stable or at risk for developmental delays or health problems. Their subsequent development and growth dictate the need for care. Early monitoring helps to identify children with significant risk factors or apparent problems requiring the expertise of pediatric therapists. Subsequent chapters will discuss how children are referred to various types of care based upon their age and the practice setting. Case studies in this book will include discussion of how decisions are made to determine optimal care for children with special needs.

VALUE OF INTERPROFESSIONAL TEAMWORK

Interprofessional teamwork refers to work involving different professionals who share a team identity and work closely together in an integrated and interdependent manner to solve problems and deliver services. Although it can be challenging to work with other team members due to the additional time and effort needed to meet, interprofessional teamwork has been shown to improve outcomes. This additional time and effort enables shared decision making, allows deeper discussion and debate of important issues, improves joint planning, and enhances communication across the team. Additionally, team members tend to adopt shared values about delivering care in an interprofessional manner.

TEAM APPROACHES USED IN VARIOUS PEDIATRIC SETTINGS

Depending upon the environment, pediatric therapists may use varying team approaches that best suit the type of care needed. These include *intradisciplinary, multidisciplinary, interdisciplinary,* and *collaborative team approaches.* The range of terms used to describe these team approaches can prove confusing for those new to a practice setting. Although similar, each approach has certain distinctions that are described here.

- *Intradisciplinary Team Approach*[27]: Team members individually conduct an examination of the child, plan an appropriate intervention, and carry out the plan with the help of therapy assistants or aides within the same discipline, as needed. This approach is more commonly seen in private practice or outpatient settings.
- *Multidisciplinary Team Approach*[27]: Team members individually conduct an examination of the child, then write a report that is shared with other team members. Meetings are held to discuss each discipline's examination and plan for treatment. Plans for intervention and the execution of each intervention are discipline specific. This approach is more commonly seen in acute care and outpatient facilities.
- *Interdisciplinary Team Approach*[27]: Although each member of the team individually examines the child, professionals share information across disciplines to develop a plan of care. Team members may incorporate some aspects of other disciplines' care plans into their own interventions. This approach is more commonly seen in school settings, some acute care hospitals, and rehabilitation facilities.
- *Transdisciplinary Team Approach*[27,28]: Team members work together to examine and evaluate the child, as well as design and plan an intervention that can be carried out by all team members. In this approach, the professional roles cross boundaries of typical disciplines and the delivery of care is consistent across care providers. This approach is more commonly seen in infant development programs, some acute care settings (especially neonatal intensive care units [NICUs]), and educational settings.
- *Collaborative Team Approach*[29]: Team members work closely together in a combination of transdisciplinary and integrated therapy approaches. Therapists might delegate the majority of intervention to a teacher or aide to be carried out when the child is in a functional setting, such as a classroom.

Regardless of the setting, interprofessional collaboration is essential for desired outcomes. Each team member can serve as a consultant, educator, team player, and advocate for each child and family. By bringing together the unique strengths of each profession and developing interprofessional competencies that strengthen collaboration, therapists can optimize care for those they serve.

SUMMARY

Interprofessional competencies are built upon key principles that are embraced by pediatric therapists. Four domains developed by the Interprofessional Education Collaborative (built upon guiding principles embraced by pediatric therapists) include (1) values and ethics, (2) roles and responsibilities, (3) communication, and (4) teamwork. A framework of interprofessional pediatric care, adapted from the National Interprofessional Competency Framework, focuses on 6 key competencies, including (1) role clarification, (2) child-/family-/school-centered care, (3) interprofessional communication, (4) conflict resolution, (5) team functioning, and (6) collaborative leadership. These competencies are essential for interprofessional collaboration in all settings, including home, community, medical and educational settings.

The delivery of interprofessional care depends upon the practice setting and the referral process but always involves collaborative teamwork for optimal outcomes. The best team approach can be determined through interprofessional communication based upon a clear understanding of legal factors dictating the priorities and delivery of care.

Section 2 provides an overview of both shared and discipline-specific frameworks used by pediatric therapists; Section 3 describes cultural competence and strategies to improve intercultural communication; Section 4 outlines typical growth and development; and Section 5 discusses how pediatric therapists manage pediatric care. The remainder of this book provides examples of teamwork in a wide range of practice settings, including the NICU; early intervention; early childhood special education; elementary, middle, and high schools; and medical settings. Each setting provides unique opportunities for pediatric therapists to optimize care through interprofessional collaboration in program development, transitions across practice settings, and advocacy for needed services.

INTERPROFESSIONAL ACTIVITY

Compare and contrast the roles of pediatric therapists and other professionals by looking at the descriptions of their practice, their educational backgrounds, and their professional websites.

Begin by reviewing descriptions in this chapter, then review professional websites, as needed, to elaborate on understanding.

Discuss the following questions:
1. What do pediatric therapists have in common? List 5 characteristics.
2. How are pediatric therapists unique and distinctive from other professionals in educational and medical settings? List at least 2 distinctions for your profession.
3. What factors may lead to conflict between professionals and families?
4. How can conflicts between professionals and families be minimized?
5. What does the term *collaborative leadership* mean to you, and how do you determine who should lead discussions with family members?
6. As a team, describe similar vs distinctive roles working with the following 2 cases:

Case 1-1: A 6-month-old girl with Down syndrome

Sandy is a 6-month-old girl with a medical diagnosis of Down syndrome.[30] Sandy is being seen in an outpatient follow-up clinic following a recent heart surgery for her atrioventricular septal defect. Sandy was identified as high risk at birth and has delayed development (motor, cognition, communication, and social-emotional). Her physical features include short stature, brachycephaly (a disproportionate shortness of head), upslanting palpebral fissures, atlantoaxial instability, a bent little finger on both hands, a surgically repaired heart defect, an enlarged tongue, generalized low muscle tone, bilateral hearing loss, risk for immune deficiency, low-set ears, a tendency to mouth breathe, a risk for polycythemia, slight seborrheic dermatitis on her scalp, single line on both palms, thickening of the skin of the palms and soles, and problems with her vision. Discuss what you think your roles would be with Sandy and her family, including what would be similar vs distinctive, based upon your professional training.

Case 1-2: A 5-year-old boy with athetoid cerebral palsy

Jason is a 5-year-old boy with a medical diagnosis of athetoid cerebral palsy.[31,32] Jason's family just moved to your town after living in a rural, underserved community with no access to therapy services. Jason just turned 5 years old and is eager to enter kindergarten. As a team, you are observing Jason for the first time. Discuss what you think your roles would be with Jason and his family, including what would be similar vs distinctive, based upon your professional training.

REFERENCES

1. Interprofessional Education Collaborative. Core Competencies for Interprofessional Collaborative Practice. American Association of Colleges of Nursing Web site. https://nexusipe-resource-exchange. s3-us-west-2.amazonaws.com/IPEC_CoreCompetencies_2011.pdf. Published 2016. Accessed May 2, 2017.
2. Dibben M, Lena M. Achieving compliance in chronic illness management: illustrations of trust relationships between physicians and nutrition clinic patients. *Health Risk Soc.* 2003;5(3)(suppl):241-259.
3. Krupat E, Bell R, Kravitz R, et al. When physicians and patients think alike: patient-centred beliefs and their impact on satisfaction and trust. *J Fam Pract.* 2001;50(12)(suppl):1057-1062.
4. Canadian Interprofessional Health Collaborative. *A National Interprofessional Competency Framework.* Vancouver, Canada: College of Health Disciplines University of British Columbia; 2010.
5. Xyrichis A, Lowton K. What fosters or prevents interprofessional teamworking in primary and community care? A literature review. *Int J Nurs Stud.* 2008;45(1):140-153.
6. Academy of Pediatric Physical Therapy. The ABCs of Pediatric Physical Therapy. Academy of Pediatric Physical Therapy Web site. https://pediatricapta.org/includes/fact-sheets/pdfs/09%20ABCs%20 of%20Ped%20PT.pdf. Published 2009. Accessed May 2, 2017.
7. American Physical Therapy Association. The Physical Therapist Scope of Practice. American Physical Therapy Association Web site. http://www.apta.org/ScopeOfPractice/. Published November 20, 2015. Accessed January 24, 2017.
8. American Occupational Therapy Association. Scope of Practice. Pacific University Web site. https://www.pacificu.edu/sites/default/files/documents/10-Scopeofpractice.pdf. Published 2005. Accessed January 24, 2017.
9. Trombly C. Anticipating the future: Assessment of occupational function. *Am J Occup Ther.* 1993;47:253-257.
10. Case-Smith J. *Occupational Therapy for Children and Adolescents.* 4th ed. St. Louis, MO: Mosby; 2001.

11. Clark GF, Chandler BE, eds. *Best Practices for Occupational Therapy in Schools*. Bethesda, MD: AOTA Press; 2013.

12. Jost M, Rohn JL. Best practices in the role of occupational therapy assistants in schools. In: Clark G, Chandler B, eds. *Best Practice for Occupational Therapy in Schools*. Bethesda, MD: AOTA Press; 2013:35-40.

13. American Speech-Language-Hearing Association. Scope of practice in audiology. *ASHA*. 1996;38(suppl 16):12-15.

14. American Speech-Language-Hearing Association. Frequently asked questions: Speech-Language Pathology Assistants (SLPAs). American Speech-Language-Hearing Association Web site. http://www.asha.org/associates/SLPA-FAQs/. Published 2017. Accessed December 28, 2017.

15. American Medical Association. Physician-led team-based care. American Medical Association Web site. https://www.ama-assn.org/delivering-care/physician-led-team-based-care. Accessed May 10, 2017.

16. American Academy of Physician Assistants. What is a PA? American Academy of Physician Assistants Web site. https://www.aapa.org/What-is-a-PA/. Accessed May 10, 2017.

17. American Speech-Language-Hearing Association. Scope of practice in audiology. American Speech-Language-Hearing Association Web site. http://www.asha.org/policy/SP2004-00192/. Published 2004. Accessed January 24, 2017.

18. Hawkins BL, Cory LA, McGuire FA, Allen LR. Considerations for therapeutic recreation practitioners, school systems, and policy makers. *J Disabil Policy Stud*. 2010;23(3):131-139.

19. The Academy Quality Management Committee and Scope of Practice Subcommittee of the Quality Management Committee. Academy of Nutrition and Dietetics: Scope of Practice for the Registered Dietitian. Idaho Academy of Nutrition & Dietetics Web site. http://www.eatrightidaho.org/app/uploads/archive/uploads/Scope-of-Practice-for-the-Registered-Dietitian.pdf. Published 2013. Accessed May 10, 2017.

20. Learn.org. What does a pediatric nutritionist do? Learn.org Web site. http://learn.org/articles/What_Does_a_Pediatric_Dietician_Do.html. Published 2017. Accessed April 24, 2017.

21. National Association of Social Workers. Social work profession. National Association of Social Workers Web site. https://www.socialworkers.org/Practice. Accessed November 18, 2016.

22. Special education terms and definitions. Understanding Special Education Web site. http://www.understandingspecialeducation.com/special-education-terms.html. Published 2016. Accessed November 18, 2016.

23. American Counseling Association. About us. American Counseling Association Web site. https://www.counseling.org/about-us/about-aca. Published 2017. Accessed January 24, 2017.

24. American Psychology Association. School psychologists. National Association of School Psychologists. https://www.nasponline.org/about-school-psychology/who-are-school-psychologists. Published 2017. Accessed May 10, 2017.

25. Adapted Physical Education National Standard. What is adaptive physical education? Adapted Physical Education National Standard Web site. http://www.apens.org/whatisape.html. Accessed May 10, 2017.

26. Center for Parent Information and Resources. IDEA—the Individuals with Disabilities Education Act. Center for Parent Information and Resources Web site. http://www.parentcenterhub.org/repository/idea/. Published September 4, 2010. Accessed May 10, 2017.

27. Stember M. Advancing the social sciences through the interdisciplinary enterprise. *The Social Science Journal*. 1991;28(1):1-14.

28. Kilgo JL. Transdisciplinary teaming from a higher education perspective. In: Kilgo JL, ed. *Transdisciplinary teaming in early intervention/early childhood special education: Navigating together with families and children*. Olney, MD: Association for Childhood Education International; 2006:77-80.

29. Bridges DR, Davidson RA, Odegard PS, Maki IV, Tomkowiak J. Interprofessional collaboration: three best practice models of interprofessional education. *Med Educ Online*. 2011;16(10). http://www.tandfonline.com/doi/full/10.3402/meo.v16i0.6035. Published April 8, 2011. Accessed February 2, 2017.

30. Asim A, Kumar A, Muthuswamy S, Jain A, Agarwal S. Down syndrome: an insight of the disease. *J Biomed Sci*. 2015;22(1):41.

31. Centers for Disease Control. Facts about cerebral palsy. Centers for Disease Control and Prevention Web site. https://www.cdc.gov/ncbddd/cp/facts.html. Published February 3, 2017. Accessed May 10, 2017.

32. Athetoid dyskinetic. BrainAndSpinalCord Web site. http://www.brainandspinalcord.org/athetoid-dyskinetic/. Published 2017. Accessed May 2, 2017.

Section 2

Interprofessional Frameworks of Pediatric Practice

Catherine Rush Thompson, PT, PhD, MS; Pamela Hart, PhD, CCC-SLP; and Ketti Johnson Coffelt, OTD, MS, OTR/L

OVERVIEW

Educational training of professionals working in pediatric practice settings share common theoretical frameworks and approaches for managing children with special needs. This section discusses the frameworks of practice commonly used by pediatric therapists and those that explain differences in perspectives when assessing and developing interventions to help children and families in need.

INTERNATIONAL CLASSIFICATION OF FUNCTIONING, DISABILITY AND HEALTH

The World Health Organization describes the International Classification of Functioning, Disability and Health (ICF) Model as "a classification of health and health-related domains, as the functioning and disability of an individual occurs in a context."[1] As a broad conceptual framework, the ICF Model is used internationally for measuring health and disability at both individual and population levels. The ICF Model categorizes the multiple factors that impact a person's ability to engage fully in life, referred to as *participation*. For example, it looks at the person's *health condition* (medical diagnoses), *body systems and body functions* impacted by that health condition, the individual's *activities* (skills or abilities), the *environment* (both physical and psychosocial) impacting the individual's ability to perform these skills, *personal factors* (such as motivation, age, gender, and lifestyle factors), and, finally, *participation* (the extent the individual is able to participate in all aspects of life) (Figure 2-1).[1]

Pediatric therapists are experts at assessing a child's abilities and skills, as well as identifying likely body structures and body functions that can impact these activities or skills. Further, therapists recognize how the environment (both physical and psychological) plays a key role in how children demonstrate certain skills and behaviors, such as how a child might behave on a public playground compared with how she plays in her own backyard. A vital feature of this framework is the concept of participation. A primary goal of all pediatric therapists is to ensure that each child has opportunities to fully participate in life. This goal includes the role of advocacy for children and their families to promote legislation and social attitudes empowering families and enabling children with special needs to access resources that enable full participation that most families enjoy.

Thompson CR. *Pediatric Therapy: An Interprofessional Framework for Practice* (pp 15-27).
© 2018 SLACK Incorporated.

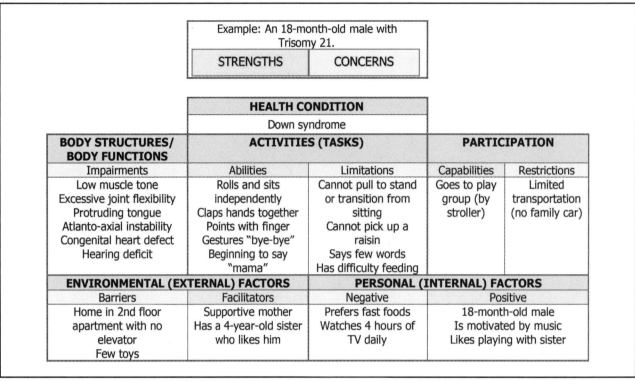

	Example: An 18-month-old male with Trisomy 21.	
	STRENGTHS	CONCERNS

HEALTH CONDITION				
	Down syndrome			
BODY STRUCTURES/ BODY FUNCTIONS	**ACTIVITIES (TASKS)**		**PARTICIPATION**	
Impairments	Abilities	Limitations	Capabilities	Restrictions
Low muscle tone Excessive joint flexibility Protruding tongue Atlanto-axial instability Congenital heart defect Hearing deficit	Rolls and sits independently Claps hands together Points with finger Gestures "bye-bye" Beginning to say "mama"	Cannot pull to stand or transition from sitting Cannot pick up a raisin Says few words Has difficulty feeding	Goes to play group (by stroller)	Limited transportation (no family car)
ENVIRONMENTAL (EXTERNAL) FACTORS		**PERSONAL (INTERNAL) FACTORS**		
Barriers	Facilitators	Negative	Positive	
Home in 2nd floor apartment with no elevator Few toys	Supportive mother Has a 4-year-old sister who likes him	Prefers fast foods Watches 4 hours of TV daily	18-month-old male Is motivated by music Likes playing with sister	

Figure 2-1. International Classification of Functioning, Disability and Health.

FAMILY-CENTERED CARE

According to the Maternal and Child Health Bureau Division of Services for Children with Special Health Needs:

> Family-centered care (FCC) assures the health and well-being of children and their families through a respectful family-professional partnership. It honors the strengths, cultures, traditions, and expertise that everyone brings to this relationship. Family-centered care is the standard of practice which results in high-quality services.[2]

Regardless of practice setting, pediatric therapists recognize the importance of involving families and empowering caretakers engaged in each child's care. This common philosophy of family-centered care is the cornerstone of early intervention provided for young children designed to empower parents to be their child's first teacher. The principles of family-centered care, developed by researchers and organizations supporting families, recognize the importance of a partnership between families and the pediatric professionals and experts serving them.[2-5] This essential partnership can be strengthened by adhering to the following principles[2-5]:

- Trust is acknowledged as fundamental a principle.
- Communication and information sharing are open and objective.

- Participants make decisions jointly.
- Family-centered care acknowledges the family as the constant in a child's life.
- Family-centered care builds on family strengths.
- Family-centered care supports the child in learning about and participating in his care and decision making.
- Families and professionals work together in the best interest of the child and the family. As the child grows, she assumes a partnership role and begins to advocate for herself.
- Everyone respects the skills and expertise brought to the cross-disciplinary relationships.
- There is an openness and willingness to negotiate.
- Family-centered care honors cultural diversity and family traditions.
- Family-centered care recognizes the importance of community-based services.
- Family-centered care promotes an individual and developmental approach.
- Family-centered care encourages family-to-family and peer support.
- Family-centered care supports youth as they transition to adulthood.

As members of an interprofessional team, pediatric therapists who embrace these principles can help to empower families as they gain the skills and knowledge to support their children with special needs. Pediatric therapists recognize their role and responsibilities for educating parents, caretakers, and other family members about each child's special needs, just as they respect the unique perspectives that families provide in assessing and addressing their concerns. Family education includes:

- Providing a rationale for assessment. For example, does the child demonstrate delayed developmental skills? The interprofessional team must explain why these issues are important for the child's development for independent function. If appropriate, the team should explain who made the referral and why. Consider a child who has difficulty copying information from the board, suggesting a wide range of sensory, motor, cognitive, and/or language problems. These problems could be further assessed using a team approach.

- Providing a rationale for treatment strategies and techniques. For example, the interprofessional team needs to educate the child who is paralyzed and his caretakers regarding the reason it is important to maintain normal joint mobility and monitor skin integrity secondary to sensory loss.

- Providing resources for support (eg, emotional, psychological, equipment needs). For example, the interprofessional team should contact support groups (eg, United Cerebral Palsy, Muscular Dystrophy Association, Spina Bifida Association, and others), local vendors of durable equipment, parent support groups, and local funding sources that can provide needed assistance.

- Consulting for comprehensive care. For example, the interprofessional team should encourage parents to actively participate in team conferences to discuss goals, progress, and modifications in treatment. Also, the team needs to maintain contacts with other professionals (eg, therapists providing services in hospital clinics, school-based therapists, home health therapists, orthotists, vendors of equipment, orthopedists, neurologists, primary care physicians) to educate them regarding the child's progress or other issues of concern.

- Recommending therapeutic activities for all environments (eg, home, school, work, recreation). For example, professionals should learn about local activities that might encourage motor skill development (eg, tell the child and families about local swimming programs, summer camps, and opportunities for hippotherapy).

- Attempting to combine individual goals together for the most meaningful function in a given context. For example, the team could have the child work on sitting balance while using augmentative communication. These skills are functional because the child can communicate while working on gross motor and fine motor skills.

- Providing reinforcement of desired behaviors for maximum function. For example, the team should give the child structured choice making throughout the therapy session, determining the child's preferred therapeutic activities and using them for reinforcing desired behaviors.

Pediatric therapists must value the family-centered care framework as they work with children with special needs from birth to adulthood. Table 2-1 lists crucial behaviors for professionals offering family-centered care.

SYSTEMS APPROACH

There are many dynamic systems theories that view changes in development from different perspectives, ranging from mathematical to movement theories.[6,7] These theories recognize multiple factors impacting child development. The impact of these biomechanical, developmental, and environmental factors lead to the dynamic changes that children experience as they grow and develop.[6,7] Pediatric therapists are trained in assessing these factors and how they change across the lifespan. For example, the changes in a child during the first year of life include growth in size; changes in the development and integration of motor, language, psychosocial, and cognitive skills; alternations in the home environment; and the emergence of a unique personality the child displays over time.

Given that infants and children grow so dramatically during the first decade of life, pediatric therapists regularly assess these dynamic changes in body systems and their functions over time. For children with special needs, each pediatric therapist attempts to positively impact the child's motor, cognitive, language, and psychosocial skills with the ultimate goal of enabling the child to participate in age-appropriate life skills and roles. As noted earlier, pediatric therapists share their knowledge and skills with family members to infuse consistency of therapeutic care during the dynamic processes of growth and development.

DEVELOPMENTAL FRAMEWORK

The *developmental framework* recognizes that each child must be embraced as a whole person who is growing and developing emotionally, socially, physically, intellectually, and culturally.[8,9] Jean Piaget is best known for his contributions to developmental psychology through his observations of child development and recognition of the various stages that typical children experience from birth through adolescence[9]:

TABLE 2-1
SIGNIFICANT BEHAVIORS FOR FAMILY-CENTERED CARE RELATED TO INTERPROFESSIONAL CARE

ROLE CLARIFICATION

- Clarify your role for all team members, especially family members and caretakers
- Share relevant information related to your expertise

COLLABORATIVE LEADERSHIP

- Recognize the expertise of team members (professional and other areas of strengths)
- Assist in identifying children's strengths
- Assist in identifying children's needs
- Consider the psychosocial needs of all team members
- Mentor and guide each other's collaborative decision making

CHILD'S AND FAMILY'S NEEDS

- Use cultural competency skills
- Recognize the family's strengths
- Distinguish the child's strengths
- Believe and trust parents
- Respect coping styles
- Collaborate with parents in decision making
- Encourage parent advocacy
- Respect and support the family
- Provide individualized services
- Provide accessible services
- Value families' routines and demanding lifestyles

INTERPROFESSIONAL COMMUNICATION

- Listen to all team members, especially family members
- Communicate clearly and concisely
- Communicate without using jargon
- Be prepared to provide examples or illustrations, as needed
- Be open to new ideas and perspectives

CONFLICT RESOLUTION

- Watch carefully for signs of conflict during verbal and nonverbal communication
- Recognize problems and negotiate to resolve conflicts as soon as possible

TEAM FUNCTIONING

- Encourage participation of all members
- Encourage use of community supports
- Respect the roles, responsibilities, and expertise of team members and stakeholders

INTERPROFESSIONAL GOALS

- Discuss the rationale for each goal
- Prioritize goals that meet the child's and family's needs
- Provide information to the family about how the team plans to reach goals

- The *sensorimotor stage*, from birth to 2 years, when the infant senses and explores the world through play and manipulation.
- The *preoperational stage*, from 2 to about 7 years, when the child begins to develop an imagination and logic through play and exploration.
- The *concrete operational stage*, from 7 to 11 years, when the child develops very concrete thinking and is capable of appreciating the thoughts of others.
- The *formal operational stage*, which begins in adolescence and spans into adulthood, when the youth is more capable of using critical thinking, logic, abstract thinking, and deductive reasoning.

Positive relationships and experiences with nurturing caregivers in the early years are critical for mental and physical health. Good nutrition and safe, healthy, and stimulating environments have a positive impact on a child's development.

Frequently, pediatric therapists rely on developmental assessments providing insight into the child's overall developmental progression. Recognizing the typical developmental milestones facilitates surveillance of healthy child development and offers an opportunity to identify possible problems early in life.

Challenges for pediatric therapists include:

- Determining what to use as a foundation for intervention: typical movement patterns as compared with atypical movements for the child with limited physical abilities.
- Determining whether the child's communication and social skills are outside the range of typical language development for her age.
- Risking the development of independence at the cost of the child's developing deformities from atypical movement patterns (eg, chronic asymmetrical use of one side of body could lead to scoliosis).
- Determining the combination of therapeutic approaches that will be optimal for the child's needs across the lifespan. The range of therapeutic approaches are discussed later in this section.
- Recognizing that perspectives on therapeutic management change as the child grows and develops new skills and interests.

Interprofessional approaches within the developmental framework help pediatric therapists collaborate with families and other disciplines to prioritize needs collectively identified and most valued by families and health care providers.

TASK-ORIENTED APPROACH

From the neuroscientific perspective, the *task-oriented approach* assumes that individuals are task or goal oriented, based upon how the brain functions and activates body systems.[10,11] This approach suggests that multiple factors work together in the growing child to produce movement and control posture that is organized by the brain to accomplish a desired task. This foundational theory of motor control views the body as mechanical systems that work together to move.[11] Pediatric therapists view this theory as foundational to understanding all the body systems and how they work cooperatively in managing internal and environmental influences for performing daily tasks. One example of the task-oriented approach would be having the child complete an obstacle course that requires cognitive and language skills as well as motor planning. According to this theory, the child should focus on completion of the obstacle course rather than focusing on the individual stimuli presented in the challenging course.

PLAY-BASED APPROACH

Play is activity engaged in for enjoyment and recreation. A child's play involves active engagement and is intrinsically motivated.[12] Although play may not have obvious extrinsic goals, it can promote a sense of wonder, exploration, investigation, and interest in a rich range of materials, resources, and opportunities. "Play provides the most natural and meaningful process by which children can construct knowledge and understanding, practice skills, immerse themselves naturally in a broad range of literacy and numeracy, and engage in productive, intrinsically motivating learning environments."[12]

The play-based approach recognizes the value of play as a vehicle for learning and development[13-16]:

Research shows that children are playing-learning individuals. In an open and tolerant atmosphere, where children are free to make their own choices, both play and learning dimensions will be present. Children do not separate play and learning unless they are influenced by adults.[16]

Furthermore, this approach employs a child's motivation to engage in experiences based upon their developmental skills, individual strengths, and unique interests. In other words, children learn by being active.[17]

Effective strategies for supporting learning through this approach encourage therapists to:

1. Balance play, noting how often the child leads or initiates play;
2. Provide needed supports to facilitate play (including toys, environmental structure, and other children, as appropriate);
3. Engage in conversations during play to engage the child individually or in group problem solving and discussion, if possible; and
4. Support the inclusion of all children in play for psychosocial benefits.

Ideally, a play-based program relies on the child's interests, routines, and creative ideas. Play can take place in a wide range of environments and incorporates all types of play, from sensory play (eg, painting with whipping cream) to constructive play (eg, building a model airplane). The interprofessional team can brainstorm with the child to identify materials, games, interests, and locations for play that address his unique abilities and learning styles. For optimal play, the team should incorporate the child's own ideas and interests into planned experiences and routines.

Play offers each child an opportunity to develop motor, cognitive, and psychosocial skills that lead to *psychological and emotional control* while exploring the environment. For this reason, play is the basis for the majority of pediatric therapy. The basic stages of play behavior through which children normally progress are listed in Table 2-2.[18,19]

Pediatric therapists are frequently asked for age-appropriate toys for children based upon their ages. In all instances, toys should be geared to the child's chronological age rather than cognitive age because motor function might limit opportunities to engage with toys offering sufficient intellectual changes for certain children. Some electronic toys can be adapted to enable children with motor dysfunction, such as those with cerebral palsy, to activate toys with a master switch or other control device. Table 2-3 lists age-appropriate toys for play-based learning.

Finally, the social aspects of play are a fundamental consideration for structuring play activities with other children.[17-19] Table 2-4 lists the typical ages at which the various types of play emerge, ranging from solitary play typically seen in infants to gang or team play typically seen as children engage in school activities.

Although play is used as the primary means of engaging children in therapeutic activities, the pediatric therapist must also consider the optimal therapeutic approach that best meets the child's medical and educational needs, ranging from helping her learn early in life to aiding in recovery from a serious accident during adolescence.

THERAPEUTIC APPROACHES

Habilitation refers to learning movements for the first time.[20] Pediatric therapists become experts at recognizing the habilitation potential of children by examining current evidence regarding realistic expectations for children with specific diagnoses. In some cases where children have congenital malformations or significant functional limitation, team members can work collaboratively to offer children opportunities for participation in a wide range of activities through creative adaptations, as needed. The habilitation approach is commonly used to help children achieve motor milestones through play-based activities that provide multiple opportunities for practicing challenging skills. The habilitation approach typically applies the progression of developmental milestones to guide therapeutic activities.

Modification occurs when the child is unable to achieve a task without adaptation. Modification allows the child to more fully participate in structured activities, resulting in self-determined or self-controlled strategies to solve motor problems.[20] For example, a child needing to perform a task, such as eating lunch, might require modifications of the eating task and specialized equipment that makes the task easier to perform. Developing appropriate modifications relies on interprofessional collaboration to determine optimal therapeutic positioning, adaptive devices, and social interaction supports for the child to successfully accomplish the task. As the child grows and develops new skills, equipment and learning materials are often modified to enable the child to gain more independent function.

Preventive care is anticipated for every child. One hallmark of preventive care is that it should be integrated into daily activities in the natural setting. Preventive care can include health recommendations (eg, immunizations, diet, sleep, nutrition), environmental changes (eg, arrangement of the physical environment, proximity of objects, space for safe movement), and behavioral changes (eg, safe transfers, training in use of devices, staff education, parent education). Everyone must be certain that each child engages in activities designed to reduce risks and to eliminate secondary complications resulting from the primary impairments, such as weakness, limited range of motion, and sensory deficits. For example, children who have difficulties moving are prone to developing contractures (limited joint movement), skin breakdown, and deformities. The interprofessional team must integrate preventive care while developing therapeutic activities to promote age-appropriate skills.

Remediation occurs when a child engages in activities designed to correct, remedy, or improve skills.[20] For example, a 1-year-old child with increased muscle tone

TABLE 2-2
STAGES OF PLAY

INFANCY (BIRTH TO 24 MONTHS)

The infant:
- Experiments with bodily sensations and movements
- Establishes important social attachments (largely by being held and matching voices to smiles and other facial expressions)
- Engages in self-discovery: playing with hands and feet
- Is attracted to toys with sharp, contrasting colors; changes in sound; or changes in texture
- Observes others in play
- Seeks objects that they can grasp, push, or pull to master motor abilities and develop coordination
- Demonstrates communicative intent through play

TODDLERHOOD (2 TO 3 YEARS)

The toddler:
- Develops independence and a sense of self through practice play and repetition
- Enjoys conversations/books
- Enjoys social games (eg, peek-a-boo and pat-a-cake)
- Learns to take turns
- Enjoys hiding games: find the object/person
- Pretend play: care for dolls, make dinner, shop
- Demonstrates a variety of communicative functions through play

EARLY CHILDHOOD (3 TO 5 YEARS)

The preschooler:
- Enjoys make-believe play and imitating others
- Love to engage in gross motor play (running, jumping, climbing, and throwing) as well as rough-and-tumble activities (especially males)
- Enjoys social interaction with peers, taking turns
- Engages in constructive play: playing with blocks and build structures; water painting; working with modeling clay, water, sand, and rice, with reports of increased mathematical scores

MIDDLE CHILDHOOD (6 TO 10 YEARS)

School-aged children:
- Enjoy competition and explicit rules that stress fair play and satisfy social and intellectual challenges; this type of play builds self-esteem, which is so important to middle childhood
- Enjoy playing games with their family
  - Games with strategy: chess and checkers
  - Games with skills: card games encourage math skills

ADOLESCENCE (11 TO 18 YEARS)

Adolescents/young adults:
- Enjoy competitive games and sports
- Enjoy computer and video games/indoors play (they foster spatial cognition skills, with reports of increased mathematical scores)
- Improve gross motor skills

Adapted from Pathways. Stages of play. Pathways Web site. https://pathways.org/blog/kids-learn-play-6-stages-play-development/. Accessed May 10, 2017.

TABLE 2-3

AGE-APPROPRIATE TOYS FOR PLAY-BASED LEARNING

AGE RANGE	APPROPRIATE TOYS AND GAMES
1 month to 6 months	The infant is visually focused, developing sensorimotor skills, and engaged in exploring the environment. Popular toys encourage reaching, grasping, holding and mouthing (eg, rattles, objects of a solid primary color hung in easy view, cradle gym or mobile, bells on an elastic band, fuzzy toys, and musical toys).
6 to 12 months	The infant is more socially aware of others and enjoys interactive games like peek-a-boo and pat-a-cake. Toy play expands to different textures and environments, including playing with floating toys, putting water in containers and pouring it out, and picking up and throwing down objects.
1 year to 1.5 years	With increasing mobility, the toddler enjoys chasing and hiding games, watching and following (imitating actions), and engaging in a wide range of motor skills (eg, walking, climbing, bending over, sitting down, turning pages in books, manipulating handling objects, scribbling, smearing, pounding, and arranging objects in order). The toddler also enjoys dancing and clapping to music.
1.5 to 2 years	As fine motor skills refine and postural control improves, the toddler enjoys creatively playing with finger paints, clay, sand, water, soap, wooden toys (cars and animals), blocks, crayons, and paper. With increased balance, the toddler enjoys rocking on a large toy and holding a book while turning pages.
2 to 3 years	The young child enjoys participating in parallel play and hearing stories over and over again. Activities that engage gross motor movements (eg, toys to push and pull, climbing, kicking and throwing) and fine motor skills (eg, taking simple things apart, building block towers, stringing beads, putting together simple puzzles, placing objects in a row, and repeatedly emptying and filling containers) amuse the child.
3 to 4 years	Social skills become more evident as the young child begins taking turns. Cognitive and motor skills are explored as the child recognize the results of efforts (eg, putting together more complex puzzles, performing imaginative block play, playing dress-up, using dress-up clothes, dropping objects through small openings, using instruments to create rhythm, rhyming, drawing, and painting). Movements involving increased coordination (eg, hopping and jumping) and motor planning (eg, maneuvering through obstacle courses) further develop.
4 to 5 years	By 4 years, the child enjoys cooperative play and begins sharing toys. Play is more constructive and creative (eg, cutting and pasting objects, building structures, and playing with a wider range of toys that refine gross and fine motor skills). The child's cognitive and emotional development is more evident (eg, she wants her creations saved and recognizes numbers and letters).
6 to 7 years	From 6 years on, the child engages in a wider range of toys and appreciates cooperative and self-directed activities (eg, playing card and board games, creating art with a range of materials, reading books, and enjoying mechanical toys). Children over the age of 6 typically love sports, including those that involve manipulation (eg, sports involving gloves, balls, and bats) and increasing coordination (eg, riding a bicycle). As children continue to develop and become exposed to the wide range of possible activities, they show greater preferences for those activities that match their abilities and interests.

Adapted from BabyCenter. Age-appropriate toys. BabyCenter Web site. https://www.babycenter.com/0_age-appropriate-toys_5.bc. Accessed May 10, 2017 and St. Louis Children's Hospital. Age-appropriate toys and activities. St. Louis Children's Hospital Web site. http://www.stlouischildrens.org/sites/default/files/wellness_development/files/SLC10659_AgeAppropriateToysBrochureR3.pdf. Accessed May 10, 2017.

TABLE 2-4
SIX TYPES OF PLAY

THE FOLLOWING 6 TYPES OF PLAY DEVELOP FROM BIRTH TO 6 YEARS:

1. **Unoccupied play (begins at birth)**

   This is the most basic type of play. The infant gains awareness of her surroundings and basically observes the environment.

2. **Independent or solitary play (emerges around 2 to 3 years)**

   The infant plays alone with her body parts, smiles at other babies, attends to other babies' cries, and begins to explore other children.

3. **Onlooker play (emerges at 2 years)**

   Two children engage in solitary play while in close proximity, exchanging toys, imitating each other, and following and chasing each other. This type of play is common among children developing their communication skills.

4. **Parallel play (emerges around 3 years)**

   Children demonstrate conscious cooperation and work together to accomplish a task (eg, building with blocks). As a child matures, the duration and complexity of the task increases. The group size also grows, so rules and laws are developed by the group to regulate behaviors.

5. **Associative play (emerges around 3 years)**

   As children develop friendships, they become more involved in group play, but their play is not well organized. In addition to their motor skills, they are engaged in more socialization, problem solving, cooperation, and use of language.

6. **Cooperative play (school age)**

   As children mature, they spontaneously form groups with membership. To show solidarity, these groups may develop nicknames for group identification.

Adapted from Gudritz L. 6 types of play important to your child's development. Healthline Web site. http://www.healthline.com/health/parenting/types-of-play. Published June 20, 2016. Accessed May 10, 2017 and Wellhousen K, Crowther I. *Creating Effective Learning Environments*. Clifton Park, NY: Cengage Learning; 2004:4-7.

might "bunny hop" (using a primitive reflex, symmetrical tonic neck reflex, for movement) rather than creep reciprocally. Encouraging the child to creep reciprocally (using verbal and/or manual assistance) helps the child to develop new strategies for movement on the floor. Remediation also involves training in the use of assistive technology and devices that enable a child to communicate and engage in purposeful classroom and functional activities.

Compensation occurs when intervention programs are designed to promote other aspects of performance or substitute a different form of action.[20] For example, children with athetosis need to stabilize their posture and extremities for more control of their movements. A child with athetosis could learn to dress herself using the wall for postural support. Similarly, this child could learn to use elbow support (eg, using a table or stabilizing her elbow against her trunk) for fine motor control. Both of these are compensatory strategies to assist with motor control.

Maintenance activities help a child retain acquired functional skills. Repetition of functional skills enables a child to maintain the ability to perform these skills over time.[20] For example, once a child learns to walk, he should be expected to walk on a regular basis. The focus of therapy would then shift from walking to walking with increased speed and endurance. Similarly, once a child learns new words or fine motor skills, the interprofessional team should encourage frequent use of these new skills to maintain their use in the child's daily routines.

Although all of the approaches discussed thus far are commonly shared by pediatric therapists, some perspectives are unique to each profession. The management of a child's care is enriched by the distinctive models and approaches that physical therapists, occupational therapists, and speech-language pathologists bring to their interprofessional teams.

PHYSICAL THERAPY: THE PATIENT/CLIENT MANAGEMENT MODEL

The Patient/Client Management Model is uniquely used by physical therapists to deliver care across all practice settings and patients/clients.[21] With a strong emphasis on growth and development, the pediatric physical therapist performs an extensive review of systems that includes the musculoskeletal, neuromuscular, cardiopulmonary, integumentary, and other body systems and relates findings to the child's growth, development, and motor control.

Examination addresses (a) aerobic capacity and endurance; (b) anthropometric characteristics; (c) assistive technology; (d) balance; (e) circulation (arterial, venous, lymphatic); (f) community, social, and civic life; (g) cranial and peripheral nerve integrity; (h) education life; (i) environmental factors; (j) gait; (k) integumentary integrity; (l) joint integrity and mobility; (m) mental functions; (n) mobility (including locomotion); (o) motor function; (p) muscle performance (including strength, power, endurance, and length); (q) neuromotor development and sensory processing; (r) pain; (s) posture; (t) range of motion; (u) reflex integrity; (v) self-care and domestic life; (w) sensory integrity; (x) skeletal integrity; (y) ventilation and respiration; and (z) work life.[21] Although all areas may not be examined in all children, these areas serve as the foundation for the management of pediatric conditions in both educational and medical settings.

According to the *Guide to Physical Therapist Practice*,[21] intervention is the "purposeful interaction of the physical therapist with an individual—and, when appropriate, with other people involved in that individual's care—to produce changes in the condition that are consistent with the diagnosis and prognosis." *Evaluation* considers examination results and interactions between the child and others. The *physical therapy diagnosis* is determined, specifying activity limitations. In pediatrics, *impaired neuromotor development* is a common physical therapy diagnosis because many children have difficulty with achieving typical developmental milestones. The *prognosis* for physical therapy is based upon the child's potential for the development of neuromotor skills and learning adaptive skills to function optimally. The *plan of care* is developed based upon an integration of the evaluation and the goals of family and other stakeholders. The *outcomes* of physical therapy are based upon objective SMART goals that are monitored closely throughout the use of evidence-based interventions.[22,23] The SMART acronym is used to ensure that goals are specific, measurable, achievable, realistic, and time sensitive.[22,23]

The evaluation process continues throughout interventions to accommodate changing environments (eg, school needs vs home needs) and the changing needs of the family and child. The desired outcome of physical therapy is to assist each child in becoming as healthy as possible (including physically, mentally, and psychosocially) and to enable each child to fully participate at home and school, in recreational opportunities, and in the community in a meaningful manner.

OCCUPATIONAL THERAPY: OCCUPATION-BASED APPROACH

The *Occupational Therapy Framework: Domain and Process (Third Edition)*[24] provides a guided outline of occupational therapy services for individuals such as a child and her family with the overall aim to develop the child's occupation participation in roles, habits, and routines. Occupational therapy practice is dependent upon the specific condition and age of the child and can occur within a variety of contexts, such as the home, a medical setting (eg, hospital, rehabilitative facility, outpatient facility), and educational classrooms (preschool through high school grades).

Occupational therapists analyze a child's occupation performance in the following areas: activities of daily living (self-feeding, functional mobility, bathroom skills, managing classroom materials); instrumental activities of daily living (bicycling, riding buses, walking); rest and sleep, education (academic, nonacademic, extracurricular, and vocational); and play and social participation (peers and others). The emphasis for occupational therapists practicing in the school learning environment is to identify factors that affect students' "learning and participation in the context of educational activities, routines, and environments."[25]

Occupational therapists observe and assess each child's performance skills of (a) cognition, (b) emotional regulation, (c) visual perceptual, (d) fine motor, (e) gross motor, (f) sensory processing, (g) sensory integration, (h) motor planning, and (i) social-emotional abilities—all of which may be limiting their occupational performance in the hallway, lunchroom, classroom, playground, and other relevant settings. Based on an analysis of the occupation, performance skills, and activity demands of the task, along with the occupational profile of the child, occupational therapists create intervention strategies to develop necessary skills and make adaptations or modifications to support the child's overall learning performance.

Drawing from theories and known evidence, occupational therapists use clinical reasoning during the occupational therapy process of evaluation and intervention planning in the development of individualized educational programming. Occupational therapists continually review programming and monitor the child's progress, assessing the effectiveness of their interventions and making changes as necessary. Occupational therapists realize that learning opportunities exist for children all day long, thus they place value in the collaborative consultation process with teachers and paraprofessional educators to exchange information, educate each other, and train skills and strategies so that children can continually practice skills and embed routines enhancing school performance.[25]

SPEECH-LANGUAGE PATHOLOGY: THE SPEECH-LANGUAGE PATHOLOGY PRACTICE FRAMEWORK

The practice of speech-language pathology is conceptualized by cardinal documents from the American Speech-Language-Hearing Association (ASHA) outlined in the Scope of Practice, Preferred Practice Patterns, Position Statements, Knowledge Guidelines, and Knowledge and Skill Statements.[26] These documents describe the depth and breadth of practice in speech-language pathology. General areas of practice for speech-language pathologists include assessment and intervention across (a) speech sound production, (b) resonance, (c) voice, (d) fluency, (e) expressive language, (f) receptive language, (g) social pragmatic skills, (h) cognition, (i) feeding and swallowing, and (j) communication modalities, including augmentative and alternative communication strategies. These broad, diverse areas of clinical knowledge and skill require an understanding of how the disorder affects the individual's ability to function in daily life. As such, the general practice framework in speech-language pathology is based on the previously described World Health Organization's ICF Model.[1] Within this framework, impairments may range from minor to major.

Relative to speech-language pathology, a client who has cerebral palsy may experience severe impairments in health conditions, specifically body functions, to the extent that she is unable to use verbal speech for communication. This same client, however, may have positive contextual factors, including family support and adequate financial resources, thus enabling access to services in a supportive environment that enables her to experience greater success. Application of this framework to speech-language pathology encourages consideration of the whole person and the ways the disability impacts various aspects of the person's life.

Also central to the practice of speech-language pathology is the use of research evidence, stakeholder perspectives, and clinical judgment as a comprehensive method of evidence-based practice.[27] It is no longer adequate to approach clinical service provision as a speech-language pathology with a philosophy of "I use this approach because it works." It is now the expectation that speech-language pathologists use their clinical judgment while including stakeholder perspectives in the development of the treatment plan. This is completed with full consideration and analysis of the related research evidence for or against the chosen intervention toward a goal of maximizing client progress in the most efficient manner as possible.[27]

All pediatric therapists are expected to engage in professional development and critical analyses of research to ensure that they offer the most contemporary and evidence-based care to meet the needs of children and their families. Interprofessional collaboration relies on this professional development for optimal outcomes in all practice settings.

WORKING IN EDUCATIONAL VERSUS MEDICAL SETTINGS

Pediatric therapists are employed in various settings, including hospitals, outpatient clinics, school systems, and community-based settings. The provision of care at each setting is contingent upon laws, regulations, and funding sources.

Subsequent sections will provide an overview of interprofessional pediatric therapy in a range of settings. Section 6 covers medical care in the neonatal intensive care unit, Section 7 discusses family-centered care in early intervention, Section 8 describes child-centered early childhood special education, Section 9 relates therapeutic supports to educational settings (elementary, middle, and high schools), and Section 10 discusses urgent care in hospital settings. Table 2-5 illustrates the range of settings that warrant different approaches of care based upon legal and financial considerations.

SUMMARY

This section provided an overview of the similarities between physical therapy, occupational therapy, and speech-language pathology in terms of the approaches used in the management of children receiving care in various practice settings. It also outlined the different perspectives each type of therapy offers to children and their families based upon the context of care and the unique needs of each child. Section 3 will discuss the cultural competency needed to address diverse needs and values of families and settings, and Section 4 will provide details regarding typical growth and development. Section 5 will describe how pediatric therapists use their expertise to manage the needs of children and their families. Sections 6 through 10 will focus on specific pediatric practice settings, providing additional details regarding the legal and ethical considerations for each setting, the populations typically served, the expected roles of health care professionals, and the focus of the interprofessional team.

TABLE 2-5			
SETTINGS FOR PEDIATRIC THERAPY			
MEDICAL	**HOME-BASED**	**EDUCATIONAL**	**OTHER**
• NICU (neonatal intensive care unit) • PICU (pediatric intensive care unit) • Inpatient • Outpatient • Rehabilitation • Outpatient clinics • Urgent care	• Early intervention (in home or early intervention programs) • Homebound • Group home	• Preschool • Elementary school • Secondary school • College	• Sports centers • Community centers • Parks • Playgrounds • Adult day programs • Shopping centers • Entertainment centers

INTERPROFESSIONAL ACTIVITY

1. Read the following case studies and consider the needs of each child across childhood and the roles and responsibilities of physical therapy, occupational therapy, and speech-language pathology in managing children with special needs.

2. Answer the following questions for each case:

    a. What would you expect in terms of this child's growth and development compared with others of the same age?

    b. What types of assessments would be commonly used across all pediatric therapies? (See Appendix B for a list of tests and measures used by pediatric therapists.)

    c. What might be distinctive assessments for physical therapy, occupational therapy, and speech-language pathology for each child and his or her family?

    d. How would you conduct an interprofessional assessment?

    e. What frameworks would you apply to your plan of care for the child and family?

    f. How would you adjust your presentation of results for the following situations:

        i. Sharing your findings with interprofessional team members

        ii. Sharing your findings with the family

        iii. Sharing your findings with Cindy's preschool teacher

        iv. Sharing your findings with Cindy's primary care physician

Case 2-1: A 4-year-old girl with myelomeningocele[28]

Cindy was diagnosed with myelomeningocele T4-T6 and obstructive hydrocephalus secondary to Chiari II malformation shortly after birth. Cindy's mother reports that she has always been healthy and never took any medications that would impact her pregnancy. After Cindy's birth, the family noted a mass growing in her upper spine, so they sought medical care, including a ventriculo-peritoneal shunt for her hydrocephalus. At age 2, Cindy had a seizure that was treated in the emergency department. At age 3, Cindy began demonstrating temper tantrums and had difficulty with her right eye and right jaw. Cindy is now 4 years old, and the interprofessional team needs to address her needs. The family just moved to your rural area, and you need to assess Cindy's abilities in the local clinic.

Case 2-2: A 10-year-old boy with autism spectrum disorder

Zachary is a 10-year-old boy who was diagnosed with autism spectrum disorder (ASD). His mother, a homemaker, reported that Zachary was born full-term with no birth complications. She added that Zachary generally met developmental milestones during his first year of life. At age 2, she began to notice that he had "awkward" movements and did not use words. She homeschooled Zachary until age 9 in an attempt to meet all of his needs. Although Zachary has been generally healthy, he has recently been diagnosed with rheumatoid arthritis and is sensitive to pain. This year he began attending school and has been receiving special education. Zachary is reportedly curious and very alert, but he is challenged by his impulsivity, poor communication, difficulty with balance and coordination, and problems with fine motor skills, such as using the computer. He also has difficulties interacting with his peers, and when he gets frustrated, he acts out with tantrums, aggressive behavior, and property destruction.

REFERENCES

1. World Health Organization. International Classification of Functioning, Disability and Health (ICF). World Health Organization Web site. http://www.who.int/classifications/icf/en/. Accessed January 24, 2017.
2. Family Voices. Family-centered care. Family Voices Web site. http://www.familyvoices.org/admin/work_family_centered/files/FCCare.pdf. Accessed January 24, 2017.
3. National Center for Family-Professional Relationships. Family-centered care. Family Voices Web site. http://www.fv-ncfpp.org/quality-health-care1/family-centered-care/. Accessed January 24, 2017.
4. US Department of Health and Human Services. Philosophy and key elements of family-centered practice. Child Welfare Information Gateway Web site. https://www.childwelfare.gov/topics/famcentered/philosophy/. Accessed January 24, 2017.
5. Forry ND, Moodi, S, Simkin S, Rothenberg L. Family-Provider Relationships: A Multidisciplinary Review of High Quality Practices and Associations with Family, Child, and Provider Outcomes, Issue Brief OPRE 2011-26a. Washington, DC: Office of Planning, Research and Evaluation, Administration for Children and Families, US Department of Health and Human Services; 2011.
6. McDaniel S, Hepworth J, Doherty WJ. *Medical Family Therapy: A Biopsychosocial Approach to Families With Health Problems*. New York, NY: Basic Books; 1992.
7. Smith L, Thelen E. Development as a dynamic system. *Trends Cogn Sci*. 2003;7(8):343-348.
8. Cherry K. Theories of development. https://www.verywell.com/theories-of-development-2795092. Verywell Web site. Accessed January 24, 2017.
9. Cherry K. Piaget's theory: The four stages of cognitive development. Verywell Web site. https://www.verywell.com/piagets-stages-of-cognitive-development-2795457. Accessed January 24, 2017.
10. Mathiowetz V, Bass-Haugen J. Motor behavior research: Implications for therapeutic implications for therapeutic approaches to CNS dysfunction. *Am J Occup Ther*. 1994;(48):733-745
11. Dickstein R, Hocherman S, Pillar T, Shaham R. Stroke rehabilitation. Three exercise therapy approaches. *Phys Ther*. 1986;66:1233-1238.
12. Walker K. *Play Matters: Engaging Children in Learning the Australian Developmental Curriculum: A Play and Project Based Philosophy*. Camberwell, Victoria: ACER Press; 2007.
13. Bodrova E, Leong DJ. Uniquely preschool: What research tells us about the ways young children learn. *Educational Leadership*. 2005;63(1):44-47.
14. Shipley D. Empowering children. *Play Based Curriculum for Lifelong Learning*. 4th ed. Toronto, Ontario: Nelson Education; 2008.
15. Siraj-Blatchford I. Understanding the relationship between curriculum, pedagogy and progression in learning in early childhood. *Hong Kong Journal of Early Childhood*. 2008;7(2):6-13.
16. Samuelsson P, Carlsson A. The playing-learning child in preschool. *Every Child*. 2003;14(2):3.
17. Samuelsson P, Carlsson A. The playing learning child: Towards a pedagogy of early childhood. *Scandinavian Journal of Educational Research*. 2008;5(6):623-641.
18. Parten MB. Social participation among preschool children. *J Abnorm Soc Psychol*. 1932;27(3):243-269.
19. Wellhousen K, Crowther I. *Creating Effective Learning Environments*. Clifton Park, NY: Cengage Learning; 2004:4-7.
20. Stucki G, Cieza A, Ewert T, Kostanjsek N, Chatterji S, Üstün T. Application of the International Classification of Functioning, Disability and Health (ICF) in clinical practice. *Disabil Rehabil*. 2002;24(5):281-282.
21. American Physical Therapy Association. Physical Therapist Examination and Evaluation: Focus on Tests and Measures. In: *Guide to Physical Therapist Practice*. Alexandria, VA: American Physical Therapy Association; 2014. http://guidetoptpractice.apta.org/content/1/SEC4.body. Accessed December 28, 2017.
22. Doran GT. There's a S.M.A.R.T. way to write management's goals and objectives. *Management Review*. 1981;70(11):35-36.
23. Davis AM, Davis S, Moss N. First steps towards an interdisciplinary approach to rehabilitation. *Clin Rehabil*. 1992;6:237-244.
24. American Occupational Therapy Association. Occupational therapy practice framework. Domain and process. 3rd ed. *Am J Occup Ther*. 2014;68(suppl 1):S1-S48.
25. American Occupational Therapy Association. Occupational therapy services in early childhood and school-based settings. *Am J Occup Ther*. 2011;65(suppl):246-254.
26. American Speech-Language-Hearing Association. Scope of practice in speech-language pathology. University of Central Oklahoma Web site. http://sites.uco.edu/ceps/files/apss/slp-asha-scopeofpractice.pdf. Published 2007. Accessed February 3, 2017.
27. American Speech-Language-Hearing Association. Evidence-based practice. American Speech-Language-Hearing Association Web site. http://www.asha.org/Research/EBP/. Accessed January 24, 2017.
28. Medscape. Spina bifida. Medscape Web site. http://emedicine.medscape.com/article/311113-overview#a4. Published 2017. Accessed May 10, 2017.

Section 3

Culturally Competent Pediatric Care

Catherine Rush Thompson, PT, PhD, MS

OVERVIEW

According to research, by 2060, 64% of children under the age of 18 in the United States are projected to belong to racial and ethnic minorities, as compared with 48% of children in 2014.[1] "Greater cultural competence of mental health service providers is associated with better overall outcomes (access, participation, satisfaction, and service outcomes) for African American youth and their families."[2] This increase in diversity in our communities necessitates preparing pediatric therapists to be culturally competent, a process that is ongoing and deliberate.

Designed to engage the learner in ongoing reflection, this section develops, refines, and grows awareness of cultural competency and cultural and linguistic diversity. It also offers options for improving cross-cultural communication and for supporting policies that facilitate culturally competent care.

ROLES OF PEDIATRIC THERAPISTS

Pediatric therapists aim to help children reach their maximum potential to function in all environments. With this effort in mind, physical therapists, occupational therapists, and speech-language pathologists play a critical role in bridging the gaps between local communities (medical, educational, and societal) and the home through education, advocacy, developmental expertise, advising, and resourcefulness. Interprofessional collaboration between stakeholders relies on the abilities of these therapists to maintain a climate of mutual respect while communicating with children, families, communities, and other health professionals in a responsive and responsible manner. Competent communication and collaboration include the provision of culturally and linguistically appropriate services. The underlying spirit of this section is based on assumptions that closely align with the principles of family-centered care outlined in an earlier section and include the following assumptions:

- Assumption #1: Every child and family with which the allied health professional will have contact is unique.

- Assumption #2: Every child's and family's values, wants, and beliefs are respected, even when in conflict with that of the allied health professional.

- Assumption #3: All children and their families are to be treated with dignity and respect.

- Assumption #4: The family is a valued member of the health care team.

Thompson CR. *Pediatric Therapy:*
An Interprofessional Framework for Practice (pp 29-42).
© 2018 SLACK Incorporated.

- Assumption #5: *Cultural competence* is not something that the individual obtains; cultural competence is an ongoing process that constantly keeps each person engaged in exploring her or his own beliefs, biases, values, and assumptions and how these ideas influence and shape interactions with other professionals, families, children, and others they aim to influence.

All pediatric therapists need to engage in ongoing efforts to increase their cultural competence to provide family-centered care that meets each child's needs in cross-cultural situations. Ultimately, the role of this developing team culture is the achievement of successful outcomes for the child, the family, and the communities in which they live. One key ingredient for achieving these team outcomes is an intentional effort to increase cultural and linguistic competence.

CULTURAL AND LINGUISTIC COMPETENCE

What is *cultural and linguistic competence*?

Cultural and linguistic competence is a set of congruent behaviors, attitudes, and policies that come together in a system, agency, or among professionals that enables effective work in cross-cultural situations. Per the Cultural Competence Continuum, this capability involves ensuring that the needs of diverse patients/clients/customers are met by health service and public health organizations based on the acquisition of specific skill sets, valuing diversity, and taking concrete steps to ensure efficacy in serving [underrepresented and/or historically marginalized populations] populations.[3]

"Cultural and linguistic competence is as important to the successful provision of services as are scientific, technical, and clinical knowledge and skills."[4] This sentiment is echoed across all professions in the United States, given the culturally diverse population of individuals from a variety of different cultural and linguistic backgrounds.

DEVELOPING CULTURAL COMPETENCE

How is cultural competence developed? The Cultural Competence Continuum, proposed by Cross et al[5] outlines the progressive development of cultural competence from cultural incapacity in its earliest stages to cultural proficiency, involving advocacy for societal changes to support cultural diversity and cultural competency. Cultural proficiency can be achieved once a therapist is able to understand, appreciate, and accept different cultures based on an in-depth knowledge of cultural variations. Ultimately,

pediatric therapists need to be able to establish and maintain partnerships with diverse constituency groups that span the boundaries of the traditional health and mental health care arenas to eliminate racial and ethnic disparities. This continuum has been used across disciplines to serve as a model of developing cultural competence, and ultimately cultural proficiency, at both the individual and institutional level (Table 3-1).

This continuum suggests that the lack of cultural competency (ie, culturally incompetent attitudes, policies, structures, and practices) can hinder the provision of care across cultures. The learner is encouraged to reflect on personal and team cultural competence: At what level are you personally? At what level on the continuum would you consider your pediatric team? One important role of pediatric therapists is to serve as facilitators in the development of cultural competence impacting families, organizations, and society at large.

In addition, helping all team members understand common terminology is a positive step toward developing cultural competency. For example, the word *culture* is thought to be synonymous with race and ethnicity; however, culture encompasses much more than just race and ethnicity and includes such aspects as nationality, religion, spirituality, and socioeconomic status. Culture is defined differently by many; however, central to the idea of culture is that it "is the shared beliefs, values, traditions, assumptions, and lifestyles of a group of people."[6] Within this definition are several variables that shape an individual's culture. For example, several different words that are associated with cultural and linguistic diversity and are encountered in pediatric settings include ethnicity, sexual identity, gender identity, nationality, poverty, race, religious orientation, and stereotyping.

What is the difference between race and ethnicity? The United States Office of Management and Budget set the standard for classifying race and ethnicity within the United States.[3] These standards were put forth in part of an effort to "collect data on the race and ethnicity of broad population groups in this country, and are not anthropologically or scientifically based."[3,7,8] Although some may disagree with these categories, they are used to describe various individuals and groups, so pediatric professionals should have familiarity with them.[3] The definitions of race, ethnicity, and nationality are provided in Table 3-2.

The various ethnicities are further delineated in Table 3-3, as defined by the United States Office of Management and Budget.[8] It should be noted, however, that there are social implications behind these categories that have a major influence on how individuals are able to participate in the societies in which they live. Although it is understood that race is a social construct, historically and contemporarily used to create a hierarchy among the races, it must also be understood that despite this absence of an anthropological and social basis for race, these identifiers are associated with

TABLE 3-1
CULTURAL COMPETENCE CONTINUUM
Cultural destructiveness is characterized by attitudes, policies, structures, and practices within a system or organization that are destructive to a cultural group.
Cultural incapacity is the lack of capacity of systems and organizations to respond effectively to the needs, interests, and preferences of culturally and linguistically diverse groups. Characteristic include, but are not limited to, institutional or systemic bias; practices that may result in discrimination in hiring and promotion; disproportionate allocation of resources that may benefit one cultural group over another; subtle messages that some cultural groups are neither valued nor welcomed; and lower expectations for some cultural, ethnic, or racial groups.
Cultural blindness is an expressed philosophy of viewing and treating all people as the same. Characteristics of such systems and organizations may include policies and personnel who encourage assimilation; approaches in the delivery of services and supports that ignore cultural strengths; institutional attitudes that blame consumers (individuals or families) for their circumstances; little value placed on training and resource development that facilitate cultural and linguistic competence; workforce and contract personnel that lack diversity (eg, race, ethnicity, language, gender, age); and few structures and resources dedicated to acquiring cultural knowledge.
Cultural precompetence suggests that an organization is aware of its strengths and areas of growth for responding to culturally and linguistically diverse populations. Characteristics include, but are not limited to, the system or organization expressly valuing the delivery of high-quality services and supports to culturally and linguistically diverse populations; commitment to human and civil rights; hiring practices that support a diverse workforce; the capacity to conduct asset and needs assessments within diverse communities; concerted efforts to improve service delivery, usually for a specific racial, ethnic, or cultural group; tendency for token representation on governing boards; and no clear plan for achieving organizational cultural competence.

(continued)

both negative (eg, disenfranchisement, marginalization, oppression) and positive (eg, healthy ethnic/racial identity development, cultural connection, tradition, and pride) factors that play into one's experiences, both perceived and real. Whether or not the impact of these experiences is in any individual's conscious awareness, it is important for the therapeutic team to be mindful of them because they will play a role in their conceptualization of the family they are treating.

The use of the terms *majority* and *minority* provide illustration of how categories can influence an individual's participation in society. These terms are sometimes used to denote the number of people; however, in the context of cultural competency, the terms majority and minority denote who holds power and privilege, and conversely who does not hold them, in a given society.[6] *Majority*, or mainstream population, is defined as "the group [who] occupies a position of power and privilege."[6] Traditional standards of "acceptable behaviors, values, and belief systems have been established by this group of people."[6] The *minority* group is defined as the "group that is considered to be in a subordinate position of prestige, power, and privilege."[6] People

belonging to a minority group are commonly excluded from full participation in the life of a society.[6,9]

Although some individuals whom the therapist will encounter continue to use the terms minority and majority, many health professionals have moved away from this language in preference for language that more specifically highlights the experience of the individual (eg, underrepresented, historically marginalized, and targeted identities). Therapists interested in learning more about these terms are directed to explore the psychology of minoritization literature.

Therapists need to be sensitive to the differences in race and ethnicity of the families and children they serve. For example, federal policy defines Hispanic not as a race, but as an ethnicity, yet 69% of young Latino adults 18 to 29 years say their Latino background is part of their racial background, as does a similar share of those in other age groups, including those 65 and older.[10] "At 54 million, Hispanics make up 17% of the nation's population, and they are projected to grow to be 29% of the U.S. population by 2060."[11] Classifications of race and ethnicity in the United States are used for interpersonal interactions, accurate documentation, and reliable research, so therapists need to be familiar with

TABLE 3-1 (CONTINUED)
CULTURAL COMPETENCE CONTINUUM

Cultural competence is demonstrating an acceptance of and respect for cultural differences, including:

1. Creating a mission statement for the organization that articulates principles, rationale, and values for cultural and linguistic competence in all aspects of the organization.

2. Implementing specific policies and procedures that integrate cultural and linguistic competence into each core function of the organization.

3. Identifying, using, and/or adapting evidence-based and promising practices that are culturally and linguistically competent.

4. Developing structures and strategies to ensure consumer and community participation in the planning, delivery, and evaluation of the organization's core function.

5. Implementing policies and procedures to recruit, hire, and maintain a diverse and culturally and linguistically competent workforce.

6. Providing fiscal support, professional development, and incentives for the improvement of cultural and linguistic competence at the board, program, and faculty and/or staff levels.

7. Dedicating resources for both individual and organizational self-assessment of cultural and linguistic competence.

8. Developing the capacity to collect and analyze data using variables that have a meaningful impact on culturally and linguistically diverse groups.

9. Practicing principles of community engagement that result in the reciprocal transfer of knowledge and skills between all collaborators, partners, and key stakeholders.

Cultural proficiency is holding culture in high esteem and using this as a foundation to guide all endeavors, including:

1. Continuing to add to the knowledge base within the field of cultural and linguistic competence by conducting research and developing new treatments, interventions, and approaches for health and mental care in policy, education, and delivery of care.

2. Developing organizational philosophy and practices that integrate health and mental health care.

3. Employing faculty and/or staff, consultants, and consumers with expertise in cultural and linguistic competence in health and mental health care practice, education, and research.

4. Publishing and disseminating promising and evidence-based health and mental health care practices, interventions, training, and education models.

5. Supporting and mentoring other organizations as they progress along the Cultural Competence Continuum.

6. Developing and disseminating health and mental health promotion materials that are adapted to the cultural and linguistic contexts of populations served.

7. Actively pursuing resource development to continually enhance and expand the organization's capacities in cultural and linguistic competence.

8. Advocating with, and on behalf of, populations who are traditionally unserved and underserved.

9. Establishing and maintaining partnerships with diverse constituency groups that span the boundaries of the traditional health and mental health care arenas to eliminate racial and ethnic disparities in health and mental health.

Adapted from Cross T, Bazron B, Dennis K, Isaacs M. *Towards a culturally competent system of care, Volume I.* Washington, DC: CAASP Technical Assistance Center, Georgetown University Child Development Center, CASSP Technical Assistance Center; 1989.

TABLE 3-2
DEFINITIONS OF RACE, ETHNICITY, AND NATIONALITY

TERM	DEFINITION
Race	Some argue that race is a biological construct describing inherited anatomical features and psychological attributes. Others argue that it is becoming a social construct. For the purpose of this book, race refers a population with shared inherited traits and attributes.
Ethnicity	The fact or state of belonging to a social group that has a common national or cultural tradition.
Nationality	The status of belonging to a particular nation. This status can be related to a place of birth or through citizenship, generally governed by where the person reside.

Information compiled from Gannon M. Race Is a Social Construct, Scientists Argue. Scientific American Web site. https://www.scientificamerican.com/article/race-is-a-social-construct-scientists-argue/. Published February 5, 2016. Accessed March 30, 2017 and Oxford Dictionary. https://en.oxforddictionaries.com/definition/ethnicity. Accessed March 30, 2017.

TABLE 3-3
CLASSIFICATIONS OF ETHNICITY IN THE UNITED STATES

ETHNICITY	DESCRIPTION
Hispanic	A person of Cuban, Mexican, Puerto Rican, Cuban, South or Central American, or other Spanish culture or origin, regardless of race; the term "Spanish origin" can be used in addition to "Hispanic or Latino"
Non-Hispanic	A person not identifying with any of the origins considered Hispanic

Adapted from Standards for Maintaining, Collecting, and Presenting Federal Data on Race and Ethnicity. Centers for Disease Control and Prevention Web site. https://wonder.cdc.gov/wonder/help/populations/bridged-race/OMB-RaceStandards1997.pdf. Published January 1, 2003. Accessed December 2, 2017.

Note: Although the terms Hispanic and Latino have been used interchangeably, Hispanic refers to individuals with heritage from the Iberian Peninsula, whereas Latinos/Latinas are generally from Mexico, Central and South America, and the Caribbean.[3]

the correct description of each. Table 3-4 provides the current classifications of race and their descriptions, and Table 3-3 provides the classifications of ethnicity. When making these designations, it is helpful to describe each term for future reference.

Assimilation and *acculturation* are words that describe how people may choose, and in some cases are forced, to incorporate themselves into different societies and cultures.[12] *Assimilation* is the process by which individuals give up their own culture in favor of assuming the attributes of another culture, and *acculturation* is the process by which individuals take on the attributes of another culture.[12] In her research, Battle[12] proposes three models that help to explain the cultural and linguistic diversity in the United States. These models of assimilation and acculturation are explained in Table 3-5.

The Conformity Model has been used throughout the history of the United States; whereas the Melting Pot Model gained traction throughout the 1960s.[12] Although some individuals continue to support the idea of the melting pot, far more identify with the idea that the United States is like a mosaic where people from different cultures come to the United States, retain much of their unique culture, and still blend into the fabric of American society to create a rich and unique culture.[6] This is more indicative of the Cultural Pluralism Model, which gained prominence in the 1990s.[12]

How, and if, a person choses to assimilate or acculturate may be influenced by several factors (eg, race, ethnicity, gender, religion).[12] Circumstances surrounding the immigration may also greatly influence how a person integrates into society.[12] Battle[12] states, for example, that people who identify as voluntary immigrants may have more time to prepare for their transition into the new culture and, therefore, may be more accepting of cultural changes that help them succeed in the new society. In contrast, involuntary immigrants and those seeking asylum may not have time to prepare and

TABLE 3-4
CLASSIFICATIONS OF RACE IN THE UNITED STATES

RACE	DESCRIPTION
American Indian or Alaska Native	A person having origins in any of the original peoples of North and South America (including Central America) and who maintains tribal affiliation or community attachment
Asian	A person having origins in any of the original peoples of the Far East, Southeast Asia, or the Indian subcontinent, including Cambodia, China, India, Japan, the Koreas, Malaysia, Pakistan, the Philippine Islands, Thailand, and Vietnam
Black or African American	A person having origins in any of the Black racial groups of Africa
Native Hawaiian or Other Pacific Islander	A person having origins in any of the original peoples of Hawaii, Guam, Samoa, or other Pacific Islands
White	A person having origins in any of the original peoples of Europe, the Middle East, or North Africa
Adopted from Standards for Maintaining, Collecting, and Presenting Federal Data on Race and Ethnicity. Federal Register Web site. https://www.federalregister.gov/documents/2016/09/30/2016-23672/standards-for-maintaining-collecting-and-presenting-federal-data-on-race-and-ethnicity. Published September 30, 2016. Accessed on December 2, 2017.	

TABLE 3-5
MODELS OF ASSIMILATION AND ACCULTURATION

MODEL	DESCRIPTION
Conformity Model	Ethnic minority group members within a larger society abandon their own social, cultural, and personal traditions to take on the characteristics and traditions of the dominant ethnic group.
Amalgamation (Melting Pot) Theory	All ethnic groups combine their traditions values and characteristics with one another to create a new group.
Accommodation (Cultural Pluralism) Theory	Ethnic groups can coexist and still maintain their culture; they can also comingle with the larger dominant group and maintain relative equality.

may even be outcast in the new society and, therefore, may be more resistant to assimilation.[12]

When pediatric therapists work with immigrant families, they must be especially resourceful exploring their native cultures to better understand their cultural beliefs, especially regarding children, families, education, and health. One of the greatest barriers to providing culturally competent care is language: speaking, listening, reading, and, most importantly, understanding the families who are seeking care.

Table 3-6 provides common terms related to culture. While not exhaustive, the list can be useful for self-development by exploring, defining, and applying these commonly encountered terms to societal issues faced in local communities Some of these terms are sensitive, and working with terms with variable definitions may be ineffective. Try to decide on a common definition for team members for improved communication and understanding among team members and those served.

DIVERSITY VERSUS CULTURAL COMPETENCY

In both health care and education, there is a push to continue to diversify the workforce in terms of race, ethnicity,

TABLE 3-6

CULTURAL TERMINOLOGY DEFINITIONS

OVERARCHING CONCEPTS	
Culture	"The set of shared attitudes, values, beliefs, goals, and practices that characterizes group or organization; the set of values, conventions, or social practices associated with a particular field, activity, or societal characteristic"
Ethnic	"Of or relating to large groups of people classed according to common racial, national, tribal, religious, linguistic, or cultural origin or background"

BACKGROUND/DEMOGRAPHICS/GENDER IDENTITIES	
Androgynous	"Having the characteristics or nature of both male and female"
Sex	"Either of the two major forms of individuals that occur in many species and that are distinguished respectively as female or male especially on the basis of their reproductive organs and structures"
Gender	"The behavioral, cultural, or psychological traits typically associated with one sex"
Generation	"A group of individuals born and living contemporaneously, eg, • Gen Z, iGen, or Centennials: Born 1996 and later • Millennials or Gen Y: Born 1977 to 1995 • Generation X: Born 1965 to 1976 • Baby Boomers: Born 1946 to 1964 • Traditionalists or Silent Generation: Born 1945 and before"

Adapted from The Center for Generational Kinetics. Generational breakdown: Info about all of the generations. The Center for Generational Kinetics Web site. http://genhq.com/faq-info-about-generations/. Published 2016. Accessed December 2, 2017.

Heritage	"Something that is handed down from the past, as a tradition: a national heritage of honor, pride, and courage; something that comes or belongs to one by reason of birth; an inherited lot or portion"
Indigenous	"Growing, living, or occurring naturally in a particular region or environment (the indigenous culture)"
Nationality	"National status; specifically, a legal relationship involving allegiance on the part of an individual and usually protection on the part of the state nationality bestowed by birth"
Race	"A family, tribe, people, or nation belonging to the same stock; a class or kind of people unified by shared interests, habits, or characteristics"

ECONOMIC STATUS	
Poverty	"The state of one who lacks a usual or socially acceptable amount of money or material possessions"
Privilege	"A right or immunity granted as a peculiar benefit, advantage, or favor"
Socioeconomic status	"One's access to financial, social, cultural, and human capital resources…the primary measurement of SES over the years has been the 'big 3' variables: (a) family income, (b) educational attainment of heads of household, and (c) occupational status of heads of household"

Adapted from Improving the Measurement of Socioeconomic Status for the National Assessment of Educational Progress: A Theoretical Foundation. https://nces.ed.gov/nationsreportcard/pdf/researchcenter/Socioeconomic_Factors.pdf. Published November 2012.

Wealth	"An abundance of valuable possessions or money"

(continued)

TABLE 3-6 (CONTINUED)	
CULTURAL TERMINOLOGY DEFINITIONS	
SEXUAL ORIENTATION	
Asexual	"A sexual orientation generally characterized by not feeling sexual attraction or a desire for partnered sexuality; asexuality is distinct from celibacy, which is the deliberate abstention from sexual activity; some asexual people do have sex"
UC Davis. LGBTQIA Resource Center Glossary. UC Davis Web site. https://lgbtqia.ucdavis.edu/educated/glossary.html. Published October 13, 2017. Accessed December 2, 2017.	
Bisexual	"Possessing characters of both sexes and especially both male and female reproductive structures; of, relating to, or characterized by sexual or romantic attraction to members of both sexes; also, engaging in sexual activity with partners of more than one gender"
Cisgender	"Of, relating to, or being a person whose gender identity corresponds with the sex the person had or was identified as having at birth"
Gay/ Homosexual	"Of, relating to, or characterized by a tendency to direct sexual desire toward another of the same sex"
Heterosexual	"Of, relating to, or characterized by a tendency to direct sexual desire toward the opposite sex"
LGBTQIA	"Lesbian, gay, bisexual, transgender, queer and/or questioning, intersex, asexual"
Adapted from UC Davis. LGBTQIA Resource Center Glossary. UC Davis Web site. https://lgbtqia.ucdavis.edu/educated/glossary.html. Published October 13, 2017. Accessed December 2, 2017.	
Transgender	"A wide range of identities and experiences of people whose gender identity and/or expression differs from conventional expectations based on their assigned sex at birth; not all trans people undergo medical transition (surgery or hormones)"
Adapted from UC Davis. LGBTQIA Resource Center Glossary. UC Davis Web site. https://lgbtqia.ucdavis.edu/educated/glossary.html. Published October 13, 2017. Accessed December 2, 2017.	

(continued)

and gender to create a workforce that looks like the clients served. However, it is important to note that a pediatric therapist working with a family from a culturally and/or linguistically diverse background from her own does not need to be a member of that group to provide services to someone of a different culture.[6] Instead, it is more important that the therapist have the skills and training necessary to deliver services in an unbiased and culturally competent manner.

Pediatric therapists need to be very familiar with the idea of *difference versus disorder*.[6] *Difference* and *disorder* are terms commonly used to describe children who are atypical or different. A child who is *different* may be atypical due to cultural variability but not developmentally abnormal or unhealthy. A child with a *disorder* may have a physical or mental condition that is not normal or healthy. The Interprofessional Activity section offers an opportunity to explore difference versus disorder in the context of cultural differences that may impact a child's developmental skills.

POLICIES, STANDARDS, AND MANDATES PROMOTING CULTURALLY COMPETENT HEALTH CARE

The importance of providing culturally competent health and educational services has been underscored by the creation and implementation of federal, state, and local government policies, accreditation standards, and other mandates aimed at reducing bias in service delivery, eliminating health disparities, and improving the health of communities at risk.[3]

Medical cultural competency legislation and regulation includes Title VI of the Civil Rights Act of 1964, a national law that protects persons from discrimination based on their race, color, or national origin in programs and activities that receive federal financial assistance.[13] In 2000, Executive

TABLE 3-6 (CONTINUED)

CULTURAL TERMINOLOGY DEFINITIONS

SOCIAL ATTITUDES/BELIEFS	
Bigotry	"Obstinate or intolerant devotion to one's own opinions and prejudices"
Classism	"Prejudice or discrimination based on class"
Equality	"The quality or state of being equal"
Hate	"Intense hostility and aversion usually deriving from fear, anger, or sense of injury; extreme dislike or disgust"
Micro-aggression	"A comment or action that subtly and often unconsciously or unintentionally expresses a prejudiced attitude toward a member of a marginalized group (such as a racial minority)"
Oppression	"Unjust or cruel exercise of authority or power"
Power	"Ability to act or produce an effect; possession of control, authority, or influence over others; physical might, mental or moral efficacy, political control or influence"
Prejudice	"Preconceived judgment or opinion; an adverse opinion or leaning formed without just grounds or before sufficient knowledge; an instance of such judgment or opinion; an irrational attitude of hostility directed against an individual, a group, a race, or their supposed characteristics"
Racism	"A belief that race is the primary determinant of human traits and capacities and that racial differences produce an inherent superiority of a particular race"
Sexism	"Prejudice or discrimination based on sex; especially, discrimination against women; behavior, conditions, or attitudes that foster stereotypes of social roles based on sex"
Stereotype	"An idea or statement about all of the members of a group or all the instances of a situation"
Religion	"A body of beliefs and practices regarding the supernatural and the worship of one or more deities"
Spirituality	"The deepest values and meanings by which people live"

Adapted from Sheldrake P. *A Brief History of Spirituality.* Hoboken, NJ: Wiley-Blackwell; 2007:1-2

Unless noted otherwise, definitions reprinted from Merriam Webster. Merriam Webster Web site. https://www.merriam-webster.com. Published 2017. Accessed December 2, 2017.

Order 13166, Improving Access to Services for Persons with Limited English Proficiency, required federal agencies to examine the services they provide, identify any need for services to those with limited English proficiency (LEP), and develop and implement a system to provide those services so LEP persons can have meaningful access to them.[13]

In 1995, the Center for Linguistic and Cultural Competence in Health Care (CLCCHC) was established to address the health needs of populations who speak limited English and helps to fulfill the requirements of PL 101-527.[14] CLCCHC is a "center without walls," encompassing all existing and new policy, partnerships, communications, service demonstrations, and evaluation activities related to cultural competency.[14]

The latest mandate to address culturally competent health care comes from the Affordable Care Act (ACA).

In 2015, the Department of Health and Human Services enacted the Nondiscrimination in Health Programs and Activities final rule that implements Section 1557 of the ACA.[15] The Department of Health and Human Services states that the "final rule prohibits discrimination based on race, color, national origin, sex, age, or disability as well as enhances language assistance for individuals with limited English proficiency and protects individuals with disabilities."[16] The final rule was implemented in an effort to improve health equity and reduce disparities in health care. Essentially, the rule helps to provide protections from discrimination in health care based on sex and provide protections and access to individuals with disabilities and individuals who have LEP.

Although these policies are currently in place, they may not be recognized and enforced in some environments. As advocates for children and their families, pediatric therapists need to ensure that families are aware of their rights and serve as advocates for support to ensure culturally competent care for all.

COMMUNICATING WITH CULTURAL COMPETENCY

Linguistics and *language* are words often used interchangeably in the cultural competence and cultural and linguistic diversity literature. In the context of diversity, linguistic diversity—or language diversity—refers to the number of languages and speakers of those languages in a given place (eg, the United States).[17] The US Census Bureau (2015) reported there to be over 350 languages spoken in the United States households.[18] Therefore, pediatric therapists should expect to encounter individuals from linguistically diverse backgrounds and be prepared to work with them.

One culture commonly encountered in pediatrics is the Deaf culture. Whereas the word deaf suggests someone with hearing impairments, the Deaf culture (with a capital "D") refers to the attitudes, values, traditions, and history shared by this culture.[19] According to the American Society for Deaf Children, ample evidence supports the benefits of using sign language with all children, regardless of their hearing status. The following are universal benefits of early visual language[20]:

- Early language learning experiences with sign language positively impact other areas of development and are critical to children's future success.

- Sign language provides the earliest possible mode through which children can learn expressive language skills.

- All children benefit from the use of sign language without any detriment to their other language skills.

Because family involvement is a critical factor in the language development of children who have complete or partial hearing loss, pediatric therapists should strive to support a home environment that is linguistically accessible to a deaf child by encouraging parental use of sign language. Therapists should also work as an interprofessional team to identify those signs that best serve the child's and family's needs. In cases where a child has cognitive and/or motor impairments, the interprofessional team can help the child and family develop adapted signs for communication.

Translation and *interpretation* have important meanings when working with families whose first language may not be English. *Interpretation* is providing a clear explanation of written words, whereas translation refers to the process of translating spoken words[3] or text from one language into another. In the provision of culturally competent services, it is important to consider delivery of information in the language and medium most conducive to the child's and family's linguistic ability. The ACA prohibits discrimination in health coverage and care based on race, color, national origin, age, disability, and sex, so health care agencies must provide appropriate interpretation and translation services when needed.[17]

Communicating with families with different languages has some ground rules that are important to consider. Here are some key considerations when considering the use of an interpreter[19]:

- Use trained interpreters. Although it may often seem easier, or even better, to have translation and/or interpretation done by a member of the family, one must not forget that the untrained person may not have been exposed to medical or health care jargon and may not be able to accurately convey the intended message; there can be variations in dialect that may cause misunderstandings. In addition to being a potential Health Insurance Portability and Accountability Act (HIPAA) violation, this practice puts both you and the family at risk for miscommunication and misinformation.

- Use the "teach back" method: (1) ask the family to repeat back what was just explained to them to assess their understanding; (2) repeat your information, clarifying as needed; then (3) ask the family to share what they heard to confirm their understanding.

- Talk directly to the family, not to the interpreter. Ask the family, "Do you...?" Speak more slowly rather than more loudly. Speak at an even pace in relatively short segments. Pause so the interpreter can interpret. Assume, and insist, that everything you say, everything the patient says, and everything that family members say is interpreted. Give the interpreter time to restructure information in his mind and present it in a culturally and linguistically appropriate manner. Speaking English does not mean thinking in English.

- Expect the interpreter to be a neutral party and to not take sides. The interpreter's role is limited to facilitating linguistic and cultural communication between you and the child and family.

- Remember the cultural differences between you and the family. A family member may not answer questions as directly or clearly as you'd like, but that may be due to cultural differences in dealing with sensitive information. Ask the family member what she believes the problem is, what causes it, and how it would be treated in their country of origin.

- Encourage the interpreter to ask questions and to alert you about potential cultural misunderstandings that may come up.

- Ask the interpreter for clarification if you are unsure as to his role.
- Recognize the limits of your bilingual skills.
- Do not ask the interpreter, "Do you think the family understood?" The interpreter is not qualified to make cognitive assessments. The interpreter's role is to only interpret, not to explain, simplify, alter, add, omit, or summarize what is said. This helps keep the provider in control.
- Do not tell the interpreter, "Don't interpret this, but...." It is a violation of his code of ethics. Remember that the interpreter is required to interpret everything that is said within the patient's earshot. If it is something an English-speaking patient would hear, the foreign language–speaking patient has the right to hear the same information.
- Do not ask the interpreter to interact with the family if you are not present.
- Avoid asking families if they understand. Individuals may be embarrassed to admit that they do not understand.
- Keep in mind that interpreters are not advocates, social workers, health care providers, or family representatives.

When therapists work cross-culturally with families, it is helpful to:
- Take a few minutes to explain our health care culture to the family.
- Speak clearly and slowly without raising your voice.
- Use Mrs, Miss, and Mr for parents. Avoid using their first names, which may be considered discourteous in some cultures. Always use the formal "usted" when addressing parents/adult Spanish-speaking patients.
- Avoid gestures: they may have a negative connotation.
- Acknowledge beliefs. Some individuals believe their child's problems are caused by supernatural or environmental factors like cold air or cold water. Do not dismiss these beliefs because they play an important role in some people's lives.

The LEARN Model

Awareness of the family's cultural background is critical to understanding the other person's point of view and relevant issues. The LEARN model, emphasizing listening and sharing similarities and differences, can be used to effectively overcome cultural communication barriers.[20] The acronym LEARN represents the following key components of the model[20]:

L = Listen with sympathy and understanding to the client's perception of the problem.

E = Explain your perceptions of the problem.

A = Acknowledge and discuss the differences and similarities.

R = Recommend a course of action.

N = Negotiate an agreement.

Using the LEARN model enables pediatric therapists to effectively communicate with each other, children, and others involved in the children's care.

The ETHNIC Model

Another model for working with families from diverse backgrounds goes by the acronym ETHNIC[21] and serves as another means of organizing cross-cultural communication:

E = Explanation: Have the person describe what he believes is the reason for the child's problems. Ask: What do you think may be the reason your child has these symptoms? What do friends and family say about these symptoms? Do you know anyone else with this problem? What have you heard on the TV or radio about the condition?

T = Treatments: Have the person share prior treatments used to manage the child's issues. Ask: What medicines, home remedies, or other treatments have been tried? Is there anything you eat, drink, or avoid to stay healthy? Please tell me about it. What treatment are you seeking?

H = Healers: Consider that many cultures value alternative therapies and inventions. Ask: Have you used alternative therapies or folk healers? Tell me about it.

N = Negotiate: Families may not be familiar with current options for addressing their concerns. At this point it is important to negotiate mutually acceptable options that incorporate the family's beliefs and those that offer the most benefit for the child.

I = Intervention: Consider how standard protocols may not be the best option for families who value alternative interventions. Determine interventions that respect the values and beliefs of each family.

C = Collaboration: Recognize the importance of interprofessional collaboration that integrates input from the child, the family, therapists, other professionals, alternative care providers, and community resources.

Pediatric therapists have the unique opportunity to meet and work with families *where they are*. This catchphrase is often used to mean that the health care team should value and respect the needs, wants, abilities, and capacities of the families they serve. Part of meeting families where they are is an understanding of the family's strengths. *Strengths-based approaches* to therapy focus on what the child and family can do rather than what they cannot do.[22-25] In the context of intervention, strengths-based approaches consider the child's skills rather than his limitations. These skills are then used as a basis for implementing compensatory strategies and interventions. In the context of families, strengths-based approaches consider what the family's abilities are in terms of caring for the child.

Finally, pediatric therapists must serve as advocates for cultural competency, ensuring that public policies and laws support access to resources that help people of all cultures who seek health care services in the United States. Listed here are resources that provide additional cultural competency information for self-assessment, professional development, population specific care, and advocacy.

RESOURCES FOR CULTURAL COMPETENCY

1. Health Resources and Service Administration: Culture, Language, and Health Literacy—This site lists essential health literacy tools and resources for distinct populations, including race/ethnicity, gender, age, and special populations. https://www.hrsa.gov/culturalcompetence/index.html

2. US Department of Health and Human Services Office of Minority Services: Cultural and Linguistic Competency—This site provides links to the National CLAS Standards, including a collective set of mandates and guidelines that inform, guide, and facilitate both required and recommended practices related to culturally and linguistically appropriate health services. It also links to the Center for Linguistic and Cultural Competency in Health Care that addresses the health needs of populations who speak limited English. https://minorityhealth.hhs.gov/omh/browse.aspx?lvl=1&lvlid=6

3. US Department of Health and Human Services: Tracking CLAS—This interactive map displays each state's efforts to promote and provide culturally and linguistically appropriate services (CLAS) through legislation, policies, and/or practices. https://www.thinkculturalhealth.hhs.gov/

4. Guide to Providing Effective Communication and Language Assistance Services—This government site features a guide designed for health care professionals, administrators, and executives who work across a broad spectrum of health care organizations. Register for this guide and additional free resources at https://hclsig.thinkculturalhealth.hhs.gov/

5. National Center for Cultural Competence—This site offers resources to increase the capacity of health care and mental health care programs to design, implement, and evaluate culturally and linguistically competent service delivery systems to address growing diversity and persistent disparities and to promote health and mental health equity. https://nccc.georgetown.edu/

6. CultureVision—A comprehensive, user-friendly database offering information about culturally competent care. http://www.crculturevision.com/

7. *Cultural Competency for the Health Professional*, by Patti R. Rose.

SUMMARY

As mentioned in earlier sections, pediatric therapists who work with family members must value family-centered care. Family-centered care respects families' values, beliefs, and ideas and attempts to integrate families' wishes and goals into therapeutic interventions to reach desired outcomes. For this reason, pediatric therapists must collaboratively work toward becoming culturally competent clinicians and educators; be open to other points of view and avoid value judgments; treat everyone with dignity and respect; and use a strengths-based approach, recognizing each family's unique strengths as a basis for assessment, intervention, and education. Also, when managing care, pediatric professionals need to be sensitive to their workplace's character and personality, also referred to as the *workplace culture*. Section 4 will discuss how the workplace culture shapes interprofessional teamwork.

INTERPROFESSIONAL ACTIVITIES

Your Cultural Identity

Reflect on your cultural competency in light of the information presented in this section.

1. What are your cultural identities, and what defines you the most? (Facets of your cultural identity may include, but are not limited to, your nationality, ethnicity, native language and other languages, race, gender, religion or spiritual beliefs, occupational status, educational status, economic status or social class, physical attributes, relationship status, age group, generation, geographical/regional residency, health status, and personality.)

2. How do your cultural identities impact how you react with others?

3. How would you rate yourself on the Cultural Competency Continuum?

Cultural Competency in Communication

Consider how diversity in families can impact how you will interact professionally with children and their families.

1. Read the following case studies and discuss how the interprofessional team can interact most effectively with the child and the family. Consider whether or not the RESPECT or ETHNIC method would be appropriate.

2. What cultural factors might influence delays in each child's development?

3. As an interprofessional team, what resources would you explore in preparation for reassessing this child's functional skills? See the resources listed in this section.

Case 3-1: A 13-month-old girl from China

Bo lived in an orphanage in Beijing, China, until she was adopted by her American parents and brought to the United States when she was 10 months old. Her parents, Mary and Suzanne, also have 3 other recently adopted children, Grace (a 5-year-old daughter from Ecuador), Bryan (a 7-year-old son from Guatemala), and Cam (a 9-year-old daughter from Vietnam). Mary is a housewife who takes care of the children, and Suzanne runs a successful business that frequently takes her out of town. Bo is currently 13 months old; however, her developmental skills are at the 6-month level of development. Both parents are interested in receiving private services for Bo to help her gain the skills needed to catch up with her peers.

Case 3-2: A 3-year-old girl with developmental delay

Maher and Aroos, Amena's father and mother, immigrated to the United States from Afghanistan when they discovered that Amena was not developing like other children her age. Both parents are professionals and very religious. As Muslims, they feared that their family would be shamed if they remained in Afghanistan, so both parents found secure jobs in technology. At 3 years, Amena is now integrated into a half-day private preschool program. Amena is able to walk but demonstrates poor balance, a wide base of support, and high guard arm position when ambulating. Amena can kick a ball, but falls once with 3 kicks. She ascends and descends stairs in marking time with both hands holding onto the rails. Amena demonstrates palmar grip around all objects. Her mother states she is left-hand

dominant, but Amena does not show any dominance when coloring. Amena uses her thumb and all 4 fingers to grasp objects and turn pages. She has difficulty following simple tasks. She does vocalize with other children at the preschool. Her developmental screens on average showed her functional skills at the 20-month developmental age when she was 36 months old. The interprofessional team is working with a private preschool to provide needed supports and equipment to ensure that Amena has what she needs to optimally learn in the preschool environment.

REFERENCES

1. Colby SL, Ortman JM. Projections of the size and composition of the US population: 2014 to 2060, Current Population Reports, P25-1143. Washington, DC: US Census Bureau; 2014. https://www.census.gov/content/dam/Census/library/publications/2015/demo/p25-1143.pdf. Published 2014. Accessed January 25, 2017.

2. Mancoske RJ, Lewis ML, Bowers-Stevens C, Ford A. Cultural competence and children's mental health service outcomes. *Journal of Ethnic & Cultural Diversity in Social Work*. 2012;21:195-211.

3. Rose PR. *Cultural Competency for the Health Professional*. Burlington, MA: Jones & Bartlett; 2013.

4. Cultural Competence. American Speech-Language-Hearing Association Web site. http://www.asha.org/PRPSpecificTopic.aspx?folderid=8589935230&section=References. Accessed February 28, 2017.

5. Cross T, Bazron B, Dennis K, Isaacs M. *Towards a culturally competent system of care, Volume I*. Washington, DC: CAASP Technical Assistance Center, Georgetown University Child Development Center, CASSP Technical Assistance Center; 1989.

6. Coleman TJ. *Clinical Management of Communication Disorders in Culturally Diverse Children*. Old Tappan, NJ: Pearson; 1999.

7. US Department of Health and Human Services Office of Minority Health. Race. United States Census Bureau Web site. https://www.census.gov/quickfacts/meta/long_RHI225215.htm. Accessed March 30, 2017.

8. Ford C, Harawa NT. A new conceptualization of ethnicity for social epidemiologic and health equity research. *Soc Sci Med*. 2010;71(2):251-258.

9. Essential principles in history. Democracy Web Web site. http://democracyweb.org/majority-rule-principles. Accessed March 30, 2017.

10. Gonzalez-Barrera A, Lopez M. Is being Hispanic a matter of race, ethnicity or both? Pew Research Center Web site. http://www.pewresearch.org/fact-tank/2015/06/15/is-being-hispanic-a-matter-of-race-ethnicity-or-both/. Published 2017. Accessed January 25, 2017.

11. US Census Bureau. 2014 National Population Projections: Summary Tables. United States Census Bureau Web site. http://www.census.gov/population/projections/data/national/2014/summarytables.html. Accessed January 25, 2017.

12. Battle B. *Communication Disorders in Multicultural Populations*. 4th ed. Maryland Heights, MO: Mosby; 2011.

13. Limited English Proficiency. Executive Order 13166. Limited English Proficiency Web site. https://www.lep.gov/13166/eo13166.html. Accessed January 25, 2017.

14. US Department of Health and Human Services Office of Minority Health. Center for Linguistic and Cultural Competency in Health Care. US Department of Health and Human Services Office of Minority Health Web site. https://minorityhealth.hhs.gov/omh/browse.aspx?lvl=2&lvlid=34. Accessed January 25, 2017.

15. US Department of Health and Human Services. Section 1557: Ensuring Meaningful Access for Individuals with Limited English Proficiency. https://www.hhs.gov/sites/default/files/1557-fs-lep-508.pdf. Published August 25, 2016. Accessed December 2, 2017.

16. US Department of Health and Human Services. Strategic Language Access Plan. Centers for Medicare & Medicaid Services Web site. https://www.cms.gov/About-CMS/Agency-Information/OEOCRInfo/Downloads/StrategicLanguageAccessPlan.pdf. Accessed January 25, 2017.

17. Rumbaut RG, Massey DS. Immigration and language diversity in the United States. *Daedalus.* 2013;142(3):141-154.

18. US Census Bureau. Census Bureau Reports at Least 350 Languages Spoken in U.S. Homes. United States Census Bureau Web site. https://www.census.gov/newsroom/press-releases/2015/cb15-185.html. Published November 03, 2015. Accessed December 28, 2017.

19. Minnesota Department of Health and Human Services. Deaf culture. Minnesota Department of Health and Human Services Web site. http://www.dhs.state.mn.us/main/idcplg?IdcService=GET_DYNAMIC_CONVERSION&RevisionSelectionMethod=Latest Released&dDocName=id_004566. Published February 11, 2013. Accessed February 28, 2017.

20. National Science Foundation. Visual and visual learning brief: advantages of early visual language. American Society for Deaf Children Web site. http://deafchildren.org/wp-content/uploads/2014/05/ASDC-Article-VL2-Advantages-of-Early-Visual-Language.pdf. Published January 2012. Accessed February 28, 2017.

21. American Translators Association. https://www.atanet.org/. Accessed January 25, 2017.

22. Welch M. *Enhancing Awareness and Improving Cultural Competence in Health Care: A Partnership Guide for Teaching Diversity and Cross-Cultural Concepts in Health Professional Training.* San Francisco: University of California.

23. Levin SJ, Like RC, Gottlieb JE. ETHNIC: A Framework for Culturally Competent Clinical Practice. In: Appendix: Useful clinical interviewing mnemonics. *Patient Care.* 2000;34(9)188-189.

24. Hoagwood KE, Olin SS, Kerker BD, Kratochwill TR, Crowe M, Saka, N. Empirically based school interventions targeted at academic and mental health functioning. *J Emot Behav Disord.* 2007;15(2):66-92.

25. Reddy LA, DeThomas CA, Newman E, Chun V. School-based prevention and intervention programs for children with emotional disturbance: A review of treatment components and methodology. *Psychology in the Schools.* 2009;46(2):132-153.

Section 4

Overview of Human Growth and Development for Pediatric Therapists

Catherine Rush Thompson, PT, PhD, MS

OVERVIEW

The developmental framework for pediatric therapy is similar across professions; however, each professional focuses on different aspects of dynamic changes in a child's growth and development. For example, when working with a child, the physical therapists might attend more closely to the growth and development of body systems and body functions, as well as the child's ability to learn and perform motor skills related to postural control and functional movements. The occupational therapist might look more closely at the child's sensorimotor integration and engagement in daily activities, such as eating and dressing, keeping in mind similar motor learning factors. The speech-language pathologist might examine the child's swallowing and communication skill development more closely. All 3 experts might observe the child's snack time with attention to different aspects of this daily activity. The physical therapist would attend to the child's posture for optimizing motor control and providing a good base of support for feeding. The occupational therapist would examine the task of feeding itself, noting fine motor and oral motor control for feeding. The speech-language pathologist would attend closely to the child's safety for oral feeding, including risk of aspiration, and would provide opportunities for communication during

feeding. Sharing a similar knowledge of typical growth and development provides a foundation for interprofessional collaboration and appreciation of each professional's expertise when caring for children and educating their caretakers. This section provides references to typical growth and development that help guide the management of children with special needs. It also offers a reference for interprofessional collaboration and sets the stage for comprehensive goals that address a child's learning and healthy development. Finally, it provides a guide to caretakers interested in providing age-appropriate stimulation for their children.

GROWTH AND DEVELOPMENT

All pediatric therapists aim to enhance children's participation in learning opportunities, social engagement, and meaningful lives. Fundamental to this goal is an understanding of typical growth and development. This knowledge helps families and professionals identify concerns and collaboratively generate interventions and resources to support the healthy growth and development of children from birth through adulthood. Although the terms *growth* and *development* are often used interchangeably, they have distinct meanings for pediatric therapists. Growth generally

Thompson CR. *Pediatric Therapy:*
An Interprofessional Framework for Practice (pp 43-70).
© 2018 SLACK Incorporated.

refers to the process of the child's body increasing in physical size, as well as the increase in structures associated with body systems. Development refers to the child's maturation, involving increasingly complex body functions and the differentiation of functional skills over time. Both growth and development must be carefully monitored to ensure that each child's environment (eg, the psychosocial and physical environment) is optimal for the development of age-appropriate skills.

PRINCIPLES OF GROWTH AND DEVELOPMENT

Physical growth occurs concurrently with the development of functional skills. Without an environment that encourages exploration, movement, and communication, a child's mental, psychosocial, and physical growth can suffer. Assuming that children are reared in healthy environments, maintain good health, and engage in physical activity, they grow in predictable patterns.[1] Using these predictable patterns to inform critical thinking, pediatric professionals can monitor growth and anticipate children's needs. These predictable patterns, commonly referred to as the *principles of growth and development*, include the following:

- *Simple to complex*: The body develops from simple, undifferentiated cells to highly differentiated organs and body structures. Likewise, a child's functional skills become more sophisticated and complex with development. For example, an infant develops basic cognitive concepts early in childhood, then later demonstrates the ability to solve problems and use abstract thinking, requiring a more sophisticated level of intellect.

- *Cephalocaudal development*: This principle states that the direction of growth and development occurs from the head downward, or head to toe. Examples of this principle include how a child gains control of movement, beginning with head control, followed by coordination of the arms, then coordination of the legs. Another example of how the body grows head to toe can be observed by the changing head proportions (eg, head circumference) with growth; the head is typically disproportionately larger as a body part in infancy. Later in childhood and adolescence, the head circumference stabilizes in size, whereas the trunk and legs grow in spurts, typically matching adult proportions by 21 years.

- *Continuous process*: The process of growth and development is continuous with a predictable sequence. Although it is continuous, there is some variation, such

as when a child experiences growth spurts. Similarly, development milestones follow a predictable pattern that is sequential, building on prior skills. However, variations in this predictable pattern can occur when a child focuses on a new milestone, sometimes causing a regression in his performance of certain earlier skills.

- *General to specific*: The principle of general to specific is seen in both growth and development. During the first months of gestation, the fetus' limbs are not well differentiated; however, the fingers and toes become clearly distinguishable as the fetus approaches full gestation. In terms of development, early movements employ larger muscle groups, resulting in inaccurate and uncoordinated movements. As the infant matures, smaller muscle groups are activated for increased control for refined movements. For example, an infant may initially swipe at a mobile but later develops the ability to accurately point at objects with a single digit, evidence of developing eye-hand coordination.

- *Proximodistal development*: This principle states that development proceeds from the center of the body outward. During growth in utero, the spinal cord begins developing before the limbs. Similarly, a child develops motor control of the trunk (proximally), then gradually refines movement at the periphery, as she demonstrates control of her fingers (distally).

- *Maturation*: This principle states that biological growth and development depend upon maturation (eg, biological growth and changes in the nervous system contribute to increasingly complex cognitive and motor skills). Maturation is innate, yet the development of skills relies upon environmental stimulation. For example, a child must mature to a certain level of readiness to talk, comprehend words, and read. Similarly, legibly writing one's name requires fine motor control that develops through experiences involving repeated motor practice.

- *Individual rates*: Perhaps the most important principle that pediatric therapists recognize is that each child is unique and, although these patterns are often observed in a sequential pattern, the rates of growth and development vary from child to child. For this reason, growth charts provide a range of normal height and weight. Similarly, motor milestones occur across a wide range of ages depending upon environmental factors, including parenting styles, lifestyle behaviors, personal factors, and environmental enrichment.

These principles are helpful for recognizing patterns of growth and development for the typical child and are clearly evident in the first year of life.

KEY FEATURES OF GROWTH IN THE FIRST YEAR OF LIFE

Growth is a dynamic process that is dependent upon a child's genetics and movement. Muscle growth and the development of muscle strength and control of joint movement are all critical for a child to fully develop motor skills for independence. With the earliest movements, the child's skeletal muscle fibrils grow by multiplication, increasing strength to meet the demands of future movement. Simultaneously, skeletal muscles lengthen or stretch in response to skeletal growth, allowing more range of motion. For children with motor problems restricting movement, skeletal muscles may not reach their full length, potentially restricting future motor development. Similarly guided by genetic codes, cells of the visceral muscles (ie, smooth, involuntary muscles lining the blood vessels, stomach, digestive tract, and other internal organs) increase in number and size throughout the growth process. The cardiac muscle, like skeletal muscle, is responsive to the body's demands for increased circulation during activity, resulting in enlargement of existing muscle fibers, particularly in ventricular muscles.

In accordance with the cephalocaudal principle of development, the infant develops functional skills for survival. From early infancy, the muscles of the face and respiration are well developed, allowing the newborn to breathe, feed, and vocalize at birth, assuming the child is born full term. Typically at birth, after spending 9 months positioned in the womb, the neonate is positioned in a predominantly flexed posture. In the womb, the fetus was not positioned to allow neck extension in the last trimester, so the strength of cervical muscles is poor. Once out of the womb, the newborn wants to see the world. As the newborn moves spontaneously and experiences the effects of gravity, the second month of life is typically characterized by decreased postural flexion and increased extension and asymmetry, generally progressing from head to toe. For example, the infant begins to raise her head against gravity to either side when placed in a prone position as she visually explores her surroundings.

During the third month of life, the infant's movements are characterized by more symmetrical movements, including the beginning of bilateral control of neck muscles, facilitating head control. At this point, the infant initiates rolling in both direction and swipes at toys held within reach. By 6 months, the infant can extend her neck against gravity when lying prone, can roll, and can sit with minimal support. By 7 months, the infant can pivot in prone using symmetrical upper-extremity movements, and by 8 months, the baby can creep as the primary means of locomotion. At 1 year, the baby is capable of rising to stand by using her developing leg muscles. Simultaneously, fine motor control progresses from mass grasp patterns to isolated finger movements, including finger opposition by 12 months. These advances are matched by increased control in oral motor skills that enable the child to first vocalize and then to utter her first words by 1 year.

During the first year of life, the infant experiences dramatic changes in growth and development, dependent upon a healthy environment, opportunities for movement against gravity, and social interactions with parents and other caretakers. The brain maturation process evolves as synapses form, nerves myelinate, and the brain's efficiency increases through synaptic pruning, improving the child's sensory integration and motor control.[2] The brain develops into separate lobes associated with specific functions, including the occipital lobes that control vision; the parietal lobes processing bodily sensations like heat, cold, pressure, and pain; and the temporal lobes involved with hearing, language skills, and social understanding, including perception of other people's eyes and faces. Finally, the frontal lobes, associated with memory, abstract thinking, planning, and impulse control, are the last to mature. These lobes include the prefrontal cortex, associated with the most advanced cognitive functions, including attention, motivation, and goal-directed behavior.[3-5]

The growth and development of body systems across infancy, childhood, and adolescence exemplify the principles of growth and development discussed previously. Whereas genes help direct newly formed neurons to their correct locations in the brain, brain connections are reinforced or modified by infant and child behavior.[6-8] During the infant's active exploration of the environment, the neurological and musculoskeletal systems work in concert to enable postural control for handling toys and uttering meaningful sounds. As early as 6 months, protective reactions emerge, and by 12 months, equilibrium reactions in an upright posture enable the infant to stand unsupported for play. By 1 year, the infant is typically able to communicate through gestures and sounds, demonstrate intent by pointing at objects, appreciate object permanence, and manually feed herself, among many other skills. Table 4-1 illustrates the growth and development of body systems in the first year of life.

GROWTH THROUGHOUT CHILDHOOD

Activities during early childhood further drive the development of body systems to respond to the stresses imposed on tissues. The child's health and growth are monitored from birth to adulthood by physiological markers, such as blood pressure and respiration, and by anthropometric measurements (eg, head circumference, height, and weight) recorded on growth charts. Table 4-2 describes the changes

TABLE 4-1

TYPICAL GROWTH AND DEVELOPMENT OF BODY SYSTEMS FROM BIRTH TO 1 YEAR

AGE	MUSCULOSKELETAL	NEUROLOGICAL/COGNITIVE	CARDIOPULMONARY	INTEGUMENTARY
Birth to 6 months	• Neonate: physiological flexion • Pronated feet • Genus valgus • Primary centers of ossification are present in all long bones • Fontanelles are present in the skull (these are non-serrated sutures) • Skull vault is large • Secondary centers of ossification present in lower end of femur, heads of femur and humerus, and upper end of tibia • Bones of the pelvis and lower limbs are less advanced as far as final size than those of the upper limbs and shoulder girdles • Ilia and sacrum are more upright, and subpubic angle is more acute so cavity of pelvis is small and funnel shaped • At 6 months, the mandibular incisors emerge • At 6 months, the secondary cervical curve has appeared • Feet are flat, soft, subtle, difficult to appreciate due to increased subcutaneous fat; lower extremity range of motion is increased	• Neonate: flexion→extension • The spinal cord is about 15 to 18 cm long • Myelinization continues in both the periphery and the cerebral cortex • Primitive (spinal cord and brainstem) reflexes are present at birth • Optical righting reflex starts to develop at 2 months • Sensorimotor integration	• Rapid heart rate, respiratory rate	• Intact • As the skin grows, the sensory endings become thinned out and not as closely packed
7 to 12 months	• The skull follows the very rapid growth of the brain • The mastoid process forms in the skull • The capitate of the wrist starts to ossify • The growth in skeletal height is approximately 20 to 22 cm/year • With walking, sacral curvature increases, ilia become thicker, and acetabula become deeper	• Protective reactions emerge at 6 months • Righting reactions develop • Equilibrium reactions develop • Beginning of speech patterns: single words repeated		

TABLE 4-2		
SKELETAL CHANGES FROM 1 YEAR TO 6 YEARS		
	1 YEAR TO 3 YEARS	**4 TO 6 YEARS**
Spine and extremities	• Leg growth accelerates in the toddler years • Height increases 5 inches in the second year and 2 inches during the third year • The structural changes of long bone are greatest at 2½ years	• Primary ossification centers appear in the patella and the carpal bones by 3 to 3½ years • Height increases from 5 to 6 cm/year
Skull	• All bones of the skull are ossified by 2 years	
Dentition		• By 6 years, the child has developed the primary dentition and has had some teeth replaced by the secondary dentition (permanent teeth)
Skeletal alignment/ curvature	• Toddler stands bow-legged (genu varus) at 18 months and nock-kneed (genu valgus) at 3 years because of remodeling of the pelvis • With increased walking, lower limbs realign, feet evert, and the angle made by the neck of the femur with the shaft gradually decreases from about 160 degrees to the adult value of 125 degrees	• At 3 years, nearly 75% of children develop genu valgum, which is resolved by 6 to 7 years

in the body alignment as a result of movement and illustrates the changes in dentition that enable eating a wider variety of foods.[7]

After the first year of life, muscles continue to grow and develop in response to activity. Muscle fibers enlarge, providing the strength needed for oral motor, fine motor, and gross motor skills. The child is able to walk, run, and jump with increasing power and endurance, speak with increased volume and clarity, and more easily manipulate objects with varying grasp patterns. These dynamic changes are not without some discomfort; children may experience growth pains during growth spurts.[7] The child also develops the power to securely grip a spoon and self-feed. At this time, the sphincter muscles develop sufficiently to allow toilet training. By 5 years, the child has adequate manipulation skills to begin handwriting, and oral motor mechanisms are developed for clear articulation and chewing (Table 4-3).

The most important system for learning is the neurological system, responsible for a child's desire to explore and to store information. Through play, the child's nervous system develops efficiency for sensory recognition, sensory integration, movement, language development, and cognitive functioning. The central nervous system and the organs of special senses grow so rapidly that they reach 90% of their adult size by 5 or 6 years.[7] Table 4-4 outlines neurological changes impacting sensory, motor, and cognitive functions from 2 to 6 years.

Adolescence is when children again undergo dramatic physical changes:

The human adolescent growth spurt is the rapid and intense increase in the rate of growth in height and weight that occurs during the adolescent stage of the human life cycle. The human adolescent growth spurt is noted in virtually all of the long bones of the body and most other skeletal elements. The major exception is the female pelvis, which follows a smooth and continuous increase in size until adulthood.[8]

During adolescence, most boys and girls reach adult height and weight, although there is considerable variation in when this occurs. In general, boys become heavier and taller than girls, but their growth is later. Adolescent males experience a growth spurt between 13 and 15½ years; a gain of 4 inches can be expected in the year of maximum growth. By 18 years, boys have about ¾ inch of growth remaining, and girls have slightly less.[8] Girls experience an earlier growth spurt between 11 and 13½ years; a gain of 3½ inches can be expected in the year of maximum growth.[8] Height

TABLE 4-3		
MUSCULAR CHANGES FROM 1 YEAR TO 6 YEARS		
	1 YEAR TO 3 YEARS	**4 TO 6 YEARS**
Skeletal muscles	• Early in this stage, the muscular strength of the trunk and lower extremities increases to support bipedal locomotion	• Creatinine in urine increases as muscle mass increases • Muscle fibers increase in diameter as strength increases • Muscle strength increases as activity increases
Cardiac muscle	• Muscles of the left ventricle of the heart grow more than the right to accommodate the increase in workload	
Sphincter muscles	• Sphincter muscles develop to allow toilet training	
Postural patterns associated with muscle development	• With continued weight bearing, the growth of intrinsic feet muscles causes the once fat, thick, and archless foot to become arched with the development of the longitudinal arch • At 2 years, the toddler displays a mature grasp pattern that enables prehension and the manual exchange of objects	• Muscle strength depends upon body proportions; adult normative values are not accurate for children. • Children may experience growth pains as muscle growth accompanies bone growth • By 5 years, children have adequate manipulation skills to begin handwriting

increases most before menstruation begins, as hormones surge to develop reproductive systems. Also, the prefrontal cortex does not fully mature until after 21 years, illustrating that executive brain function (associated with the highest levels of planning, critical thinking, and problem solving) lags behind body growth. Table 4-5 outlines how body systems change from adolescence into adulthood.[6]

Knowledge of how the body systems grow and mature provides a basis for understanding how the child is capable of achieving the typical motor milestones throughout childhood. The next section provides an overview of how skills needed for functional independence are typically developed and sequenced from birth to adulthood.

DEVELOPMENTAL MILESTONES

A child's development is appraised through observations of social interactions and achievement of developmental milestones. Even before birth, a mother should feel the fetus kicking and moving in her womb, an early indicator of healthy growth and development.

At birth, typically following 40 weeks' gestation, the newborn engages in interactions with the external world that promote social engagement, movement, and play. Pediatric therapists carefully note these developmental milestones as an indirect means of assessing the child's neuromuscular function and potential for learning.

A newborn's development is reliant upon her ability to engage with the environment. How early is the newborn able to interact with the environment for learning? This question can be answered by looking at studies on the development of *perception*, or the ability to be aware of sensory input. Studies on hearing have shown that the fetus can perceive her mother's voice while in utero.[9,10] This perception of hearing is hypothesized as the reason that a newborn tends to turn her head toward the source of sounds and distinguishes her mother's voice.[9,10] Young infants also have a keen sense of smell and can distinguish pleasant vs unpleasant smells, preferring honey or chocolate to rotten eggs or fish.[11] Similarly, newborns can differentiate salty, sour, bitter, and sweet tastes, favoring sweets at birth, then preferring salty tastes at 4 months.[12] Prenatal flavor experiences

	1 YEAR TO 3 YEARS	**4 TO 6 YEARS**
Structure of the brain and spinal cord	• The brain growth spurt ends between 2 to 4 years, and, by the end of the second year it has doubled its birth weight	• Nerve conduction rates increase as nerve fibers increase in diameter • Peripheral nerves grow to keep pace with growing bones and muscles • Cortex modifies synapses as cognitive function increases • Little change in the cortical thickness takes place after 4 years
Myelinization	• During this stage, the motor (pyramidal) tracts become completely myelinated	
Sensory	• At 2 years, the auditory pathways become myelinated	• The central nervous system and the organs of special senses growth pattern is so rapid that they reach 90% of their adult size by 5 or 6 years
Motor	• The child is able to control eye movements to track objects	• Coordination improves as the cerebellar function develops
Cognition	• By 3 years, the child has a vocabulary of approximately 900 words	

TABLE 4-4

NEUROLOGICAL CHANGES FROM 2 TO 6 YEARS

enhance the acceptance and enjoyment of similarly flavored foods during weaning.[13,14]

Touch is a sensation that relies on the sensory receptors in the skin, the largest sense organ and the first to develop.[15] The fetus receives sensory input from the maternal womb, demonstrating increased activity when stimulated by the mother's abdominal wall.[15,16] The sense of touch is integral to breastfeeding and handling, especially skin-to-skin contact between the mother and child, as facilitated in *kangaroo care*.[17] Touch can also be used to communicate, conveying different emotions, not unlike facial and vocal expressions.[17,18] Touch deprivation in newborns and young infants, whether caused by time spent isolated in the neonatal intensive care unit or by a mother experiencing postpartum depression, can lead to later cognitive and neurodevelopmental delays.[19,20] These delays resulting from touch deprivation appear to persist for many years.[21]

Vision is the least mature of all the senses at birth due to the lack of visual stimulation in utero prior to birth. Although vision is limited at birth, by 6 months, the infant's visual acuity approaches 20/25 and reaches adult visual acuity (20/20) by 1 year.[22] At birth, infants have the greatest sensitivity to intermediate wavelengths (yellow/green) and less to short (blue/violet) or long (red/orange) wavelengths. Whereas newborns can perceive only a few colors, by 3 to 4 months, they are able to see the full range of colors.[22]

Visual perception is key to the eye-hand coordination that the newborn begins to develop at birth. Through the integration of sensorimotor experiences, the infant demonstrates visually directed movements to explore her environment through vision, touch, smell, hearing, and taste. This early play lays the foundation for the development of spatial orientation, conceptualization, reading, spatial transformation, and adult cognition.

Language development is complex but, in general, follows a predictable, sequential pattern. However, although the pattern is predictable, there is a wide range of what is considered typical development during infancy and the toddler years. Beginning in infancy, children learn language through a social context. While in the uterus, all the infant's needs are met by the body of the mother. Upon birth, however, infants are dependent on caregivers to interpret nonlinguistic cues such as crying, yawning, and other reflexive sounds to have their needs met. Gradually over the first year, infants develop intentional communication and ultimately verbal language, but this is largely influenced by the environment (including caregiver responsiveness to these early nonlinguistic cues).[23]

TABLE 4-5

GROWTH DURING ADOLESCENCE

STAGE	MUSCULOSKELETAL	NEUROLOGICAL/ COGNITIVE	CARDIOPULMONARY	INTEGUMENTARY	OTHER SYSTEMS
Adolescent	• Growth spurts: males as early as 11, typically 13 to 15½; females as early as 9, typically 11 to 13½	• Development: prefrontal cortex continues to develop through the 20s	• Slowing of heart rate and respiratory rate	• Intact	• Development of reproductive systems: hormonal surge
Adult	• Mature system: function contingent upon fitness	• All neurological functioning mature	• All systems mature	• Intact	

During the first years of life, in addition to learning the specific language spoken by the family, children also learn the contexts in which communication occurs. During the first 2 months, infants typically express themselves by babbling for pleasure and making their first vowel sounds at the front of their mouth. By 3 months, infants can comprehend pleasure, anger, and fear by listening to the intonational patterns of their parents and caretakers, depending upon the situation in which the sounds are heard. Vocalizations might reflect similar intonations, but expressions in these early months are often limited, and the infant may use any variety of cries to communicate needs. By 6 months, infants are typically able to respond to words with some vocalizations that approximate words, and, by 8 months, they begin to use increased inflection in vocal play, use elaborate jargon, and make fluent sounds. At 8 months, infants are becoming more intentional with gestural communication, but it is not until 10 to 12 months that infants usually speak their first words.[23] It is believed that infants watch others carefully and make sounds that approximate what they hear. Language growth occurs by leaps and bounds following their first words; by 18 months, most have a vocabulary of 50 words and may be starting to combine words into phrases.[23]

The development of language, both *receptive language* (understanding what others say) and *expressive language* (the ability to express information to others through words, gestures, or writing), is foundational to understanding a child and appreciating her needs. Delays in language development can have a profound impact on psychosocial function and family relationships. Because the fetus hears sounds in the womb during its last trimester, some researchers believe that receptive language may begin before birth. If there is a hearing loss, however, language may be delayed. Fortunately, infants are usually screened for hearing loss at birth; if not, the average age of detection of significant hearing loss is approximately 14 months.[9] Table 4-6 provides the typical sequence of language development.

Underlying the development of functional skills throughout infancy and early childhood are developmental reflexes[24] that facilitate the development of motor skills. Pediatric therapists should be familiar with each of these reflexes, which are indicators of an infant's neurological development and how the body responds to stimuli from the environment. Terms used to describe the developmental reflexes include the following:

- *Reflex*: A reflex is an involuntary response. This type of response occurs when a stimulus activates what is considered an innate or involuntary movement associated with nervous system function.

- *Reaction*: A reaction may be demonstrated spontaneously by the infant, child, or adult and may also be elicited by external stimuli. This response is a coordinated pattern of movement involving multiple joints and muscles co-contracting.

- *Early reflexes:* This is a category of developmental reflexes that are apparent in fetal life that may contribute to movements that contribute to the development of motor functions, such as sucking and grasping objects.

- *Attitudinal reflexes*: Attitudinal reflexes produce persisting changes in body posture that result from a change in head position.

- *Postural reflexes*: Postural reflexes enable an infant to increase muscle activation for support of body weight against gravity.

- *Righting reactions*: Righting reactions allow the child to bring the head and trunk into normal position in space and in relation to the ground.

- *Equilibrium reactions:* These automatic reactions help the child maintain or control the center of gravity.

- *Protective reactions*: These are reactions to protect the body when falling or when the head is placed in jeopardy for injury.

- *Tilting reactions*: These automatic reactions tend to preserve the equilibrium of the body under conditions of instability of the supporting base.

- *Postural fixation reactions*: These reactions automatically sustain and balance the person as a whole. The child's body parts (head, trunk, and extremities) are in positions appropriate to the activity of the movement and to any external forces that may be acting on them.

- *Integration of a reflex*: Typically, early reflexes, including the tonic attitudinal reflexes and the postural reflexes, become integrated. In other words, the stimulus does not elicit a stereotypical or predictable response consistently. The integration of a reflex, noted when it is not predictable and consistently elicited, allows the individual to move more voluntarily.

- *Obligatory response*: This type of response is a persistent, stereotypic response to a stimulus that should be integrated, suggesting atypical neuromotor development. An obligatory response is a developmental red flag.

Appendix A includes a detailed list of these developmental reflexes commonly used to assess neuromotor development.[24]

The development of skills that are commonly used to assess infants and young children is outlined in Table 4-7. These skills include gross motor skills, fine motor skills, oral motor skills associated with feeding and communication, social and emotional skills, and cognitive skills. Pediatric therapists should be familiar with all of these skills, recognizing the expertise of team members to assess areas of concern and to provide transdisciplinary care for comprehensive management of each child. It is also imperative to educate

TABLE 4-6

NEUROLOGICAL CHANGES FROM 2 TO 6 YEARS

AGE	RECEPTIVE LANGUAGE	EXPRESSIVE LANGUAGE
5 mos	• Listens to voices and watches face of speaker	• Begins socialized vocalization with cooing sounds
6 mos	• Begins to understand highly familiar words (mommy, daddy) in context	• Babbles with reduplicated sounds: "ba ba ba," "da da da"
9 mos	• Understands the meanings of many words	• Babbling becomes more complex with varying sounds such as "ba da ba"
10 mos		• Uses jargon that sounds like words with intonation and inflection • First word may begin to emerge • Uses intentional gestures to communicate
12 mos	• Understands simple questions: "Where's Mommy?" • Responds to simple commands such as "No"	• Uses a few words (2 to 6) consistently • Uses both words and gestures
15 mos	• Comprehends about 50 words	• Expressive vocabulary of 10 words • Indicates refusal by bodily protest
18 mos	• Listens to stories • Points to familiar named objects in the environment and in books	• Expressive vocabulary of 50 words • Begins to produce 2-word utterances • Verbalizes ends of actions: "bye-bye," "all gone"
21 mos		• Asks for food, bathroom, and drink • Repeats words or short phrases
2 yrs	• Understands "what" questions • Points to common objects when described: "What do you use to brush your teeth?"	• Expressive vocabulary of 200 to 300 words • Asks, "What's that?" • Speech accompanies activities • Verbalizes immediate experiences

(continued)

TABLE 4-6 (CONTINUED)		
NEUROLOGICAL CHANGES FROM 2 TO 6 YEARS		
AGE	RECEPTIVE LANGUAGE	EXPRESSIVE LANGUAGE
2½ yrs		• Begins to produce 3-word phrases when approximately half of utterances consist of 2-word phrases • Demands to do things by self • Gives full name • Elicits: "Look at me!"
3 yrs	• Follows 2-step directions • Begins to understand most "wh" questions	• Begins to produce 4-word phrases when approximately half of utterances consist of 3-word phrases • Expressive vocabulary of 1000 words • Interested in conforming: "Is that right?" • Expresses limitations by "can't" or "I don't know"
4 yrs	• Understands most of what is said in conversation	• Talks about everything • Plays with words • Questions persistently • Elaborates simple responses into long narratives • Able to take turns in conversation • Can tell a story combining real and unreal features • Tendency toward self-praise: "I'm smart," "I know everything" • Bosses and criticizes others
5 yrs	• Understands instructions given by unfamiliar people • Understands the meaning of stories • Understands how things are same or different • Follows 3-step directions	• Expressive vocabulary of 2200 to 2500 words • Begins to be aware of social standards and limitations with respect to language use • Adjusts language based on context and situation (may talk more slowly to a younger child)
6 yrs	• Normal comprehension of everyday language (slightly immature)	• Uses most grammatical morphemes (eg, plurals, possessives, past tense) appropriately • Speech production is mostly adult-like, with few developmental articulation errors remaining

		TABLE 4-7		
	DEVELOPMENT OF FUNCTIONAL SKILLS/ABILITIES FROM BIRTH TO 6 YEARS			
	GROSS MOTOR	**FINE MOTOR**	**ORAL MOTOR AND FEEDING**	
Birth to 2 mos	• Physiological flexion (birth) • Holds head up • Begins to push up when lying on tummy • Makes smoother movements with arms and legs	• Visual tracking • Begins to follow things with eyes • Recognizes people at a distance • Palmar grasp • Traction reflex	• Rooting reflex • Suck reflex • Bite reflex	
4 mos	• Holds head steady, unsupported • Pushes down on legs when feet are on a hard surface • May be able to roll over from tummy to back • When lying on stomach, pushes up to elbows	• Can hold a toy and shake it and swing at dangling toys • Brings hands to mouth		
6 mos	• Rolls over in both directions (front to back, back to front) • Begins to sit without support • When standing, supports weight on legs and might bounce • Rocks back and forth, sometimes crawling backward before moving forward • Muscle tone is neither stiff nor floppy		• Brings things to mouth	
9 mos	• Stands holding on • Can get into sitting position • Sits without support • Pulls to stand • Crawls	• Moves things smoothly from one hand to the other • Picks up things like cereal o's between thumb and index finger	• Puts things in her mouth	

TABLE 4-7

DEVELOPMENT OF FUNCTIONAL SKILLS/ABILITIES FROM BIRTH TO 6 YEARS

	ORAL MOTOR AND COMMUNICATION	SOCIAL AND EMOTIONAL	COGNITIVE
	• Birth: Cries • 2 mos: Coos, makes gurgling sounds • Turns head toward sounds	• Erikson: Basic trust vs mistrust • Begins to smile at people • Can briefly calm himself (may suck on hand) • Tries to look at parent	• Pays attention to faces • Begins to act bored (cries, fussy) if activity doesn't change • Watches things move • Responds to loud noises • Learns about self and environment through motor and reflex actions • Derives thought from sensation and movement
	• Begins to babble • Babbles with expression and copies sounds he hears • Cries in different ways to show hunger, pain, or being tired	• Smiles spontaneously, especially at people • Likes to play with people and might cry when playing stops • Copies some movements and facial expressions, like smiling or frowning	• Lets you know if she is happy or sad • Responds to affection • Reaches for toy with one hand • Uses hands and eyes together, such as seeing a toy and reaching for it • Follows moving things with eyes from side to side • Watches faces closely • Recognizes familiar people and things at a distance
	• Responds to sounds by making sounds • Strings vowels together when babbling ("ah," "eh," "oh") and likes taking turns with parent while making sounds • Responds to own name • Makes sounds to show joy and displeasure • Begins to say consonant sounds (jabbering with "m," "b")	• Knows familiar faces and begins to know if someone is a stranger • Likes to play with others, especially parents • Responds to other people's emotions and often seems happy • Likes to look at self in a mirror	• Looks around at things nearby • Shows curiosity about things and tries to get things that are out of reach • Begins to pass things from one hand to the other
	• Understands "no" • Makes a lot of different sounds like "mamamama" and "babababababa" • Copies sounds and gestures of others • Uses fingers to point at things	• May be afraid of strangers • May be clingy with familiar adults • Has favorite toys	• Watches the path of something as it falls • Looks for things he sees you hide • Plays peek-a-boo • Looks where you point • Responds to own name

(continued)

TABLE 4-7 (CONTINUED)			
DEVELOPMENT OF FUNCTIONAL SKILLS/ABILITIES FROM BIRTH TO 6 YEARS			
	GROSS MOTOR	**FINE MOTOR**	**ORAL MOTOR AND FEEDING**
1 yr	• Gets to a sitting position without help • Pulls up to stand, walks holding on to furniture (cruising) • May take a few steps without holding on • May stand alone • Begins to walk with support; wide-based gait	• Brushes hair • Bangs 2 things together • Explores things in different ways, like shaking, banging, throwing • Pokes with index (pointer) finger • Puts things in a container, takes things out of a container • Uses pincer grasp	• Drinks from a cup
18 mos	• Walks alone • May walk up steps and run • Pulls toys while walking	• Can help undress herself	• Drinks from a cup • Eats with a spoon

TABLE 4-7 (CONTINUED)		
DEVELOPMENT OF FUNCTIONAL SKILLS/ABILITIES FROM BIRTH TO 6 YEARS		
ORAL MOTOR AND COMMUNICATION	**SOCIAL AND EMOTIONAL**	**COGNITIVE**
• Responds to simple spoken requests • Uses simple gestures, like shaking head "no" or waving "bye-bye" • Makes sounds with changes in tone (sounds more like speech) • Says "mama" and "dada" and exclamations like "uh-oh!" • Tries to say words you say • Says "bye-bye"	• Is shy or nervous with strangers • Cries when mom or dad leaves • Has favorite things and people • Shows fear in some situations • Hands you a book when he wants to hear a story • Repeats sounds or actions for attention • Puts out arm or leg to help with dressing • Plays games such as "peek-a-boo" and "pat-a-cake"	• Finds hidden things easily • Looks at the right picture or thing when it's named • Copies gestures • Lets things go without help • Follows simple directions like "pick up the toy" • Gestures by waving or shaking head
• Says several single words • Says and shakes head "no" • Points to show someone what he wants	• Likes to hand things to others as he plays • May have temper tantrums • May be afraid of strangers • Shows affection to familiar people • Plays simple pretend, such as feeding a doll • May cling to caregivers in new situations • Points to show others something interesting • Explores alone but with parent close by	• Knows what ordinary things are for (eg, telephone, brush, spoon) • Points to get the attention of others • Shows interest in a doll or stuffed animal by pretending to feed • Points to one body part • Scribbles on his own • Can follow 1-step verbal commands without any gestures (eg, sits when you say "sit down")

(continued)

TABLE 4-7 (CONTINUED)			
DEVELOPMENT OF FUNCTIONAL SKILLS/ABILITIES FROM BIRTH TO 6 YEARS			
	GROSS MOTOR	**FINE MOTOR**	**ORAL MOTOR AND FEEDING**
2 yrs	• Stands on tiptoe • Kicks a ball • Begins to run • Climbs onto and down from furniture without help • Walks up and down stairs holding on • Throws ball overhand	• Makes or copies straight lines and circles	• Refined spoon feeding: holds spoon with radial grasp • Finger feeds appropriate foods • Licks upper lip with tongue • 2½ yrs: eats with a fork by holding it in fist • Drinks from a plastic straw
3 yrs	• Climbs well • Runs easily • Pedals a tricycle (3-wheel bike) • Walks up and down stairs, one foot on each step	• Dresses and undresses self • Works toys with buttons, levers, and moving parts • Copies a circle with pencil or crayon • Builds towers of more than 6 blocks • Screws and unscrews jar lids or turns door handle	• Stabs with a fork and uses fork for solids • Serves self at table

TABLE 4-7 (CONTINUED)

DEVELOPMENT OF FUNCTIONAL SKILLS/ABILITIES FROM BIRTH TO 6 YEARS

ORAL MOTOR AND COMMUNICATION	SOCIAL AND EMOTIONAL	COGNITIVE
• Points to things or pictures when they are named • Knows names of familiar people and body parts • Says sentences with 2 to 4 words • Follows simple instructions • Repeats words overheard in conversation • Points to things in a book	• Early childhood: autonomy vs shame • Copies others, especially adults and older children • Gets excited when with other children • Shows more and more independence • Shows defiant behavior (doing what he has been told not to) • Plays mainly beside other children but is beginning to include other children, such as in chase games	• Finds things even when hidden under 2 or 3 covers • Begins to sort shapes and colors • Completes sentences and rhymes in familiar books • Plays simple make-believe games • Builds towers of 4 or more blocks • Might use one hand more than the other • Follows 2-step instructions such as, "pick up your shoes and put them in the closet" • Names items in a picture book, such as a cat, bird, or dog
• Follows instructions with 2 or 3 steps • Can name most familiar things • Understands "in," "on," and "under" • Says first name, age, and sex • Names a friend • Says "I," "me," "we," and "you" and some plurals (eg, cats, dogs) • Intelligible speech • Converses using 2 to 3 sentences	• Copies adults and friends • Shows affection and concern for friends • Takes turns • Understands the idea of "mine" and "his" or "hers" • Shows a wide range of emotions • Separates easily from Mom and Dad • May get upset with changes in routine	• Begins to use symbols to represent objects • Plays make-believe with dolls, animals, and people • Understands what "two" means • Turns book pages one at a time • Does puzzles with 3 or 4 pieces • Is oriented to the present • Has an egocentric perspective

(continued)

TABLE 4-7 (CONTINUED)			
DEVELOPMENT OF FUNCTIONAL SKILLS/ABILITIES FROM BIRTH TO 6 YEARS			
	GROSS MOTOR	FINE MOTOR	ORAL MOTOR AND FEEDING
4 yrs	• Hops and stands on one foot up to 2 seconds • Catches a bounced ball most of the time • Gallops	• Draws a person with 2 to 4 body parts • Uses scissors • Starts to copy some capital letters	• Pours, cuts with supervision, and mashes own food
5 yrs	• Stands on one foot for 10 seconds or longer • Hops; may be able to skip • Can do a somersault • Swings and climbs	• Can use the toilet on her own • Can draw a person with at least 6 body parts • Can print some letters or numbers • Copies a triangle and other geometric shapes	• Uses a fork and spoon and sometimes a table knife • Cuts and spreads with knife

families and caregivers about typical growth and development, encouraging them to be alert to possible delays. Ideally, parents, caretakers, and professionals should observe children in spontaneous play to observe preferred activities and strategies for movement. Parents' reports on the child's activities at home tend to be accurate and can help identify areas of strength and areas of concern.

As the child matures and goes through puberty, pediatric therapists need to gauge their interactions and interventions to best match each individual child's skills, including social skills. Table 4-8 illustrates the range of functional skills that adolescents achieve as they mature into adulthood.

DEVELOPMENTAL RED FLAGS

As an interprofessional team, therapists should recognize typical development and make referrals to others when delays in one or more areas are suspected. Red flags that warrant close attention include the following:

- Birth history risk factors: Prematurity, difficult delivery, congenital conditions
- Medical history risk factors: Genetic and congenital conditions
- Family history risk factors: Genetic conditions, familial risk factors
- Environmental factors: Diet, home environment (eg, allergens, pets, smoke), lack of stimulation

TABLE 4-7 (CONTINUED)

DEVELOPMENT OF FUNCTIONAL SKILLS/ABILITIES FROM BIRTH TO 6 YEARS

ORAL MOTOR AND COMMUNICATION	SOCIAL AND EMOTIONAL	COGNITIVE
• Knows some basic rules of grammar, such as correctly using "he" and "she" • Sings a song or says a poem from memory such as "The Itsy Bitsy Spider" or "The Wheels on the Bus" • Tells stories • Can say first and last names • Language is well established	• 4 to 5 yrs: Initiative vs guilt • Enjoys doing new things • Plays "Mom" and "Dad" • Is more creative with make-believe • Would rather play with other children than by herself • Cooperates with other children • Often can't tell what's real and what's make-believe • Talks about what she likes and what she is interested in	• Names some colors and some numbers • Understands the idea of counting • Starts to understand time • Remembers parts of a story • Understands the idea of "same" and "different" • Names 4 colors • Plays board or card games • Tells you what he thinks is going to happen next in a book
• Speaks very clearly • Tells a simple story using full sentences • Uses future tense (eg, "Grandma will be here") • Says name and address	• Wants to please and be like friends • More likely to agree with rules • Likes to sing, dance, and act • Shows concern and sympathy for others • Is aware of gender • Can tell what's real vs make-believe • Shows more independence but adult supervision is still needed • Is sometimes demanding vs cooperative	• Counts 10 or more things • Knows about things used every day, like money and food

- Poor quality of movements: Lack of movement; tremors; difficulty alternating movements; poorly coordinated movement; problems with strength, endurance, and power
- Persistent asymmetry observed in relation to movements, postures, responses to developmental reflexes, and head positioning
- Sensory disturbances: Lack of response or hypersensitivity in one or more sensory modalities (ie, auditory, olfactory, gustatory, tactile, visual, and movement)
- Delays in preacademic skills: Eye contact, attention to task, compliance, ability to follow directions, memory, imitation skills, copy skills, bilateral coordination, motor planning ability, crossing midline, interaction with other children, use of receptive and expressive language

The environment for healthy growth and development is a critical consideration. Last year, 3.6 million cases of child abuse and neglect were reported to state and local agencies in the United States, involving 6.6 million children (reports can include multiple children).[23-25] The United States has one of the worst records among industrialized nations, losing more than 4 children on average every day to child abuse and neglect. Children who experience child abuse and neglect are approximately 9 times more likely to become involved in criminal activity.[25,26] It is the second most common cause of deaths, second only to accidents.[25]

	GROSS MOTOR	FINE MOTOR	ORAL MOTOR AND FEEDING	

TABLE 4-8

DEVELOPMENT OF FUNCTIONS FROM 6 YEARS TO ADOLESCENCE

	GROSS MOTOR	FINE MOTOR	ORAL MOTOR AND FEEDING	
6 to 9 yrs	• 6 years: Refines skills for postural control and mobility • Has a narrow base of support with arm swing • 7 years: Is able to move more gracefully and quickly • Enjoys team sports that incorporate intermittent running and require a moderate level of coordination • 8 years: Plays ball (kicking and throwing); can skillfully climb • 9 years: Has adult-level skills	• 6 years: Has adult feeding skills • 7 years: Handwriting is much more legible • 8 years: Clearly prints all the letters and numbers • 9 years: Has adult level fine motor coordination	• Has adult oromotor skills	
10 to 18 yrs	• May appear clumsy secondary to a growth spurt (especially feet and hands that grow before long bones) • With adaptation to growth spurt motor performance is perfected: increased motor control, endurance, speed, reaction time, coordination, balance	• Adult abilities	• Adult abilities	
Over 18 yrs	• Optimal speed and endurance	• Optimal speed and accuracy • Power grasp	• Optimal speed and accuracy	

People causing child abuse and neglect include natural parents, adoptive or foster parents, babysitters, siblings, and others (teachers, relatives, other adults).[25] Working closely with families, therapists need to be alert to the possible risk of child abuse and neglect. *Child abuse* is the nonaccidental injury of a child, and *child neglect* is the failure to provide the necessities of life for a child (eg, medical care, nourishment, appropriate clothing, supervision, and adequate housing). Pediatric therapists are legally responsible to report suspected child abuse or neglect; however, it is important to make the distinction between willful neglect and impoverishment. Signs of possible abuse or neglect are listed in Table 4-9. If a professional suspects a child is in immediate danger, he should contact law enforcement as soon as possible.

Finally, it is important to recognize and understand terminology commonly used by fellow therapists for interprofessional discussions about a child's growth, functional skills, and therapeutic needs. Table 4-10 lists terms commonly used to describe the development of communication and language.

Similarly, occupational and physical therapists use terms commonly used in pediatric care. Table 4-11 lists terms that are helpful for describing the sensorimotor development of a child.

The terminology used to describe cognitive and intellectual development in early childhood is most commonly used in educational settings because physical therapists, occupational therapists, and speech-language pathologists all strive to improve a child's ability to learn and function as independently as possible. This independence relies upon a child's ability to process information and use it in an adaptive manner for problem solving in the real world. The key terms that all professionals should recognize are listed in Table 4-12.

When using professional terminology with others, jargon should be avoided or explained, as needed. For example, parents may need to understand the cognitive and motor

TABLE 4-8

DEVELOPMENT OF FUNCTIONS FROM 6 YEARS TO ADOLESCENCE

ORAL MOTOR AND COMMUNICATION	SOCIAL AND EMOTIONAL	COGNITIVE
• Industry vs inferiority	• 7 years: Selects toys and activities based on desire to interact with peers • 9 years: Values competition	• Developing ability to think abstractly • Starts making rational judgments about concrete or observable phenomena
• Develops adult vocabulary (contingent upon education)	• Identity vs role confusion	• Capable of hypothetical and deductive reasoning • Able to consider many possibilities from several perspectives
• Optimal skill	• Young adulthood: Intimacy vs isolation	• Optimal speed and endurance

abilities of their child to buy appropriate toys. In addition to discussing their child's developmental abilities and therapeutic activities, therapists can provide evidence-based, family-friendly websites featuring developmental milestones and play activities. See Appendix B for a list of websites featuring helpful resources for professionals and families.

SUMMARY

Sharing a similar knowledge of typical growth and development provides a foundation for interprofessional collaboration and appreciation of expertise when caring for children and educating their caretakers. Furthermore, it sets the stage for interprofessional goals for learning and healthy development for children and their families. It also allows therapists to recognize typical patterns of growth and development vs those that warrant closer examination. Based upon the common foundations described in prior sections, Section 5 will discuss interprofessional management care by pediatric therapists.

INTERPROFESSIONAL ACTIVITY

Performing Developmental Reflex Testing

This learning experience involves working as a team with a child under 1 year.

1. As a team of pediatric therapists, perform developmental reflex testing on an infant.
2. First, interview the infant's caretaker to assess possible maternal, congenital, medical, or birth-related risk factors.
3. Observe the child's spontaneous behaviors.

TABLE 4-9
RED FLAGS FOR CHILD ABUSE AND NEGLECT

TYPE OF ABUSE	PHYSICAL SIGNS	BEHAVIORAL SIGNS	CAREGIVER SIGNS
Physical	Look for age-inappropriate injuries, injuries that appear to have a pattern such as marks from a hand or belt, or a pattern of severe injuries.	Signs of physical abuse may be subtle. The child may be fearful, shy away from touch, or appear to be afraid to go home. A child's clothing may be inappropriate for the weather, such as heavy, long-sleeved pants and shirts on hot days.	Physically abusive caregivers may display anger management issues and excessive need for control. Their explanation of the injury might not ring true or may be different from an older child's description of the injury.
Emotional	Because emotional child abuse does not leave concrete marks, the effects may be harder to detect. Look at the child's behavior.	Is the child excessively shy, fearful, or afraid of doing something wrong? Behavioral extremes may also be a clue. A child may be constantly trying to parent other children, for example, or, conversely, exhibit antisocial behavior such as uncontrolled aggression. Look for age-inappropriate behaviors as well, such as an older child exhibiting behaviors more commonly found in younger children.	Does a caregiver seem unusually harsh and critical of a child, belittling and shaming him in front of others? Has the caregiver shown anger or issues with control in other areas? A caregiver may also seem strangely unconcerned with a child's welfare or performance. Keep in mind that there might not be immediate caregiver signs. Tragically, many emotionally abusive caregivers can present a kind face to the outside world, making the abuse of the child all the more confusing and scary.

(continued)

4. Take turns performing the developmental reflexes, selecting those that best match your area of expertise.

5. As a team, document the infant's responses to each stimulus.

6. Discuss the infant's responses and how they reflect the child's overall growth and development.

7. Discuss the infant's physical, mental, and psychosocial development in terms of developmental milestones observed while testing the child.

Discussing the Impact of Growth and Development on a Child

1. As a team, review the following case of the child with spastic cerebral palsy.

2. Discuss the changes in growth and skill development across domains that may impact a team's focus as the child ages from birth through adolescence.

3. Collaborate as a team to do the following:

   a. Develop questions to ask the child, family, and other shareholders about their needs and concerns.

   b. Determine the roles and responsibilities interacting with shareholders for your team meeting about issues considering a child at 11 years (current age) and following her growth spurt.

   c. Develop a team plan to discuss recommendations for assistive technology when the child is 11 vs 18 years.

		TABLE 4-9 (CONTINUED)	
RED FLAGS FOR CHILD ABUSE AND NEGLECT			
TYPE OF ABUSE	PHYSICAL SIGNS	BEHAVIORAL SIGNS	CAREGIVER SIGNS
Sexual	A child may have trouble sitting or standing or have stained, bloody, or torn underclothes. Swelling, bruises, or bleeding in the genital area is a red flag. A sexually transmitted disease or pregnancy, especially under 14 years, is a strong cause for concern.	Does the child display knowledge or interest in sexual acts inappropriate to her age, or even seductive behavior? A child might appear to avoid another person or display unusual behavior, either being very aggressive or very passive. Older children might resort to destructive behaviors to take away the pain, such as alcohol or drug abuse, self-mutilation, or suicide attempts.	The caregiver may seem to be unusually controlling and protective of the child, limiting contact with other children and adults. Again, as with other types of abuse, sometimes the caregiver does not give outward signs of concern. This does not mean the child is lying or exaggerating.
Neglect	A child may consistently be dressed inappropriately for the weather or have ill-fitting, dirty clothes and shoes. He might have consistently bad hygiene, appearing very dirty, having matted and unwashed hair, or having noticeable body odor. Another warning sign is untreated illnesses and physical injuries.	Does the child seem to be unsupervised? Schoolchildren may be frequently late or tardy. The child might show troublesome, disruptive behavior or be withdrawn and passive.	Does the caregiver have problems with drugs or alcohol? Most of us have a little clutter in the home, but is the caregiver's home filthy and unsanitary? Is there adequate food in the house? A caregiver might also show reckless disregard for the child's safety, letting older children play unsupervised or leaving a baby unattended. A caregiver might refuse or delay necessary health care for the child.

Case 4-1: An 11-year-old girl with spastic cerebral palsy

Mary is an 11-year-old with spastic cerebral palsy presenting with intermittent hypertonicity of all extremities and hypotonicity of her head, neck, and trunk. She has obligatory tonic reflexes (R>L) and poor gross motor control. Mary has fair fine motor control when she is therapeutically positioned for postural support. When positioned properly, she is able to reach and touch large targets with some accuracy.

Although her cognition is normal, her speech is severely dysarthric, making her communication a concern. She is unable to assume sitting or standing and cannot maintain sitting without support. Her mother or aide pushes her around in a manual wheelchair, a chair she has outgrown. Mary currently has a normal body mass index as she approaches her adolescent growth spurt. She likes to read and talk to her friends on the phone. She will be going to a new school and needs adaptive equipment to function in the school setting. Her mother would like recommendations for therapeutic positioning to prevent deformities during her anticipated growth spurt.

TABLE 4-10
COMMUNICATION TERMINOLOGY

TERM	DEFINITION
Communication	Ability to make information understood by others; ability to exchange messages
Language	A code in which arbitrary symbols stand for real things, ideas, and events
Receptive language	Decoding aspect of communication; receptive language precedes expressive language in both development and complexity
Expressive language	Encoding of communication
Articulation	Sensorimotor process or producing the language code
Respiration	Act of breathing; inhaling and exhaling (a fundamental process of life)
Phonation	Utterance of sounds by means of the vocal cords
Vocalization	Any sound a person produces using his organs of speech
Articulation	Distinct connected speech or enunciation

TABLE 4-11	
TERMINOLOGY FOR PERCEPTION AND MOTOR CONTROL	
TERM	**DEFINITION**
Activity tolerance	Sustaining a purposeful activity over time
Bilateral integration	Interacting with both sides of the body in a coordination manner during activity
Body scheme	Acquiring an internal awareness of the body and the relationship of body parts to each other
Crossing the midline	Moving the limbs and eyes across the sagittal plane of the body
Depth perception	Determining the relative distance between objects, figures, or landmarks and the observer
Endurance	The ability to perform a skill over an increased time period
Figure ground	Differentiating between foreground and background forms and objects
Fine motor coordination	Using small muscle groups for controlled movements, particularly in object manipulation
Form constancy	Recognizing forms and objects as the same in various environments, positions, and sizes
Graphesthesia	Identifying letters or numbers drawn on the skin
Gross motor coordination	Using the large muscle groups for controlled movement
Kinesthesia	Identifying the excursion and direction of joint movement
Laterality	Using a preferred unilateral body part for activities requiring a high level of skill
Left-right discrimination	Differentiating on side of the body from the other
Motor control	Ability to activate and coordinate the muscles and limbs involved in the performance of a motor skill
Motor learning	Process of acquiring a skill by which the learner, through practice and assimilation, refines and makes automatic the desired movement.
Oral-motor coordination	Coordinating oropharyngeal musculature for controlled movements
Perception	The process of interpreting or giving meaning to an experience
Position in space	Determining the spatial relationships of figures and objects to self or other forms and objects
Power	Ability to use strength in a short time frame, resulting in greater force
Praxis	Conceiving and planning a new motor act in response to an environmental command
Spatial orientation	Ability to maintain the body orientation and/or posture in relation to the surrounding environment (physical space) at rest and during motion
Strength	Ability to move a joint actively
Stereognosis	Identifying objects through the sense of touch
Topographical orientation	Determining the location of objects and settings and the route to the location
Visual closure	Identifying forms or objects from incomplete presentations
Visual motor integration	Coordinating the interaction of visual information with body movement during activity

TABLE 4-12	
TERMINOLOGY ASSOCIATED WITH COGNITIVE AND INTELLECTUAL DEVELOPMENT IN EARLY CHILDHOOD	
TERM	**DEFINITION**
Accommodation	The establishment of a new schema or the modification of an old schema; this results in a change in, reorganization of, or development of cognitive structures (schemata)
Adaptive behavior	Behavior that fosters appropriate individual interaction with the environment
Assimilation	The cognitive process by which the person integrates new perceptual matter or stimulus events into existing schemata or patterns of behavior
Attention span	The ability to focus on a task over time
Behavior	The way in which an individual acts or performs
Behavior modification	Giving reinforcement to specific behaviors to encourage or discourage the repetition of those behaviors
Categorization	The ability to identify similarities of and differences between environmental information
Cognition	The process or act of knowing; our reception of raw sensory information and our transformation, elaboration, storage, recovery, and use of this information; the operation of the mind process by which we become aware of thought and perception, including all aspects of perceiving, thinking, and remembering; involves sensing, perceiving, recognizing, conceiving, judging, reasoning, and imagining
Concept formation	The ability to organize a variety of information to form thoughts and ideas
Conceptualization	The action or process of forming a concept or idea of something
Conditioning	The process whereby individuals, as a result of their experience, establish an association or linkage between 2 events
Contingent behavior	Actions that are dependent upon a specific stimulus
Dishabituation	The discrimination between to similar stimuli that causes a response
Equilibration	The result of balance between the processes of assimilation and accommodation; when disequilibrium occurs, it provides motivation for the individual to assimilate or to accommodate further

(continued)

TABLE 4-12 (CONTINUED)	
TERMINOLOGY ASSOCIATED WITH COGNITIVE AND INTELLECTUAL DEVELOPMENT IN EARLY CHILDHOOD	
TERM	**DEFINITION**
Generalization of learning	The ability to apply previously learned concepts and behaviors to similar situations
Habituation	Repeated presentation of a stimulus that causes reduced attention to the stimulus
Imitation	Performing an activity after having a model of the activity
Intellectual operations in space	The ability to mentally manipulate spatial relationships
Level of arousal	Demonstrating alertness and responsiveness to environmental stimuli
Memory	The retention of information over time: • Short-term: Recall information for brief periods of time (15 to 30 seconds) • Long-term: Recall information for long periods of time • Remote: Recall events from the distant past • Recent: Recall events from immediate past • Declarative memory: Memory of knowledge • Procedural memory: Memory of how to do a task
Object permanence	Recognition that objects have an independent existence
Orientation	The ability to identify person, place, time, and situation
Problem solving	The ability to recognize a problem, define a problem, identify alternative plans, select a plan, organize steps in a plan, implement a plan, and evaluate the outcome
Recognition	Ability to identify familiar faces, objects, and other previously presented materials
Schema	A cognitive structure with specific kinds of situations in their environment
Schemata	Plural of schema
Sequencing	Place information, concepts, and actions in order
Spatial transformation	A mapping function that establishes a spatial correspondence between all points in an image and its counterpart

REFERENCES

1. Ruffin N. Human growth and development—A matter of principles. https://pubs.ext.vt.edu/350/350-053/350-053_pdf.pdf. Published 2013. Accessed January 25, 2017.
2. Carter R, Aldridge S, Page M, Parker S. *The Human Brain Book*. New York, NY: DK Publishing; 2009.
3. Durston S, Casey BJ. What have we learned about cognitive development from neuroimaging? *Neuropsychologia*. 2006;44:2149-2157.
4. Holmboe K, Pasco Fearon RM, Csibra G. Freeze-frame: a new infant inhibition task and its relation to frontal cortex tasks during infancy and early childhood. *J Exp Child Psychol*. 2008;100:89-114.
5. Skaliora I. Experience-dependent plasticity in the developing brain. *International Congress Series*. 2002;1241:313-320.
6. Kagan J, Herschkowitz N, Herschkowitz E. *A Young Mind in a Growing Brain*. Mahwah, NJ: Lawrence Erlbaum Associates; 2005.
7. Sinclair D, Dangerfield P. *Human Growth After Birth*. 6th ed. New York, NY: Oxford University Press; 1998.
8. Bogin B. *Patterns of Human Growth*. Cambridge, UK: Cambridge University Press; 1999.
9. Partanen E, Kujala T, Näätänen R, Liitola A, Sambeth A, Huotilainen M. Learning-induced neural plasticity of speech processing before birth. *Proceedings of National Academy of Sciences*. 2013;110(37):15145-15150.
10. Kisilevsky BS1, Hains SM, Lee K, et al. Effects of experience on fetal voice recognition. *Psychol Sci*. 2003;14(3):220-224.
11. Moon C. Language experienced in utero affects vowel perception after birth: a two-country study. *Acta Paediatrica*. 2013;102(2):156-160.
12. Mennella JA, Beauchamp GK. Infants' exploration of scented toys: Effects of prior experiences. *Chem Senses*. 1998;23:11-17.
13. Rosenstein D, Oster H. Differential facial responses to four basic tastes in newborns. *Child Dev*. 1988;59:1555-1566.
14. Mennella JA, Jagnow CP, Beauchamp GK. Prenatal and postnatal flavor learning by human infants. *Pediatrics*. 2001;107(6):E88.
15. Montagu A. *Touching: The Human Significance of the Skin*. New York, NY: Columbia University Press; 1971.
16. Dieter JN, Field T, Hernandez-Reif M, Emory EK, Redzepi M. Stable preterm infants gain more weight and sleep less after five days of massage. *J Pediatr Psychol*. 2003;28:403-411.
17. Lagercrantz H, Changeux JP. The emergence of human consciousness: From fetal to neonatal life. *Pediatr Res*. 2009;65:255-260.
18. Ferber SG, Feldman R, Makhoul IR. The development of maternal touch across the first year of life. *Early Hum Dev*. 2008;84:363-370.
19. Chugani HT, Behen ME, Muzik O, Juhasz C, Nagy F, Chugani DC. Local brain functional activity following early deprivation: A study of post-institutionalized Romanian orphans. *Neuroimage*. 2001;14:1290-1301.
20. MacLean K. The impact of institutionalization on child development. *Dev Psychopathol*. 2003;15:853-884.
21. Beckett C, Maughan B, Rutter M, et al. Do the effects of early severe deprivation on cognition persist into early adolescence? Findings from the English and Romanian adoptees study. *Child Dev*. 2006;77:696-711.
22. Kellman P J & Arterberry ME. *The Cradle of Knowledge: Development of Perception in Infancy*. Cambridge, MA: MIT Press; 1998.
23. Tamis-LeMonda CS, Bornstein MH, Baumwell L. Maternal responsiveness and children's achievement of language milestones. *Child Dev*. 2001;72(3):748-767.
24. US National Library of Medicine. Infant reflexes. United States National Library of Medicine Web site. https://medlineplus.gov/ency/article/003292.htm. Published December 5, 2017. Accessed December 8, 2017.
25. US Department of Health and Human Services, Administration for Children and Families. Child Maltreatment 2013. Administration for Children and Families Web site. http://www.acf.hhs.gov/sites/default/files/cb/cm2013.pdf. Published January 15, 2015. Accessed March 2, 2017.
26. US Department of Health and Human Services, Children's Bureau. Child maltreatment. Administration for Children and Families Web site http://www.acf.hhs.gov/programs/cb/research-data-technology/statistics-research/child-maltreatment. Published 2016. Accessed March 2, 2017.

Section 5

Interprofessional Management of Pediatric Care

Catherine Rush Thompson, PT, PhD, MS and Grace McConnell, PhD, CCC-SLP

OVERVIEW

This section provides an overview of the workplace culture and key competencies for the interprofessional management of care, including selecting appropriate tests and measures, interpreting results, developing an interprofessional plan of care, and providing age-appropriate interventions to optimize an individual's inclusion in education, social activities, and work.

WORKPLACE CULTURE

When managing care, pediatric professionals need to be sensitive to their workplace's character and personality, also referred to as the *workplace culture*. Workplace culture relates to the values, beliefs, behaviors, and interactions that can impact interprofessional collaboration. For example, pediatric professionals typically share child- and family-centered approaches to care; however, each person brings a unique cultural and perspective to the workplace. Similarly, each workplace embraces values that impact policies, procedures, and interprofessional behaviors (eg, for profit vs nonprofit settings).

The workplace culture can impact the extent of interactions and communication between professionals, families, referral sources, and those responsible for payment. Pediatric professionals need to be sensitive to the needs of families as well as the workplace culture when managing care; they should support a workplace culture that encourages *lateral leadership* (providing peer guidance and encouragement), *openness to new ideas, clear communication, professionalism*, and *interprofessional competency*. For example, the neonatal intensive care unit (NICU) focuses on intensive medical attention to stabilize a neonate's physical health, so medical team members use specialized care and technology to manage the newborn's body systems and body functions.[1] The NICU is a protective environment designed to address the multiple threats to a newborn's life while supporting the parents' need to bond with their child. In programs offering early intervention, the focus is on family education, so parenting skills and play activities are highly valued.[2] As the child grows to school age, the focus shifts to the child's participation in learning and social activities.[2] Although each workplace culture varies, key interprofessional competencies for effective management are consistent. Each team member should take the time to understand each workplace culture in terms of what is expected and what is needed for optimal care. Similarly, pediatric therapists need to be especially

Thompson CR. *Pediatric Therapy:*
An Interprofessional Framework for Practice (pp 71-83).
© 2018 SLACK Incorporated.

aware of the home environments where they provide services, recognizing the intimacy and trust that is required to open one's home to others.

KEY INTERPROFESSIONAL COMPETENCIES FOR EFFECTIVE MANAGEMENT

As described in Section 1, the key principles for interprofessional practice include the following:

1. Sharing common values and ethics for interprofessional practice;

2. Using the knowledge of one's own role and those of other professions to appropriately assess and address the health care needs of the children and families served;

3. Communicating with children, families, communities, and other health professionals in a responsive and responsible manner that supports a collaborative team approach for the maintenance of health and the treatment of disease; and

4. Building relationships for effectively planning and delivering customized care that is safe, timely, efficient, effective, and equitable.

Following these principles, caring professionals can more effectively work as a team for case management. By definition, *teamwork* includes "the interrelated set of specific knowledge (cognitive competencies), skills (affective competencies), and attitudes (behavioral competencies) required for an interprofessional team to function as a unit."[3] Although professionals value teamwork and interprofessional collaboration, many experience barriers to these efforts. Reported barriers include limited time for interactions, lack of receptiveness to ideas shared, lack of adaptability to recommendations made, poor written communication skills (ie, lack of clear information), poor verbal communication skills, poor listening skills, conflict(s) with coworkers, limited resources (eg, guidelines, training, counseling for interpersonal reactions), and lack of interprofessional training.[3] According to one study, the majority of interprofessional communication problems resulted from misunderstandings, followed by personality differences, lack of follow-through, and poor compliance with rules and regulations.[4] Coworkers reported that they best managed interpersonal conflict through keeping communication open, being patient/taking time, collaborating with others, and focusing on the problem rather than the individual.[4]

Teams can work together most effectively if they come well prepared for focused discussion. The information needed for each meeting should be clearly laid out in an agenda

that all can view. The agenda should describe details of what will be discussed, who is responsible for leading the discussion, and the order of discussion. For example, if the goal of the meeting is to plan an assessment of a child, a designated team leader or case manager could create an agenda that lists relevant items for discussion. Table 5-1 illustrates an agenda that would be shared with all meeting participants.

The first agenda item is typically to review the *minutes* from the previous meeting, ensuring that the information is clear and accurate. If any errors exist, changes are made to the prior minutes, then the minutes from the prior meeting are approved. This approval is noted under *Action*, providing a record of the previous meeting. During the meeting, the subsequent item is then addressed, ideally within the allotted time. Notes of the *discussion* are written on the agenda form to keep minutes or a record of the current meeting and decisions made. Minutes can be written by a *designated recorder or secretary*. Any decisions that require follow-up are written under Action. Whereas the discussion can be written without specifying who made specific comments, the Action items need to be written so that someone is held accountable for ensuring that each task is addressed and reported at the following meeting.

PREPARATION FOR TEAM MEETINGS

In preparation for discussion, team members could bring the tools they would recommend for the assessment, based upon prior review of information from the child's medical and/or educational history and parental interview. Table 5-2 provides a helpful list of questions to seek in medical records, ask of a caretaker, or seek from other sources prior to conducting a comprehensive assessment of an infant or preschool child.[5]

Interview responses offer the team members a preview of the family's concerns and the relative abilities of the child to be examined. This type of preliminary information provides a general focus for the team members, reducing the chance of redundancy and ensuring the best use of time during the assessment process for each team member. Then, team members will be better acquainted to probe further into areas of expertise and to explain their selection and rationale for tests and measures suggested.

TEST SELECTION

Team discussions rely on active listening and relationship building for effective interprofessional collaboration. If the physical therapist, occupational therapist, and speech-language pathologist each administer separate assessments, the total time for examination could take over 3 hours and

TABLE 5-1
AGENDA FOR TEAM MEETINGS

AGENDA

Date: February 26, 2017

Meeting Leader (can be rotated): Nancy Moore (Case Manager)

Team Members: Cary Jones (PT), Jennifer Dawson (OT), Emily Morrison (SLP)

Present: All   Absent: None   Excused: None

ITEM	DISCUSSION	ACTION
Approval of Minutes	*Discuss minutes from prior meeting, if applicable. Make changes in minutes, as needed.*	*Approval of minutes with changes, if needed.*
Discussion		
PT	Facilitator: Carrie J. Time allotted: 5 min.	
Discussion		
OT	Facilitator: Jennifer D. Time allotted: 5 min.	
Discussion		
SLP	Facilitator: Emily M. Time allotted: 5 min.	
Discussion		
Selection of Assessments	Facilitator: Nancy Time allotted: 15 min.	
Discussion		
Reports	Facilitator: Nancy Time allotted: 10 min.	
Discussion		
Next Meeting	*Note the date, time, and place for the next scheduled meeting.*	

Respectfully submitted by:_____
(Rotate the person submitting completed minutes. Copies of completed minutes need to be shared before the next meeting.)

TABLE 5-2
COMPREHENSIVE CHILD DEVELOPMENTAL AND OCCUPATIONAL HISTORY

Child's name:_____ Mother's name:_____ Occupation:_____

Child's birth date:_____ Father's name:_____ Occupation:_____

Child's age:_____ Today's date:_____

Child's prematurity is adjusted on tests up to age 2.

PART I: Prenatal History—Questions related to mother's pregnancies and this delivery

Have you been pregnant before? *(Follow-up asking about previous pregnancies)*

If you have been pregnant before, how many times?

Were there problems during other pregnancies? If so, please specify:

(eg, preeclampsia, ectopic pregnancy, complications with umbilical cord)

What was the length of this pregnancy?_____weeks *(Full term pregnancy, 40 weeks; premature, < 38 weeks)*

Duration of labor for this child:_____ *(Prolonged labor can increase risk for hypoxia)*

Type of delivery: vaginal?____ C-section?____ Any complications? *(eg, breech delivery, forceps)*

Were there any maternal problems during this pregnancy? If so, please describe:

PART II: Child's Early History—Questions about this child's early development

What was the condition of your child at birth? *(eg, healthy, at risk, requiring neonatal intensive care)*

What problems were evident at birth? *(eg, Rh incompatibility = need for blood transfusion)*

Were you aware of any problems before your child's birth?

What was your child's Apgar score at 1 minute? *(8-10 is normal; 0-3 risk)*

What was your child's Apgar score at 5 minutes? *(0-3 risk)*

What was your child's birth weight? *(low birth weight < 1500 gm; track growth)*

What was your child's height at birth? *(see birth chart for normal vs abnormal)*

BEHAVIORS

SLEEP

What were your child's sleep patterns after birth?

Where does your child sleep?

In what position(s) does your child sleep?

Has your child had any problems with sleep since birth?

(continued)

TABLE 5-2 (CONTINUED)
COMPREHENSIVE CHILD DEVELOPMENTAL AND OCCUPATIONAL HISTORY

NUTRITION AND DENTITION

What is your child's typical diet?

Does your child have any problems with feeding or eating habits?

Does your child have allergies and/or diet restrictions? (specify): *(common allergies: milk, peanut products, seafood)*

Is your child teething now? *(teething is often accompanied by drooling and continual crying)*

ELIMINATION

Does your child have any problems with bowel or bladder *(eg, constipation, diarrhea)*

Is your child toilet trained? *(typical age = 18 mos to 2 yrs)*

Are there any problems related to your child's toileting? *(eg, possible problems with sphincter control, possible emotional problems)*

PHYSICAL ACTIVITY

What is your child's favorite activity? *(identifies reinforcers; eg, favorite toys/activities)*

How does your child react to movement? *(lack of movement suggests poor muscle tone)*

MEDICAL HISTORY

Has your child been hospitalized since birth? (specify): *(note specifics: date, location, surgery, physician, outcomes)*

Does your child have a history of ear infections? (specify): *(follow-up with screening for hearing and language development)*

Does your child have any other medical problems or had medical tests to rule out possible medical problems? *(if medical history, request release of information for complete medical records)*

DEVELOPMENTAL MILESTONES

Check milestones that have been met:

☐ Maintains eye contact with parent *(normally by 2-3 mos; red flag for autism)*
☐ Holds head upright while supported *(2 mos)*
☐ Sits alone *(6-7 mos)*
☐ Crawls on all fours *(8-9 mos)*
☐ Babbles *(normally before 9 mos; red flag for autism)*
☐ Gestures: waving, pointing, and showing *(normally before 9 mos; red flag for autism)*
☐ Pulls to stand through half-kneel *(10-11 mos)*
☐ Walks alone *(12 mos)*
☐ Picks up objects from floor *(13-18 mos)*
☐ Creeps upstairs *(13-18 mos)*

(continued)

TABLE 5-2 (CONTINUED)

COMPREHENSIVE CHILD DEVELOPMENTAL AND OCCUPATIONAL HISTORY

☐ Creeps downstairs *(18-24 mos)*
☐ Runs *(18-24 mos)*
☐ Catches a large ball *(4-5 yrs)*
☐ Uses single words *(13-18 mos)*
☐ Understands and follows simple commands *(13-18 mos)*
☐ Shakes head "no" *(13-18 mos)*
☐ Points to body parts
☐ Uses 2-word sentences *(18-24 mos)*
☐ Uses 3- to 4-word sentences *(24-36 mos)*
☐ Asks questions *(24-26 mos)*
☐ Drinks from a cup *(10-12 mos)*
☐ Dresses self *(3 yrs)*
☐ Uses a spoon *(10-12 mos)*
☐ Uses a knife *(3-5 yrs)*
☐ Uses markers or crayons *(scribbles; 18-24 mos)*
☐ Kicks ball *(24-36 mos)*
☐ Tells a short story *(1 to 2 events) (27 mos and older)*
☐ Retells a short story *(30-36 mos)*

PART III: Present Status—Current care, concerns, and management

1. Parent(s) current concerns: *(eg, vision, hearing, antigravity movement, behavior [irritable, lethargic])*
2. Current medications:
3. Current illnesses and management:

HOME – FAMILY SUPPORT

Family support:

Names and ages of siblings:

Are the other siblings in good general health? If not, please describe:

4. Interaction with other children (siblings/peers):
5. Attendance at day care, playgroups, other (specify):
6. Physician's name:
7. Physician's address:
8. Physician's phone:
9. Names of other specialists working with your child:
10. What is the family's history since the birth of this child *(note moves, changes, significant traumas, or other problems)*
11. Other comments:

_____   _____
Team Members   Date

the child's performance would likely deteriorate over time. The interprofessional team should talk with those staff who know the child and family to prioritize tests and measures, determine the possibility of testing over several sessions, consider the urgency for test results, and ensure that resources are available for test administration. Other considerations could include the following:

- Variability in performance based upon the time of day (eg, nap and meal times)
- Limited language skills of a younger child/the primary language of the child
- Family's culture and ethnicity
- Child's endurance and risk for fatigue
- Child's separation anxiety (after 9 months)
- Child's attention span/distractibility
- Child's comfort
- Child's compliance
- Family's transportation needs
- Privacy and who should be present during testing
- Most recent concerns, issues, and complaints by the child, family, and caretakers
- Primary desires/needs of the family and child, including language preferences and cultural preferences that impact service delivery
- Child's current health status (eg, changes in medical diagnoses, recent clinical tests, current anthropometrics)
- Child's current medications
- Planned/upcoming medical interventions for the child
- Performance limitations as related to the individual disease, disorder, and/or condition

This information should be reviewed in light of criteria for selecting specific tests and measures during assessment, as outlined in Table 5-2. Scheduling a series of tests and measures at the child's optimal time of day may yield the best results.

The team is charged with determining the child's and family's needs and concerns, and the focus of intervention will be to meet the needs of the child and the family while empowering them to manage health concerns. Additionally, it is important to address any issues raised by referral sources.

Before quality intervention and instruction can be delivered, appropriate assessments of a child's current level of functioning must be completed. Moreover, assessments of a child's potential for learning can aid in more accurately determining prognosis, possible additional assessments, therapy goals, intervention strategies, potential length and trajectory of therapy, and benchmarks for completion of services.

Environmental assessments (both physical and psychosocial environments) should also be considered across practice settings. For the younger child, an informal environmental assessment may address activities in the home, social activities such as athletics and social groups, and school functioning. For the adolescent with special needs, the environmental assessment may also include a job site, social activities with peers (such as church events and shopping), and ongoing therapies at a local rehabilitation facility. The individual's functioning may vary across sites because the demands upon a child are quite different when in the classroom, in the cafeteria, in music class, and so on. With so much at stake, a complete picture of the child's strengths and weaknesses/concerns needs to be developed.

Tests and measures, sometimes referred to as assessments, are designed to help professionals gather relevant knowledge about the child, family, and various environments for integrated clinical decision making. Assessment is an ongoing, dynamic process, with no, one protocol or test meeting the needs of every child, regardless of age. The interprofessional team needs to bring sensitivity for individual needs, flexibility, clinical judgment, and research support into the design of an assessment strategy. For a more complete picture of the child's level of performance, potential for growth, and personal needs, many measures and perspectives need to be brought in for consideration. An individual's needs for target performance are impacted by social and cultural norms. Therefore, no standard set of tests and measures will work for every individual. As a result, the interprofessional team needs to follow a collaborative system of selecting appropriate assessments for each individual client.

As mentioned earlier, a thorough case history, including past and present concerns, can lay the basis for understanding relevant problems. An understanding of the family and its social patterns help contribute to understanding their priorities, routines, and needs. The interprofessional team can interview both the individual (if the child is able to respond) and others who interact regularly with that child. Team members should also perform their own observations of the individual in multiple settings. This information is crucial in describing practical levels of performance, as well as identifying projected needs across environments.

Interprofessional team members may also choose to administer a variety of standardized assessments to supplement their interviews and observations. Standardized assessments need to be sensitive and selective. Most importantly, the child should be represented in the population used for the test interpretation of the standardized assessment. Table 5-3 describes key psychometric properties that can be used for selecting an appropriate standardized test.[6]

Norm-referenced tests rely on comparisons of the child's performance to the performance of other typical children with similar demographics. Screenings are usually done with norm-referenced tests. These tests can compare children to others of comparable age to determine whether there is a developmental delay in one or more areas of function. If the

---

TABLE 5-3

SELECTING A STANDARDIZED TEST

Developmental testing is most accurate when using standardized tests with strong psychometric parameters. Below are criteria that can be used to select an appropriate standardized test in pediatrics.

- Validity: The extent to which measurements are useful for making decisions relevant to a given purpose. Validity refers to the appropriateness, truthfulness, authenticity, and effectiveness of the test. Does the test measure what it was intended to measure?
  - Domain validity: This type of validity refers to the relationship of this test to other tests measuring the same domain or a similar construct.
  - Construct validity: This type of validity refers to the hypothetic construct or domain you intend to study. It defines what you intend to measure. The test content matches descriptors of the same concept described in research studies.
  - Face validity: The test makes sense to the person to whom it is administered. The individual "accepts" the test.
  - Content validity: The content of the test is narrowed to specific items or content that is essential for the domain that is being measured.
  - Concurrent validity: The results of this test concur with findings from other tests examining the same construct at the same time on the same individual.
  - Predictive validity: The test is able to predict future events or behaviors.
- Reliability: Will the test give the same results if used under the same circumstances?
  - Interobserver reliability: Does changing observer change the test score?
  - Decision-consistency reliability: Stability of decisions.
  - Test-rest reliability: Stability of individual scores when the test is given by a different examiner.
  - Intrarater reliability: This type of reliability refers to the consistency of test scores when the same examiner gives the same test. It indicates the stability of the measure.
  - Test-retest reliability: This type of reliability refers to the accuracy of the same test used in repeated measures for the same construct.

---

child is delayed, a more thorough examination could include *criterion-referenced tests*. Criterion-referenced tests assess a child's task performance in relation to specific task criteria. Although criterion-referenced tests are helpful, reports must clearly state the limitations of the test results. Table 5-4 provides a helpful comparison of norm-referenced vs criterion-referenced tests.[7]

Often standardized assessments target discrete skills that may not translate into the overall skills needed by the child to successfully function in the home, school, and other social environments. Children from linguistically and culturally diverse groups benefit from alternate methods of assessment. Even for children who are within the mainstream culture, standardized assessments may reveal mainly what a child does not know and not necessarily what a child knows or is capable of learning. *Dynamic assessment* (DA), designed using Vigotsky's model of cognitive development, can provide information about the child's ability to respond to new learning experiences, revealing the child's potential

to learn.[8,9] DA has also been shown to be a sensitive measure for children from culturally and linguistically diverse backgrounds.[10] Assessments can be devised to reveal important aspects of learning, including the child's (1) ease at learning a new skill, (2) ability to focus attention on a task, (3) ability to complete a task, (4) ability to transfer skills to new tasks, (5) persistence, (6) enthusiasm, (7) planning skills, and (8) self-regulation.

Dynamic assessments are generally developed using a test-teach-retest model, using graduated prompting to see how much support the child requires to learn a new skill. With this mediated learning experience (MLE), the examiner can judge how much effort the child and teacher must expend for the child to learn a new task.[11] If the child learns a new skill easily, possibly more exposure is needed, not necessarily intervention. However, if intervention is indicated, the learning strategies and prompts that are most effective when working with the child can be identified.[10,11]

	TABLE 5-4	
	NORM-REFERENCED AND CRITERION-REFERENCED TESTS	
	NORM-REFERENCED	**CRITERION-REFERENCED**
Purpose	To examine individual performance in relation to a representative group. Used for diagnosis and placement.	To examine an individual performance in relation to a criterion or external standard. Used for evaluation and program planning. These tests help demonstrate the effectiveness of intervention.
Test construction	Items developed from activities hypothesized to test specific skills or performances.	Items developed from task analysis related to an objective that can be accomplished through intervention.
Administration	Standardized administration.	May or may not be standardized.
Scoring	Based on standards relative to a group or normal distribution. There may be variability in scores with means and standard deviations.	Based on absolute standards. There is no variability in scores because mastery of each skill is desired.
Psychometric properties	Test should demonstrate reliability and validity	Test should demonstrate reliability and validity
Reference points or standards	Standards represent a range of performances with an average score used as a standard for comparison.	Standards are established by the consensus of experts.
Comparisons made or evaluation standard	The individual's performance is compared with the group norm.	The individual's performance is compared with a fixed standard. The individual is subsequently compared with herself.
Relationship to intervention	May or may not relate to intervention. Is generally not very sensitive to impact of intervention. Does not necessarily measure the mastery of performance.	Is specific to interventional content. Has a high overlap with interventional objectives. Identifies levels of mastery for a specific performance and guides level of instruction.
Variability	Variability is expected as scores should represent a normal distribution curve.	Variability is not expected; mastery of a skill is expected. Narrowly samples a specific domain.
Reporting results	Interpretation is based upon comparison with a specific population. Results provide a summary of overall performance in a domain.	Interpretation is based upon mastery of skills. Reports relate specific and detailed information about the individual's performance.

CONDUCTING INTERPROFESSIONAL ASSESSMENTS

After prioritizing the tests and measures the team will administer, they must consider a strategy to get the child's performance in the most economical fashion. Ideally, the team should avoid tests that might cause discomfort or distress until the end of the testing session (eg, pain sensation). Also, for the sake of efficiency, team members should work cooperatively before the actual assessment to identify appropriate resources to meet anticipated needs. Oftentimes, families appreciate readily available educational, medical, and financial resources that might be needed for the child's optimal development and equipment needs.

The team should set up an optimal test environment before the child enters. The space should be comfortable (temperature), controlled for distracting sounds or activity, and ready with equipment and markers for tests and measures. With young children, all activities for testing need to be prepared and within reach, but out of the child's reach or eyesight. It is helpful to ask the parent or caretaker to bring the child's favorite toys and to have age-appropriate popular toys on hand for use, if needed.

Interpersonal interactions are key to successful teamwork. Recognizing that the family member or caretaker is a part of the team, all professionals should introduce themselves to the parent and the child, explaining the purpose of selected tests and measures. The physical therapist, occupational therapist, and speech-language pathologist should also attempt talking to the child to gain as much information as possible directly from the child, including capabilities and interests.

Observations of spontaneous behaviors give a window of insight into the child's natural behavior. The team members should ask the child to perform a specific task that is reportedly something he or she can successfully perform. While interacting with the child, the team should take note of the child's responsiveness, changes in posture, fine and gross motor movements (including preferential use of extremities), attempts to communicate verbally and nonverbally, general mood, level of energy, and general appearance. Many times, team members use observations and knowledge of neurodevelopment to ascertain functional skills when children are unable to perform standardized or criterion-referenced assessments.

For younger children, it is often necessary to motivate the child using a goal-directed task or game or an age-appropriate toy. The team may incorporate toys into the testing situation as appropriate (eg, asking a 3-year-old child to reach for a See 'n Say toy that is activated when the child successfully touches the toy).

Team members can help caretakers appreciate *learned helplessness* so they understand why therapists require children to perform tasks with no prompting.[12] Caretakers must realize that children learn very quickly that someone else will perform a task for them if they hesitate or do not perform the task correctly on the first trial, leading children to act helpless when they may be capable of performing a task. Allowing trial and error as much as possible enables children with impairments the rare opportunity of struggling through the physical and mental challenges of new activities. Team members may offer assistance in performing tasks (only as needed and allowed by the tests) by using (1) *verbal cues or gestures*, (2) *graded manual assistance* (physical prompts that are graded from minimal to maximum assistance), and (3) modeling to allow the child to imitate certain skills.

Team members should be prepared for documenting the session, using appropriate forms and technology (eg, videotaping or recording) to best capture the child's performance. Through collaborative efforts and using test batteries that incorporate multiple assessments, team members can aid in data collection as needed.

Analyses of data in conjunction with the child's history and interviews of caretakers and others provide the essential information for developing a plan of care. The plan of care may include (1) retaining the child/family for intervention, (2) consulting with and/or referring to other health care practitioners to address issues out of the team's scope of practice or expertise, (3) addressing risk factors and risk-reduction needs through consultation, and (4) recommending activities and resources to promote the child's needs for healthy growth and development.

DEVELOPING INTERPROFESSIONAL PLANS OF CARE

When developing a child's plan of care, the team must consider legislative guidelines that dictate what the team is legally able to offer children and their families. Based upon legal and financial considerations, schools typically provide different health care and educational resources than what medical centers offer.

The School Environment

In today's schools, from pre-kindergarten through high school, all students, regardless of any disabilities, are included in the educational process. Federal laws, such as the Individuals with Disabilities Education Act,[1] and state laws, mandate the provision of services to student with special needs. To serve the needs of this population, a diverse range of professionals are required. Collaboration lessens the overlap of services and improves outcomes for the children they serve. By professionals sharing assessment and intervention responsibilities, more critical eyes can be brought to observe students' performance in a multitude of environments. With this interprofessional input, students have the opportunity to have instruction, reinforcement, and practice in their needed skills over a variety of environments and with a variety of individuals. This coordinated effort can result in quicker, more efficacious results and greater generalization of skills due to the more consistent and more frequent reinforcement.

The composition of the interprofessional team in school depends upon the dynamic needs of the student. Some representatives from different professions may interact more during assessments but may only provide consultation services or no interventions, depending on the student's needs. The overarching mantra for team members must be open and regular communication about the child's level of functioning and progress toward achieving educational goals. The provision of interprofessional collaboration in educational environments is discussed in greater detail in Sections 8 and 9.

The Medical Environment

Team-based care in the medical environment typically involves treating children with acute or chronic conditions. Inpatient and outpatient medical care are both designed to help families manage the health conditions that restrict the child's ability to live at home, attend school regularly, and/or engage in regular activities. Most pediatric hospitals offer specialty clinics to address specific needs, such as burn and trauma care, weight management, immunology, asthma, adolescent medicine, Down syndrome, wheelchair seating, orthotics, and abdominal pain.

Just as teams within a culture must be sensitive to the many factors influencing the delivery of care within a setting, so must professionals sensitively communicate between medical and school settings to ensure continuity of care and collaborative management to best meet the child's and family's needs. Because the regulations governing care varies between settings, Section 10 will provide examples of common health conditions and how they are managed in medical settings.

DEVELOPING AN INTERPROFESSIONAL PLAN OF CARE

Pediatric therapists can use the International Classification of Functioning, Disability and Health (ICF) Model as one method for developing goals and intervention strategies, addressing equipment needs, considering appropriate

motivational toys and games, and providing comprehensive care.[13] Goals are most easily measured with the use of the SMART acronym: specific, measurable, achievable, realistic, and timely goals.[14] Table 5-5 illustrates an outline for developing an interprofessional plan of care based upon the ICF Model.

PREVENTIVE CARE FOR HEALTHY GROWTH AND DEVELOPMENT ACROSS PRACTICE SETTINGS

Interprofessional teams must serve as a safety net in both medical and educational settings where care may be compartmentalized. Genetics or inherited characteristics play a key role in an infant's physical and psychological makeup; however, physical activity and other environmental factors can *nurture* a child, greatly influencing her healthy growth and proper development, increasing fitness, and emergent wellness. Combinations of genetic and environmental factors, including stressors the family may be encountering, play key roles in these maturational processes. Certain aspects of growth are more strongly influenced by genetic factors, including dental development, the sequence of bone ossification, and sexual differentiation during puberty, but all are shaped by environmental factors. The interprofessional team should offer health promotion education and resources that help families deal with daily challenges, as well as stress the importance of healthy lifestyle choices (eg, sleep, nutrition, fitness, hydration, immunizations, stress management) that can provide the most positive impact on their children.

SUMMARY

Physical therapists, occupational therapists, and speech-language pathologists can work alongside others in medical, educational, and community settings in a collaborative effort to promote healthy growth and development of children in their care. In the community, health care providers can provide screenings for children in daycares, schools, and community centers. In the medical setting, pediatric therapists can more carefully examine children with special needs, offering suggestions for individualized care that promotes healing and reduces the risks of future injury or illness. All health professionals need to work with families to help their children achieve functional goals and healthy bodies. Similarly, teachers and school-based professionals can collaborate with pediatric therapists to identify children at risk for developmental or learning disabilities that can impact them throughout their lives. Through early

TABLE 5-5		
DEVELOPING A PLAN OF CARE BASED ON THE INTERNATIONAL CLASSIFICATION OF FUNCTIONING, DISABILITY, AND HEALTH MODEL		
PLAN OF CARE		
Child's Name: Joey Age: 3 years Health Condition: Cerebral palsy, hypotonia		
Team Members: Date:		
ACTIVITY LIMITATIONS	**HYPOTHESES FOR ACTIVITY LIMITATIONS**	**SMART GOALS, INTERVENTION STRATEGIES (ACTIVITIES, EQUIPMENT, MOTIVATION GAMES OR TOYS)**
• Nonverbal • Poor postural control • Dependent in all mobility • Dependent in all self-care, including feeding • Unable to sit for 2 sec • Holds head for <2 sec • Unable to maintain attention to tasks	**Body Structure/Body Function** • Growth: low body mass index • Neuromuscular system: low muscle tone, sensory dysfunction, delayed developmental reflexes • Musculoskeletal system: decreased strength, range of motion, endurance, flexibility • Cardiopulmonary system: short of air, poor endurance • Integumentary system: poor skin integrity • Other body systems: abdominal pain from constipation **Environmental Factors** • To be determined **Personal Factors** • Poor motivation, fatigues easily • ↑ fatigue **Participation** • Not socially engaged in activity with others	

detection, risk management, and collaborative teamwork, therapists can offer their expertise to enhance the well-being of children and their families.

Each section of this manual goes into greater detail regarding how therapists can work collaboratively with families, teachers, and others to provide a health safety net for families. By promoting healthy lifestyles, offering health education, engaging children and their families in therapeutic play and leisure skills based upon dynamic assessment, challenging children with activities that enhance creativity and problem solving, and creating psychosocial environments that are supportive of learning and inclusion in the community, pediatric therapists manage essential elements of interprofessional care that can significantly impact a community's well-being.

INTERPROFESSIONAL ACTIVITY

Case Management

Use the following case study to discuss interprofessional management of care.

1. Use interprofessional collaboration to plan a child's assessment:
   a. Identify *agenda* items to include in your preassessment meeting.
   b. Take turns facilitating discussion for each agenda *item*.
   c. Discuss factors the team should consider when administering tests and measures.
   d. Discuss factors impacting goal development for the child.
   e. Ensure that information is documented on the agenda by a *designated reporter*.
   f. Complete the meeting with *action* items listing at least one person responsible for follow-up of each item.
   g. Approve *minutes* from your meeting (with changes, if needed).
2. As a team, discuss how you plan to share your assessment results with various stakeholders, as appropriate:
   a. Family
   b. Referral source
   c. School
   d. Physician

Case 5-1: An 18-month-old girl with CHARGE syndrome

Your team is asked to perform an assessment of a new child who will be coming to your community-based private practice next week. Jessie is an 18-month-old girl with hearing, speech, visual (left eye coloboma), and motor problems associated with her diagnosis of CHARGE syndrome.[15] She squints and has spontaneous nystagmus, facial asymmetry, polydactyly, atresia of the choanae (blocked nasal breathing passages), a cleft palate, and sensorineural hearing loss on both sides. She reportedly also has a minor atrial septal defect. She is in the 10th percentile for height, weight, and head circumference. She crawls but is unable to pull to stand or walk. You have no information from the family.

REFERENCES

1. Stanford Children's Health. The neonatal intensive care unit (NICU). Stanford Children's Health Web site. http://www.stanfordchildrens.org/en/topic/default?id=the-neonatal-intensive-care-unit-nicu-90-P02389. Accessed February 14, 2017.
2. US Department of Education. Individuals with Disabilities Education Act. US Department of Education Web site. https://www2.ed.gov/about/offices/list/osers/osep/osep-idea.html. Accessed February 14, 2017.
3. Salas E, Diaz Granados D, Weaver SJ, King H. Does team training work? Principles for health care. *Acad Emerg Med*. 2008;15:1002-1009.
4. Thompson CR. *Perceptions of Interprofessional Collaboration in Special Education* [research forum]. Missouri: Rockhurst University; 2017.
5. Thompson CR. Developmental history. In: *Prevention Practice and Health Promotion: A Health Care Professional's Guide to Health, Fitness, and Wellness*. 2nd ed. Thorofare, NJ: SLACK Incorporated; 2015:347-349.
6. University of California at Davis. Reliability and validity. University of California at Davis Web site. http://psc.dss.ucdavis.edu/sommerb/sommerdemo/intro/validity.htm. Accessed February 14, 2017.
7. Montgomery PC, Connolly BH. Norm-referenced and criterion-referenced tests. Use in pediatrics and application to task analysis of motor skill. *Phys Ther*. 1987;67(12):1873-1876.
8. Vygotsky LS. *Thought and Language*. Cambridge, MA: MIT Press; 1986.
9. Peña E, Quinn R, Iglesias A. The application of dynamic methods to language assessment: A nonbiased procedure. *Journal of Special Education*. 1992;26:269-280.
10. Gutiérrez-Clellen VF, Peña E. Dynamic assessment of diverse children: A tutorial. *Lang Speech Hear Serv Sch*. 2001;32:212-224.
11. American Speech-Language-Hearing Association. Position statement: Social dialects. American Speech-Language-Hearing Association Web site. http://www.asha.org/policy/PS1983-00115.htm. Accessed February 14, 2017.
12. Tennen H, Eller SJ. Attributional components of learned helplessness and facilitation. *J Pers Soc Psychol*. 1977;35:265-271.
13. World Health Organization. International Classification of Functioning, Disability and Health (ICF). World Health Organization Web site. http://www.who.int/classifications/icf/en/. Accessed February 14, 2017.
14. Doran GT. There's a S.M.A.R.T. way to write management's goals and objectives. *Management Review*. 1981;70:35.
15. Genetics Home Reference. CHARGE syndrome. Genetics Home Reference Web site. https://ghr.nlm.nih.gov/condition/charge-syndrome. Published February 14, 2017. Accessed February 14, 2017.

Section 6

Interprofessional Care of
High-Risk Infants

*Pamela Hart, PhD, CCC-SLP; Carol Koch, EdD, CCC-SLP; and
Catherine Rush Thompson, PT, PhD, MS*

OVERVIEW

This section provides an overview of the interprofessional care of high-risk infants typically seen in the neonatal intensive care unit (NICU). Information in this section addresses foundational concepts for clinical practice in the NICU, including characteristics of the high-risk neonate; risk factors that influence the infant's growth and development; the unique roles and responsibilities professionals who provide care to high-risk infants and their families; terminology related to the care of high-risk infants; the family systems theory approach and how it relates to the management of care for high-risk infants; and the important ethical considerations that team members must face when providing care to high-risk infants. Upon completion of this unit, the learner will be able to (1) discuss critical periods in prenatal growth and development, (2) describe risk factors associated with the high-risk infant, including prematurity and low birth weight, (3) distinguish the roles and responsibilities of professionals working with high-risk infants, (4) describe tests and measures commonly used for pregnant mothers and their newborns, (5) discuss interprofessional collaboration in the development of goals and interventions for high-risk infants and their families, including preventive care, (6) discuss current, evidence-based resources for families and other caretakers, (7) demonstrate clinical reasoning skills,

including ethical considerations, to address common problems faced in working with families of high-risk infants, (8) describe preventive care for mothers seeking to become pregnant in the future, and (9) discuss the process that facilitates the transition of the family with a high-risk infant to early intervention.

CRITICAL PERIODS IN PRENATAL GROWTH AND DEVELOPMENT

Infants may be born prematurely, full-term, or post-term, depending upon genetic and environmental factors. Although clinicians have little impact on genetic factors, they can influence environmental factors. *What could these environmental factors include?* In the case of the fetus, environmental factors could include the mother's nutrition and alcohol intake, which can potentially impact prenatal growth and development in utero. To best understand the differences between these populations and the impact of possible environmental factors, therapists should be familiar with prenatal growth and development, appreciating how body systems function, grow, and mature in utero. One of the earliest-born fetuses that has survived was born at 21 weeks' and 5 days' gestation, a figure equal to approximately

Thompson CR. *Pediatric Therapy:
An Interprofessional Framework for Practice* (pp 85-99).
© 2018 SLACK Incorporated.

TABLE 6-1		
CRITICAL PERIODS OF FETAL DEVELOPMENT		
BODY SYSTEM	CRITICAL PERIODS DURING GESTATION	CONTINUED RISK
Central nervous system/brain prenatal development 4 to 24 weeks Neuronal proliferation 6 to 30 weeks Neuronal differentiation 8 to 30 weeks Neuronal migration 10 weeks on Synapse formation 20 weeks on Programmed cell death 18 weeks on Synaptic pruning 30 weeks on Myelinization	4 to 8 weeks	Postnatal, through to adulthood
Heart	5 to 9 weeks	12th week
Upper limbs	6 to 10 weeks	12th week
Eyes	6 to 10 weeks	Term
Lower limbs	6 to 10 weeks	12th week
Teeth	9 to 11 weeks	Term
Palate	9 to 11 weeks	16th week
External genitalia	9 to 11 weeks	Term
Ears	6 to 11 weeks	13th week
Adapted from The Endowment for Human Development. Prenatal Summary. The Endowment for Human Development Web site. https://www.ehd.org/prenatal-summary.php. Published 2017. Accessed December 5, 2017.		

6 months of pregnancy.[1,2] A fetus born before 24 weeks of pregnancy has a low chance of survival, and those who do survive often suffer from some type of disability. In reviewing embryological and fetal development, consider the risks of a premature infant born as early as 6 months' gestation.

The germination period begins at conception and lasts approximately 2 weeks, at which point the embryonic period begins. During the embryonic period, lasting until 8 weeks' gestation, the fetus forms from the undifferentiated embryo to a human fetus with distinguishable body structures, a process of organ formation described as *organogenesis*. At 8 weeks, the fetal period begins and typically lasts until 38 to 42 weeks (full-term), when the neonate is equipped to leave the womb. This gestational period is divided into 3 trimesters, each lasting a period of approximately 3 months. Gestational age (GA) is measured in weeks from the first day of the woman's last menstrual cycle to the current date and is commonly used to describe a premature infant's age at birth. For example, a neonate born 4 months early would typically have a GA of 6 months.

Every fetus experiences *critical periods* in utero as it grows and develops. These critical periods are when genetic or maternal effects can significantly influence the developmental process. Negative influences throughout pregnancy, depending upon their timing, severity, and duration, can cause major congenital malformations incompatible with life or can significantly limit the structural and functional integrity of a newborn. Table 6-1 illustrates the critical periods in development when negative influences can have the greatest impact on the fetus' health.

Researchers have identified a range of negative influences on fetal development. *Teratogens* are harmful agents that can enter the womb, typically through maternal experiences, and result in birth defects.[3,4] Teratogens include radiation, chemicals, environmental pollutants, and infections. See Table 6-2 listing well-known teratogens. Depending upon the time and duration of exposure to these teratogens, they could have a significant impact on the infant's mental and physical health.

TABLE 6-2

TERATOGENS

DRUGS AND CHEMICALS	IONIZING RADIATION (X-RAYS)
Alcohol	**HYPERTHERMIA**
Aminoglycosides (Gentamicin)	
Aminopterin	**INFECTION MICROORGANISMS**
Antithyroid agents (PTU)	Coxsackie virus
Bromine	Cytomegalovirus
Cigarette smoke	Herpes simplex
Cocaine	Parvovirus
Cortisone	Rubella (German measles)
Diethylstilbesterol (DES)	*Toxoplasma gondii* (toxoplasmosis)
Diphenylhydantoin	
Heroin	**MATERNAL METABOLIC CONDITIONS**
Lead	Autoimmune disease (eg, Rh incompatibility)
Methylmercury	Diabetes
Penicillamine	Dietary deficiencies, malnutrition
Retinoic acid (Isotretinoin, Accutane)	Phenylketonuria
Streptomycin	
Tetracycline	
Thalidomide	
Trimethadione	
Valproic acid	
Warfarin	

Adapted from Gilbert-Barness E. Teratogenic Causes of Malformations. *Ann Clin Lab Sci.* 2010:40;99-114.

Note: This list includes known and possible teratogenic agents and is not exhaustive.

A mother's prenatal care is essential for assuring an optimal environment for the fetus' healthy growth and development. *What are common maternal risk factors contributing to a high-risk pregnancy?* Some maternal risk factors are controllable; that is, they are factors that are commonly addressed in prenatal care, including unhealthy lifestyle behaviors, such as cigarette smoking, drug abuse, or alcohol use, and exposure to infectious agents (eg, sexually transmitted infections and cytomegalovirus).[1] For example, heavy and prolonged drinking by an expectant mother can cause fetal alcohol syndrome, a cluster of abnormalities that affect both the infant's mental and motor functions. In some cases, risk factors are less controllable. Living in poverty is associated with increased incidents of illness, malnourishment, young teenage mothers, and stressful lifestyles; which all contribute to increased risk for the infant. If the mother is older than 35 or if she has pre-existing health conditions, such as asthma, diabetes, obesity, high blood pressure, anemia, or epilepsy,

she also puts the growing fetus at increased risk during pregnancy.[1] Other less controllable risk factors involve genetic conditions, such as single gene disorders (eg, cystic fibrosis or sickle cell disease) and chromosomal disorders (eg, Down syndrome).[5,6]

Pregnancy itself can pose risks, including problems with the uterus, cervix, placenta, or amniotic fluid; incompatible blood groups; and multiple births. Also, the birth process or delivery itself may be prolonged or traumatic, with risks including fetal distress, breech position, placenta previa, meconium aspiration, nuchal cord, and cephalopelvic disproportion.[5,6] Finally, a family's history of pregnancy complications or death of a baby during or following birth not only increases the risk to the health of subsequent children but also creates an additional emotional strain on the experience of bringing a new baby into the world.[5,6] Pediatric therapists must be mindful of these additional stressors that families face when dealing with their high-risk infants.

PREMATURITY AND
LOW BIRTH WEIGHT

A high-risk infant, whether put at risk by maternal or other factors, is a neonate who, regardless of gestational age, birth weight, or size, is judged to have a greater-than-average chance of morbidity particularly within the first 28 days of life.[5,6] Risk factors are varied and include preconceptual, prenatal, natal, or postnatal conditions or circumstances that interfere with the normal birth process or impede adjustment to extrauterine growth and development.[6]

Factors commonly putting neonates at risk include *prematurity* and *low birth weight*. Prematurity is defined as any birth occurring prior to 38 weeks' GA.[7] The shorter the infant's GA, the greater the neonate's risks for medical complications that impact brain development, health, and subsequent developmental outcomes.[8] This prematurity deprives the neonate of maternal support systems that allow essential body systems to develop and mature. Underdevelopment of key body systems jeopardize brain development and/or health outcomes, potentially diminishing the infant's ability to fully develop skills and enjoy a high quality of life.[9]

Low birth weight is defined as any neonate born weighing less than 5 pounds (2500 grams), with very low birth weight defined at 3.3 pounds (1500 grams), and extremely low birth weight defined at 2.2 pounds (1000 grams).[10] Premature infants with low birth weight face a myriad of challenges, including elevated risks for sudden infant death syndrome,[11] heart and lung problems,[12] intraventricular hemorrhage,[13] developmental impairments such as cerebral palsy,[14] problems with feeding,[15] behavioral disorders,[16] impaired cognitive skills,[17] chronic health problems (eg, asthma),[18] and problems with vision and hearing.[19] In general, the risks of these complications increase as GA at birth decreases. Some risk factors affect survival of the infant and must be addressed immediately, whereas others may not be as identifiable until the child starts school and experiences learning challenges.

IDENTIFYING HIGH-RISK INFANTS

Given these potential problems, infants deemed high-risk undergo additional screening at birth. These tests are most commonly performed on mothers who are older than 35 with (1) a family history or other child with chromosomal abnormalities, (2) a known risk for a disorder that can be diagnosed in the fetus, and (3) children with neural tube defects or abnormal maternal serum alpha-fetoprotein.[5] These tests include the following[5]:

- *Amniocentesis*: A low-risk prenatal diagnostic procedure to determine the fetal age and genetic characteristics after 4 months' gestation
- *Fetal ultrasound*: A diagnostic procedure producing an image of the fetus
- *Chorionic villi sampling or chorionic villus biopsy*: A biopsy at 9 to 12 weeks to detect chromosomal and metabolic abnormalities of the fetus
- *Fetoscopy*: A procedure used to sample tissue for laboratory testing for potential metabolic and/or genetic abnormalities
- *Cordocentesis*: A test involving percutaneous umbilical blood sampling and analysis
- *Cervical length measurement*: A measurement to assess fetal growth
- *Lab testing for fetal fibronectin*: A lab test associated with preterm labor
- *A biophysical profile*: An assessment that combines fetal heart rate monitoring (nonstress test) and fetal ultrasound

At birth, every neonate is screened using simple tests that quickly identify infants who are an increased risk. The *Apgar score* is used to score the newborn's appearance, pulse, responsiveness, muscle activity, and breathing.[20] Each category is scored with 0, 1, or 2 (2 being the highest rating and healthiest score), depending on the observed condition. The 1-minute score determines how well the neonate tolerated the birthing process, and the 5-minute score indicates how well the neonate is surviving outside of the womb. The 1-minute Apgar score typically determines the need for immediate medical help. A score between 7 and 10 is normal. Scores between 4 and 6 generally indicate the need for some help breathing, such as suctioning the nostrils or giving the newborn oxygen. Scores of 3 or less may indicate the need for immediate lifesaving measures, such as resuscitation. Babies born prematurely or delivered by Cesarean section often have lower-than-normal scores, especially at the 1-minute testing. A 5-minute Apgar score of 6 or less indicates the need for additional medical attention. Table 6-3 lists the criteria used for the Apgar score.

A baby with a low Apgar score may need attention, such as stimulation, to get the heart beating at a healthy rate, supplemental oxygen, or help clearing out the airway to improve breathing. Oftentimes, a low score at 1 minute is near normal by 5 minutes. Also, a lower Apgar score does not necessarily predict long-term health problems for the

TABLE 6-3
APGAR SCORING

Activity (muscle tone)

0 — Limp; no movement

1 — Some flexion of arms and legs

2 — Active motion

Pulse (heart rate)—a critical test

0 — No heart rate

1 — Fewer than 100 beats per minute

2 — At least 100 beats per minute

Grimace (reflex response to an irritating stimulus)

0 — No response to airways being suctioned

1 — Grimace during suctioning

2 — Grimaces and pulls away, coughs, or sneezes during suctioning

Appearance (color)

0 — Whole body is completely bluish-gray or pale

1 — Good color in body with bluish hands or feet

2 — Good color all over

Respiration (breathing)

0 — Not breathing

1 — Weak cry; may sound like whimpering, slow or irregular breathing

2 — Good, strong cry; normal rate and effort of breathing

child. However, if the newborn needs ongoing care, she is placed in the NICU for close monitoring and technological support designed to stabilize the newborn's physiological status.

Premature infants are medically fragile because of their underdeveloped body structures and body functions. For example, 90% of body weight is gained after 5 months' GA, with 50% of that weight gained in the final 2 months, so premature infants commonly appear very thin, wrinkled, and fragile with underdeveloped body features. Similarly, the newborn will have lower muscle tone than the typical full-term infant who has more fully developed and active muscles. With this in mind, expectations for sensorimotor function should be adjusted to the infant's GA rather than chronological age.

ROLES OF PROFESSIONALS WORKING WITH PREMATURE AND HIGH-RISK INFANTS

Professionals who work with these vulnerable neonates and their families must have excellent interprofessional knowledge and skills, focusing on their abilities to provide care centered on each family's needs. In addition to discipline-specific skills, these professionals have shared knowledge across embryology and genetics, typical and atypical infant development, ethical decision making, effective interdisciplinary teamwork, and family-centered care.[21] In addition to their shared knowledge, each professional contributes unique knowledge and skills to facilitate the best possible outcomes for these most fragile clients.

Because the care of high-risk infants may be complex and demanding, teams often comprise a variety of medical and rehabilitation professionals, including neonatologists, nurses, respiratory therapists, speech-language pathologists, occupational therapists, physical therapists, lactation consultants, and social workers (Table 6-4).

THE NEONATAL INTENSIVE CARE UNIT

The NICU offers a safe environment for the high-risk infant and family. At birth, the neonate's failure of any body system must be addressed with technology to replace vital functions, such as air exchange, circulation, digestion, excretion of waste, and immunologic functions. The NICU combines advanced technology and trained professionals to provide specialized care for these vulnerable neonates designed to manage the needs of the family and newborn. Tests commonly administered in the NICU include the following:

- Blood tests for anemia, high levels of bilirubin (possible jaundice), low blood sugar, chemical imbalance, infection, and blood gases
- Computed tomography (CAT or CT) scan
- Echocardiogram
- Hearing test (brainstem auditory-evoked response test) problems
- Magnetic resonance imaging (MRI)
- Newborn screening test (phenylketonuria [PKU] or newborn screening [NBS] test)
- Test for retinopathy of prematurity (ROP)
- Ultrasound
- Urine tests for kidney function
- Weight
- X-rays
- Tests for neurological maturation, such as the Milani-Comparetti Motor Development Screening Test

Pediatric therapists with expertise in the NICU work as a team to ensure that the neonate has sufficient stimulation for optimal growth and development but avoids overstimulation to the newborn's underdeveloped central nervous system. Other roles include the following[22,23]:

- Screening neonate to determine needs for referral
- Assessing the neonate's body structures, body functions, and neurodevelopment
- Developing and implementing a plan to prevent neurobehavioral disorganization and complications of prematurity in multiple systems

- Designing, implementing, and evaluating the efficacy of intervention plans in collaboration with the family and medical team
- Developing and implementing discharge plans in collaboration with the family, medical team, and community resources
- Consulting with providers of specialized equipment or services in preparation for community-based care
- Consulting and collaborating with health care professionals, families, policy makers, and community organizations to advocate for services to support the development of the neonate
- Incorporating evidence-based literature into neonatal practice
- Communicating, demonstrating, and evaluating neonatal care procedures with NICU professionals and other caregivers
- Developing an interprofessional risk management plan
- Evaluating the effectiveness of a neonatal program
- All professionals working in the NICU should be familiar with common terminology to enhance interprofessional communication. Table 6-5 lists terms associated with care of the high-risk infant. Table 6-6 lists the types of care typically provided by pediatric therapists.

The team approach to all of these issues surrounding high-risk infants is paramount to the successful management of care. All team members must be mindful of the daily demands of an infant and family in the NICU. This awareness includes assessment of the neonate's state of arousal, sleep cycles, and the sensory environment (eg, light, sound, tactile input by caregivers, machinery in NICU). Additional considerations for collaboration involves recognizing stressors of the neonate, the family, and other caregivers; addressing their concerns; and providing needed education. Education may relate to proper handling, emotional bonding, addressing the newborn's neurodevelopment, and therapeutic positioning (eg, swaddling, kangaroo care, position changes). The NICU environment, associated with extensive monitoring devices and tubes, and medical interventions impact the newborn's sensorimotor function, so special attention is needed to prevent secondary complications associated with these factors.

The challenge of oral feeding is a specific example of the need for interprofessional management. Physicians, speech-language pathologists, lactation consultants, occupational therapists, physical therapists, and nurses work together to ensure the safety of oral nutrition for the infant and to develop treatment plans working toward sufficiency of oral nutrition as a long-term goal.

TABLE 6-4		
INTERPROFESSIONAL TEAM MEMBER ROLES IN THE CARE OF HIGH-RISK INFANTS		
PROFESSION	**ROLES AND RESPONSIBILITIES IN THE CARE OF HIGH-RISK INFANTS**	**REQUIRED TRAINING**
Genetic counselor	This professional offers genetic testing, education, and counseling to patients and their families	Master's degree and licensure in some states
Neonatologist	This medical doctor provides critical care to neonates and support to parents and other physicians in the care of high-risk infants	Degree in medicine with completion of a 3-year pediatric residency followed by a 3-year residency in neonatal specialization
Registered nurse	This professional is responsible for evaluating, coordinating, and administering health care plans that may involve administering medications and nutrients, monitoring of vital signs, providing specialized respiratory care, and monitoring equipment used on the infants	Bachelor's degree in nursing
Speech-language pathologist	This professional evaluates and implements treatment plans to address communication, cognition, feeding, and swallowing in the developing infant within the context of the family	Master's degree in speech-language pathology
Occupational therapist	This professional assists each family and infant to foster optimal infant development across appropriate occupations, sensorimotor processes, and neurobehavioral organization	Master's degree or doctorate in occupational therapy
Physical therapist	This professional diagnoses and manages movement dysfunction and enhances physical and functional abilities, including preventing the onset, symptoms, and progression of impairments, functional limitations, and disabilities that may result from diseases, disorders, conditions, or injuries and advising families regarding optimal positioning for sleeping, handling, and feeding	Doctorate in physical therapy
Respiratory therapist	This professional manages respiratory support and care for infants with compromised respiratory status	Associate's degree in respiratory care
Lactation consultant	This consultant assesses and implements strategies to support the needs of the nursing mother and infant and assists other health care providers with the feeding needs of the infant	There are several pathways to becoming an International Board-Certified Lactation Consultant, but in general, medical course-work and clinical preparation are required
Social worker	This professional provides support to families in areas such as environmental stress, physical illness, and interpersonal conflicts and also performs interdisciplinary team management, collaboration, and discharge planning	Bachelor's degree in social work
Child life specialist	This specialist provides educational and emotional support for families while also working to enhance development for children in challenging situations such as hospitalization	Bachelor's degree in child psychology (or a related field) and certification by the Child Life Council

TABLE 6-5
HIGH-RISK INFANT CARE TERMINOLOGY

TERM	DEFINITION
Adjusted age	Also known as corrected age. This is the child's chronological age minus the number of weeks early he was born.
Apnea	A pause in breathing lasting 20 seconds or longer. Also known as an apneic episodes or apneic spell.
Apgar score	A numerical summary of a newborn's condition at birth based on 5 different scores, measured at 1 minute and 5 minutes.
Bilirubin	Yellow chemical that is a normal waste product from the breakdown of hemoglobin and other similar body components. When bilirubin accumulates, it makes the skin and eyes look yellow, a condition called jaundice.
Bronchopulmonary dysplasia (BPD)	A chronic lung disease of babies, when the lungs do not work properly and the babies have trouble breathing.
Brainstem auditory evoked response test	A hearing test where a tiny earphone is placed in the baby's ear to deliver sound. Small sensors taped to the baby's head send information to a machine that measures the electrical activity in her brain in response to the sound.
Developmentally delayed/disabled	A term used to describe infants and toddlers who have not achieved skills and abilities that are expected to be mastered by children of the same age.
Extremely low birth weight (ELBW)	A baby born weighing less than 2 pounds, 3 ounces (1,000 grams).
Gastroesophageal reflux (GER)	Contents of the stomach coming back up into the esophagus, which occurs when the junction between the esophagus and the stomach is not completely developed or is abnormal.
Gavage feeding	Feeding a baby through a nasogastric (NG) tube. Also called tube feeding.
Gestation	The period of development from the time of fertilization of the egg until birth. Normal gestation is 40 weeks; a premature baby is one born at or before the 37th week of pregnancy.
Hydrocephalus	Abnormal accumulation of cerebrospinal fluid within the ventricles of the brain.
Intrauterine growth retardation (IUGR)	A condition in which the fetus doesn't grow as big as it should while in the uterus. These babies are small for their gestational age, and their birth weight is below the 10th percentile.
Low birth weight (LBW)	A baby born weighing less than 5.5 pounds (2500 grams) and more than 3 pounds, 5 ounces (1500 grams)

TABLE 6-6	
INTERPROFESSIONAL CARE BY PEDIATRIC THERAPISTS IN THE NEONATAL INTENSIVE CARE UNIT	
DISCIPLINE	**ROLES AND RESPONSIBILITIES**
Shared knowledge	• Understands medical terminology, pathophysiology, diagnostics, equipment, infection control, lab tests used in the NICU, and medical precautions postsurgery • Knows prenatal development and risk factors following premature birth (including risks of the NICU environment) • Appreciates the roles and responsibilities of team members in the NICU • Embraces the philosophy of family-centered care • Applies the International Classification of Functioning, Disability and Health (ICF) Model to examination and intervention • Engages in interprofessional collaboration, group dynamic processes, and family education • Values ethical practice
Interprofessional skills	• Communicates and collaborates interprofessionally and with others involved in the infant's care • Determines optimal times for interactions (eg, screenings, examinations, and interventions) based upon the neonate's tolerance and family routines • Screens for need for needed services (eg, physical therapy, occupational therapy, speech-language pathology) • Incorporates evidence-based literature in neonatal practice • Monitors and evaluates impact of recommended interventions • Instructs, consults, and communicates with family members, caregivers, team members, and community, as appropriate, during stay in NICU and after discharge • Embraces family-centered care and cultural competency • Consults in areas of expertise and collaborates with health care professionals, families, policy makers, and community organizations to advocate for services to support families and their infant • Advocates for families and their infants and help families become self-advocates • Provides documentation that is objective, interpretive, thorough, and concise

(continued)

INTERPROFESSIONAL MANAGEMENT OF FEEDING

One example of high-risk infant care that requires a coordinated team effort is feeding. Optimum nutrition is a critical factor in managing the medical needs of extremely low birth weight, very low birthweight, and low birth weight preterm infants. The oral, pharyngeal, and digestive tract structures and functions have not fully developed sufficiently to support oral intake. In addition to prematurity, other medical conditions may necessitate alternate means of nutrition for newborns.

The complexity of care involved in addressing feeding issues is best addressed through a highly coordinated team effort. Team members are often defined based on the etiology of the feeding issues and contributing medical conditions. At the core of this team is the family, the significance of which is highlighted in the next section. Medical personnel, including the neonatologist, speech-language pathologist, occupational therapist, physical therapist, nutritionist, and lactation consultant, function as a team to coordinate the feeding and nutritional needs of the infant and family. An infant experiencing significant respiratory problems may benefit from having the respiratory therapist on the team. A cardiologist would be a key member of the multidisciplinary team for an infant with cardiac issues. Because

TABLE 6-6 (CONTINUED)	
INTERPROFESSIONAL CARE BY PEDIATRIC THERAPISTS IN THE NEONATAL INTENSIVE CARE UNIT	
DISCIPLINE	**ROLES AND RESPONSIBILITIES**
Physical therapy	• Interviews the family for family history and observes infant-parent caregiving patterns to determine need for additional support • Examines and evaluates the neonate using standardized tests and measures and assess the various aspects outlined in the ICF Model (eg, Test of Infant Motor Performance, Neonatal Behavioral Assessment Scale, Premature Infant Pain Profile, General Movement Assessment, Hammersmith Neonatal Neurological Examination) (see Appendix B for a more comprehensive list) • Develops and implements a plan to prevent neurobehavioral disorganization and complications of prematurity in multiple systems • Using clinical reasoning, designs, implements, and evaluates plans of care and therapeutic strategies appropriate to the infant's physiological, motor, and state regulation strengths and vulnerabilities and neurodevelopmental risk in collaboration with the family and NICU team; interventions may include handling, hydrotherapy, splinting, taping, range of motion, therapeutic positioning, soft tissue mobilization, adaptive equipment use, and developmental activities and strategies to prevent deformities, increase function, and optimize environmental support • Monitors autonomic, behavioral state, motor stability, skin integrity, equipment safety, pain, and vital signs • Develops and implements discharge plans, including consultation with providers of specialized equipment or services in preparation for community-based care, and educates families, caregivers, and community members about potential risks and injuries related to toys and equipment (eg, seating devices, walkers), risks for deformity (eg, asymmetrical head positioning), and risks for developmental delays (consistent supine positioning)

Adapted from American Physical Therapy Association. Neonatal physical therapy practice: Roles and training. American Physical Therapy Association Web site. http://www.apta.org/NICU/NeonatalPractice/RolesandTraining/PDF/. Accessed March 22, 2017 and Sweeney JK, Heriza CB, Blanchard Y. Neonatal physical therapy; part I: clinical competencies and neonatal intensive care unit clinical training models. *Pediatr Phys Ther.* 2009;21(4):296-307.

(continued)

gastrointestinal issues are common among high-risk infants, a gastroenterologist may be a member of an infant's team. Therefore, the care team for an infant will comprise professionals from many disciplines. The team is determined specifically according to an infant's specialized care needs. This highly specialized team will determine how to best meet the infant's nutritional needs in light of physiologic state, respiratory status, cardiac status, and ability to be fed orally. Research suggests that the prognosis for a high-risk infant to develop independent feeding skills is highly dependent on the maturation of the reflexive actions involved in respiratory coordination during feeding, pharyngeal, and glottal closure reflexes for airway protection and esophageal reflexes. Additionally, cardiac and respiratory challenges such as apnea or bradycardia can result in delays in establishing oral feeding. These challenges are met by the team, including pediatric therapists who address the functional and structural needs of the growing and developing premature infant.

Many high-risk infants require mechanical ventilation and gavage feedings to support growth and maturation. Addressing the feeding and nutritional needs of high-risk infants is integral for supporting physical growth, neurodevelopmental maturation, and addressing comorbid conditions. The impact of poor nutritional status and failure of growth can be devastating and have long-term consequences. Therefore, the well-coordinated collaboration of a dedicated team is critical for advancing the best possible outcome for high-risk infants and their families.

TABLE 6-6 (CONTINUED)	
INTERPROFESSIONAL CARE BY PEDIATRIC THERAPISTS IN THE NEONATAL INTENSIVE CARE UNIT	
DISCIPLINE	**ROLES AND RESPONSIBILITIES**
Occupational therapy	• Selects and administers formal and informal assessment procedures to identify developmental abilities, vulnerabilities, and limitations in daily life activities and occupations as they are influenced by medical status and neurobehavioral organization, sensory development and processing, motor function, pain, daily activity (eg, feeding), and social-emotional development, physical environment, caregiving practices, positioning, and nurturance on the infant's neurobehavioral organization, sensory, motor, and medical status • Formulates an individualized therapeutic intervention plan that supports the infant's current level of function and facilitates optimal social-emotional, physical, cognitive, and sensory development of the infant within the context of the family and the NICU • Modifies sensory aspects of physical environment according to infant sensory threshold • Participates with the infant and caregivers in occupational therapy interventions that reinforce the role of the family as the constant in the life of the infant and support the infant's medical and physiological status to enhance infant neurobehavioral organization; facilitate social participation; promote optimal infant neuromotor functioning and engagement in daily life activities; promote developmentally appropriate motor function and engagement in daily life activities through the use of biomechanical techniques, when appropriate; and facilitate well-organized infant behavior through adaptation of infant daily life activities • Incorporates the occupational therapy program into NICU routines
Adapted from American Occupational Therapy Association. Specialized knowledge and skills for occupational therapy practice in the neonatal intensive care unit. American Occupational Therapy Association Web site. http://www.aota.org/-/media/corporate/files/practice/children/browse/ei/official-docs/specialized%20ks%20nicu.pdf. Accessed March 22, 2017.	
Speech-language pathology	• Conducts clinical assessment of the infant and family for communication, cognition, feeding, and swallowing problems • Conducts instrumental evaluation of the infant for feeding and swallowing problems • Provides support and intervention/treatment for the infant's communication, cognition, feeding, and swallowing problems (eg, facilitate nutritive sucking process in the development of bottle feeding and breastfeeding) • Establishes an intervention plan with the parent and caregiver training to facilitate the development of safe feeding and swallowing skills • Provides education, counseling, and support to families, other caregivers, and staff regarding preferred practices in the NICU to support current and future communication, cognition, feeding, and swallowing skills
Adapted from American Speech-Language-Hearing Association. Knowledge and skills needed by speech-language pathologists providing services to infants and families in the NICU environment. American Speech-Language-Hearing Association Web site. http://www.asha.org/policy/KS2004-00080/. Accessed March 23, 2017 and Garcia-Tormos LI, Garcia-Fragoso L, Garcia-Garcia IE. Role of the speech pathologist: language in the neonatal intensive care unit. *Bol Asoc Med P R.* 2013;105(4):56-59.	

FAMILY SYSTEMS THEORY AND HIGH-RISK INFANTS

The NICU environment places unanticipated and stressful demands on parents and families of high-risk infants. Parents may have to deal with not being able to see or touch the infant for extended periods of time while the infant receives life-sustaining care.[24] When they are able to see and hold the infant, parents are often surprised by the environment of the NICU and the appearance of the infant, who may be connected to specialized equipment such as incubators, feeding tubes, and respiratory support systems. Bonding and attachment in this type of environment is a challenge, and the negative impact of the situation on mothers and fathers has been well documented by researchers.[25-27]

One method of analyzing the ways that families manage the myriad of challenges for an infant with severe disabilities is through use of a *family systems theory approach*. Family systems theories recognize the complexity of relationships and how one family member's problem(s) or change(s) can impact others in a family. Highlighted by these theories is the knowledge that families are more than the sum of their parts. To fully understand the family as a system, one must look at the whole. Although various systems theories related to families exist, one theory (proposed by Turnbull et al[28]), offers a way to explore families from a strengths-based rather than problem-based perspective. This approach emphasizes resources used by the family rather than problems experienced by the family, thus accentuating the strengths of the family.[29] The 4 components of this framework include (1) family structure, (2) family interaction, (3) family life cycle, and (4) family functions[29]:

- *Family structure* includes the number and type of family members; individual characteristics of family members across cognitive skills, coping strategies, and health needs; and the cultural and ethnic components of the family. Exploration of family structure includes the members' values, customs, and other cultural beliefs.

- *Family interaction* encompasses marital, parental, sibling, and extrafamilial subsystems. The contributions of siblings or grandparents as resources for parents of high-risk infants are valuable assets. Likewise, the stress related to siblings of children with special needs (eg, siblings' feelings of being forgotten or overlooked) are important considerations in this family systems model. The ways that members of a family relate to each other are important aspects of family interactions. As parents become older, siblings may adjust to more of a primary caregiver role for both the parents and the individual with special needs.

- *Family life cycle* includes changes of time that occur within families. These changes can be structural (eg, the addition of family members) or developmental (eg, a sibling reaching an independent or rebellious age). As individuals within the family age, this can have an important impact on the resources available for managing the needs of a child with special needs.

- *Family functions* consist of the various individual needs of each member. Functions are varied and include everything from health care resources to money or warmth between family members. These are the things that each member needs to thrive and be successful. Too many unmet needs may result in significant stress for the family members, whereas adequate management of family function resources may be an area of strength.

Use of this approach is critical because it sets the stage for future interactions with professionals that families will encounter as their infant grows. Developing a relationship of trust and respect with the family reaps rewards for ongoing collaborative care.

ETHICAL CONSIDERATIONS

The NICU represents a medical environment that has experienced growing medical and legal ethical dilemmas and pressures related to the care of medically fragile, high-risk infants. Medical advances in neonatal technology and pharmacology have significantly improved the survival rates of preterm, high-risk infants. These advances have raised ethical considerations related to the family role in decision making, informed consent, and the extent to which medical intervention will be delivered.[30-34]

The care of high-risk infants involves complex and critical decision making. There are different models that range along a continuum from medical provider autonomy to family-directed decision making.[33] Medical professionals and families face the challenge of balancing the family role with medical expertise. To fully participate in decision making, families need sufficient information. Yet while navigating the emotional and physical demands of caring for a sick infant, families may struggle with the amount of information and the complexity of technical medical information to sufficiently offer informed consent. In facilitating informed consent, physicians may also face the dilemma of attempting to determine the family's readiness for information. Additionally, medical providers may face challenges in determining whether to provide neutral, objective prognostic information that allows families to make decisions or to provide recommendations that allow families to make choices. Families will process information within the context of their religious and cultural beliefs. Each family will have a unique perspective for how technical, medical, and prognostic information is combined with religious and cultural beliefs and practices for making informed decisions.

Advances in care options supported by medicine and technology have greatly increased the viability of extremely preterm infants. As such, decisions related to administering or withholding treatment for infants at the limits of viability presents one example of an ethical dilemma. In addition to the ethical dilemma, there are legal and emotional challenges for the medical team and the families. Therefore, decision making related to treatment options or related to the withholding or withdrawing of treatment is a complex process that is guided by diagnosis and prognosis, informed consent with considerations for futility of treatment, quality of life, and parental-caregiver counseling.

Medical providers and families engaging in shared decision making may find that roles shift depending on the critical nature or urgency of a decision. Decisions in intensive care units often involve critical life-or-death circumstances. Convening a team and family for information sharing and collaborative decision making may not always be an option. In such cases, the ethical practice guidelines that govern medical providers will support critical decision making.

PREVENTIVE CARE

Some families raise questions about the risks of having additional children with similar problems. This presents an opportunity for the interprofessional team to share information with families regarding prenatal care to minimize the risk to their future newborns. Within the role of professionals promoting health, therapists should provide information about the following:

- Seeking prenatal care as soon as possible in the pregnancy
- Engaging in healthy lifestyle practices (eg, proper diet, adequate sleep, managing stress, stopping smoking, avoiding alcohol)
- Discussing the benefits and risks of over-the-counter medications, prescription medicines, vitamins, and supplements
- Discussing the benefits and risks of assisted reproductive technology (ART) because multiple pregnancies carry a higher risk of preterm labor
- Suggesting ways to reduce maternal exposure to teratogens, including insecticides, solvents, lead, mercury, paint (including paint fumes), and animal urine and feces

This is a good opportunity to emphasize the importance of maintaining lifelong health, fitness, and wellness habits to ensure optimal health for the infant and the entire family.

TRANSITIONING FROM THE HOSPITAL TO EARLY INTERVENTION

Once the neonate with special needs has stabilized physiologically, she can be discharged to the home and receive follow-up care, as needed. The transition from the hospital to the home can be challenging for many parents but can be facilitated by professional guidance. The Division for Early Childhood (DEC) of the Council for Exceptional Children provides helpful interprofessional guidelines to ease the transition[35]:

1. Communicate with the family about early intervention (EI) options and determine if they are ready for a referral.

2. Communicate between the hospital team and the EI team about the infant's developmental/health status and discharge plan, following parental consent to release information.

3. Ask the family for their preferences for the time and location of the first visit.

4. Describe early intervention as a system of family- and child-centered supports, services, and resources designed to assist parents in helping their child infant grow and learn. This explanation includes information about the Program for Infants and Toddlers with Disabilities (Part C of IDEA), a federal grant program that assists states in operating a comprehensive statewide program of EI services for infants and toddlers with disabilities (birth through 2 years) and their families.

5. Talk to the family members about their experiences, concerns, and priorities as they transition to EI.

6. In preparation for the evaluation and assessment that precedes the initiation of EI services, ask family members about how they would like to participate in the process and share this information with EI services.

7. Encourage families to engage in support groups and services that ease this transition process.

SUMMARY

Pediatric therapists working with high-risk infants may encounter these newborns and their families while working in the NICU or after their transition to EI services, if needed. Professionals working in this setting must be knowledgeable about prenatal growth and development, highly skilled in NICU care, and able to work collaboratively with others to ensure that the family and newborn are given high-quality care. The roles of professionals, although distinct, may overlap when offering collaborative care based upon a family systems theory approach. Additional considerations must be given to the ethical issues unique to infants who are physiologically unstable and in critical condition. Each pediatric therapist, whether working in the NICU or not, needs to be an advocate for prenatal health to reduce the risk of high-risk pregnancies.

INTERPROFESSIONAL ACTIVITIES

Teamwork in the Neonatal Intensive Care Unit

1. Review the terminology, roles, and issues in the following case study.
2. Distinguish the roles and responsibilities related to assessments, including your choices of assessment selection.
3. As a team, determine a plan of care that addresses key concerns.

Case 6-1: A 1-month-old girl born with myotonic muscular dystrophy and cleft palate

Meredith is a 1-month-old girl born with myotonic muscular dystrophy and cleft palate. When her mother, Sara, was 7 months pregnant, she was at work as a librarian when she suddenly felt ill and became concerned about her unborn child. She called her husband, James, a police officer, telling him she was heading to the hospital and to meet her there. Once they both arrived at the hospital, Sara was admitted to labor and delivery. After several unsuccessful attempts to stop the progression of labor, baby Meredith was born weighing 3.5 pounds and showing signs of distress, including bradycardia and respiratory distress. Meredith was admitted to the NICU with an Apgar score of 3 out of 10 at 5 minutes after delivery. Sara and James were inconsolable, faced with what felt like an insurmountable task of being with their baby in the NICU and an uncertain future. Immediately, the NICU team (involving neonatologists, respiratory therapists, nurses, and pediatricians) stabilized Meredith's respiratory status, determined the best methods for providing nutrition to Meredith, and further examined Meredith to discover an incomplete unilateral cleft palate. Meredith was not yet stable enough for her parents to be involved in her care, and they felt helpless to do anything. Given Meredith's respiratory status, cleft palate, and prematurity, she was given a nasogastric tube for nutrition. The speech-language pathologist consulted with the parents regarding Meredith's cleft palate. Over the next several days, additional concerns arose regarding Meredith's hypotonia and lack of improvement in respiratory status. The NICU team collaborated, discussing lab tests, tests of motor function, and observations to determine what else was affecting Meredith. Eventually, a geneticist determined the diagnosis of myotonic muscular dystrophy, a progressive disease that eventually destroys the ability of the muscles to function. Meredith's parents were advised that Sara was probably the carrier of the disease and they should strongly consider not having additional children. Her parents are preparing to transition from the NICU to the home setting.

Working With the Family of a High-Risk Infant

Watch the movie *little man* (http://www.littlemanthe-movie.com). After watching the movie, answer the following questions as a team:

1. Characterize the strengths and needs of each family member.
2. Discuss your respective roles in the NICU vs in the home setting.
3. Discuss family stressors witnessed throughout the film.
4. Collaborate on resources to help the family.
5. Describe potential conflicts observed between the family members and professionals and ways to reduce conflict.
6. Work together to formulate a plan to meet the needs of the child and the family in the NICU and the home setting for therapeutic positioning, feeding, and family engagement, and/or other identified needs.

Case 6-2: A high-risk infant transitioning to his home

The movie *little man* presents the story of a boy with multiple impairments transitioning from the NICU environment to the home environment. Clips of *little man* by Nicole Conn are available on YouTube, and the entire movie is available on demand at Vimeo (https://vimeo.com/ondemand/littleman). According to the site:

> *little man* is Nicole Conn's award-winning documentary about her micro-preemie son, Nicholas, born 100 days early, as he struggles for survival. When Nicholas is born 100 days early, he weighs only one pound and faces impossible odds for survival. As he struggles for life, so struggle his two mothers: out lesbian filmmaker Nicole Conn and political activist Gwen Baba, to keep their family from disintegrating under the unrelenting stress and chaos of hospitals, emergency medical crises and a crushing blow to trust. The winner of 12 Best Documentary awards at film festivals across the country, *little man* explores the core of the human spirit as a family realizes that they are capable of enduring what they never thought possible.

REFERENCES

1. Rochman B. A 21-week-old baby survives and doctors ask, how young is too young to save? Time Web site. http://healthland.time.com/2011/05/27/baby-born-at-21-weeks-survives-how-young-is-too-young-to-save/. Published May 27, 2011. Accessed January 24, 2016.

2. Flanders N. Born at 22 weeks, youngest premature baby to survive in Israel leaves hospital. Liveaction Web site. http://liveactionnews.org/born-22-weeks-youngest-premature-baby-survive-israel-leaves-hospital/. Published September 5, 2016. Accessed January 24, 2016.

3. Gilbert-Barness E. Teratogenic Causes of Malformations. *Ann Clin Lab Sci.* 2010;40;99-114.

4. Gilbert S. Environmental disruption of normal development. In: *Developmental Biology.* 6th ed. Sunderland, MA: Sinauer Associates; 2000. https://www.ncbi.nlm.nih.gov/books/NBK9998/. Accessed January 24, 2017.

5. Mayo Clinic. High risk pregnancy: know what to expect. Mayo Clinic Web site. http://www.mayoclinic.org/healthy-lifestyle/pregnancy-week-by-week/in-depth/high-risk-pregnancy/art-20047012. Published February 20, 2015. Accessed January 12, 2017.

6. Britton JR. The transition to extrauterine life and disorders of transition. *Clin Perinatol.* 1998;25:271-94.

7. World Health Organization. Preterm birth. World Health Organization Web site. http://www.who.int/mediacentre/factsheets/fs363/en/. Published November, 2017. Accessed on December 28, 2017.

8. Hack M, Taylor H, Klein N, Mercuri-Minich N. Functional limitations and special health care needs of 10- to 14-year old children weighing less than 750 grams at birth. *Pediatrics.* 2001;106:554-560.

9. Campbell D, Fleischman A. Limits of viability: dilemmas, decisions, and decision makers. *Am J Perinatol.* 2001;18:117-128.

10. Gavhane S, Eklave D, Mohammad H. Long term outcomes of kangaroo mother care in very low birthweight infants. *J Clin Diagn Res.* 2016;10(12):SC13-SC15.

11. Malloy MH. Prematurity and sudden infant death syndrome: United States 2005-2007. *J Perinatol.* 2013;33:470-475.

12. Baraldi E, Filippone M. Chronic lung disease after premature birth. *N Engl J Med.* 2007;357(19):1946-1955.

13. Stewart AL, Reynolds EO, Lipscomb AP. Outcome for infants of very low birthweight: Survey of world literature. *Lancet.* 1981;1(8228):1038-1040.

14. Kulak P, Macjorkowska E, Goscik E. Selected risk factors for spastic cerebral palsy in a retrospective hospital-based case control study. *Progress in Health Sciences.* 2014:4.

15. Jadcherla SR, Wang M, Vijayapal AS, Leuthner SR. Impact of prematurity and co-morbidities on feeding milestones in neonates: A retrospective study. *J Perinatol.* 2010;30:201-208.

16. Klein VC, Gaspardo CM, Martinez FE, Grunau RE, Linhares MB. Pain and distress reactivity and recovery as early predictors of temperament in toddlers born preterm. *Early Hum Dev.* 2011;85:569-576.

17. Milner KM, Neal EFG, Roberts G, Steer AC, Duke T. Long term neurodevelopmental outcome in high-risk newborns in resource limited settings: A systematic review of the literature. *Paediatric International Child Health.* 2015;35:227-242.

18. Laughon M, Allred EN, Bose C, et al. Patterns of respiratory distress in the first two postnatal weeks of extremely premature infants. *Pediatrics.* 2009;123(4):1124-1131.

19. Thompson LC, Gillberg C. Behavioural problems from perinatal and neonatal insults. *Lancet.* 2012;379(9814):392-393.

20. Medline Plus. Apgar score. Medline Plus Web site. https://medlineplus.gov/ency/article/003402.htm. Published November 20, 2014. Accessed January 27, 2017.

21. American Speech-Language-Hearing Association. Knowledge and skills needed by speech-language pathologists providing services to infants and families in the NICU environment. American Speech-Language-Hearing Association Web site. www.asha.org/policy/KS2004-00080/. Published 2004. Accessed May 1, 2017.

22. Sweeney JK, Heriza CB, Blanchard Y. Neonatal physical therapy; part I: clinical competencies and neonatal intensive care unit clinical training models. *Pediatr Phys Ther.* 2009;21(4):296-307.

23. Sweeney JK, Heriza CB, Blanchard Y, Dusing SC. Neonatal physical therapy; part II: practice frameworks and evidence-based practice guidelines [erratum in: Pediatr Phys Ther. 2010;22(4):377]. *Pediatr Phys Ther.* 2010;22(1):2-16.

24. Patterson D, Barnard K. Parenting of low birth weight infants: A review of issues and interventions. *Infant Mental Health Journal.* 1990;11:37-56.

25. Phillips S, Tooley G. Mothers' and fathers' experiences of complicated childbirth. In: Kostanski M. *The Power of Compassion: An Exploration of the Psychology of Compassion in the 21st Century.* New Castle, England: Cambridge Scholars Publishing; 2009:110-119.

26. Phillips S, Tooley G. Improving child and family outcomes following complicated births requiring admission to neonatal intensive care units. *Sexual and Relationship Therapy.* 2005;20:431-442.

27. Dudley M, Gyler L, Blinkhorn S, Barnett B. Psychosocial interventions for very low birthweight infants: Their scope and efficacy. *Aust N Z J Psychiatry.* 1993;27(1):74-85.

28. Turnbull AP, Summers JA, Brotherson MJ. *Working with families with disabled family members: A family systems perspective.* Lawrence, KS: University of Kansas; 1984.

29. Ronnau J, Poertner J. Identification and use of strengths: A family systems approach. *Children Today.* 1993;22:20-23.

30. Alderson P, Hawthorne J, Killen M. Parents' experiences of sharing neonatal information and decisions: Consent, cost, and risk. *Soc Sci Med.* 2006;62(6):1319-1329.

31. da Costa DE, Ghazal H, Khusaiby SA. Do not resuscitate orders and ethical decisions in a neonatal intensive care unit in a Muslim community. *Arch Dis Child Fetal Neonatal Ed.* 2002;86:F115-F119.

32. Payot A, Gendron S, Lefebvre F, Doucet H. Deciding to resuscitate extremely premature babies: How do parents and neonatologists engage in the decision? *Soc Sci Med.* 2007;64(7):1487-1500.

33. Orfali K. Parental role in medical decision-making: fact or fiction? A comparative study of ethical dilemmas in French and American neonatal intensive care units. *Soc Sci Med.* 2004;58(10):2009-2022.

34. Walther FJ. Withholding treatment, withdrawing treatment, and palliative care in the neonatal intensive care unit. *Early Hum Dev.* 2005;81:965-972.

35. Early Childhood Technical Assistance Center. Transition from Hospital to Early Intervention Checklist. Early Childhood Technical Assistance Center Web site. http://ectacenter.org/~pdfs/decrp/TR-1_Hosp_to_EI_2017.pdf. Published 2017. Accessed on December 5, 2017.

Section 7

Teamwork in Early Intervention

Catherine Rush Thompson, PT, PhD, MS and Lauren Little, PhD, OTR/L

OVERVIEW

Children younger than 3 who are at risk for developmental problems benefit from *early intervention* (EI), a federally funded, coordinated system of therapeutic services that supports families in the prevention of developmental delays.[1] This section discusses how children qualify for EI and how interprofessional teams in the EI setting serve families. There are 2 overarching topics included in this section: (1) an overview of the *Individuals with Disabilities Education Act* (IDEA), including interprofessional screening tools and practices, and the *Individualized Family Service Plan* (IFSP), and (2) a discussion about working with parents and caregivers in EI, including parent advocacy, parental strain, parenting styles, promoting parent responsiveness and play, and supporting families transitioning from EI to school-age programs.

NUTS AND BOLTS OF EARLY INTERVENTION SETTINGS

The Individuals with Disabilities Education Act

The Individuals with Disabilities Education Act (IDEA), first enacted in 1997, ensures that all children with disabilities are entitled to a free appropriate public education to meet their unique needs and prepare them for further education, employment, and independent living.[1,2] IDEA has 4 distinct sections; A, B, C, and D, with Part A laying out the basic foundation for the rest of the Act[1]:

- Part A is titled "General Provisions, Definitions and Other Issues" and describes the purpose and provisions of the law.
- Part B is titled "Assistance for Education of All Children with Disabilities" and provides services and funding for children with special needs, generally beginning at age 3.

Thompson CR. *Pediatric Therapy: An Interprofessional Framework for Practice* (pp 101-114). © 2018 SLACK Incorporated.

- Part C is titled "Infants and Toddlers with Disabilities." Part C, most relevant to the provision of EI services, defines an "at-risk infant or toddler" as a child under 3 years of age who is at risk of experiencing a substantial developmental delay if EI services were not provided.[1,2] As such, Part C addresses the needs of families of children with special needs through a comprehensive child find system and the *Individual Family Service Plan* (ISFP) to reduce the effects of developmental conditions through coordinated EI services.

- Recognizing the importance of ongoing research and quality improvement, Part D of IDEA focuses on the need to improve special education programs, prepare personnel, disseminate information, support research, and apply research to special education.

Individuals with Disabilities Education Act Part C

IDEA Part C mandates that all states must provide EI services for at-risk children from birth to their third birthday.[2] The range of EI services provided by federal law includes support to address potential problems with physical, cognitive, communication, adaptive and social, or emotional development. IDEA Part C further mandates that EI services must be provided by qualified personnel, in natural environments, and at no cost to families (except in states that provide for a system of payment, such as a sliding scale).[2]

Families are eligible for physical therapy, occupational therapy, and speech-language pathology services.[1-3] Additionally, families are eligible for the following[1]: (1) *audiological services* to identify children with issues related to hearing; (2) *medical diagnostic services* and *nursing and health services* to manage health problems and promote healthy development; (3) *nutrition services* to address issues related to feeding, including food habits and food preferences; (4) *psychological services* to assess and help manage issues such as the child's behavior, learning, and mental health; (5) *service coordination* to coordinate programs and therapies, based upon family needs; (6) *social services* to provide an assessment and resources for managing the social and emotional needs of the family; (7) *special education* for learning activities that the family can use to promote the child's development; (8) *vision services* to assess and serve children with visual impairments; and (9) *funding* to support transportation costs needed for families who must travel for needed services. Table 7-1 lists the interprofessional care typically provided by pediatric therapists in EI.

EI services are provided in the child's natural settings that best meet the needs of the family. The EI team needs to be aware of the many options for service delivery and work together collaboratively to offer the most comprehensive

and efficient EI services to each family.[2,3] Options for these services may include a wide range of sites,[2,3] including the home and community, as well as specialized center-based programs, including EI centers, clinics, and hospitals offering specialized family services for young children. Families may benefit from EI services across a variety of programming sites. For example, therapists may work with families in the home, consult with the infant's day care provider, engage with grandparents in their home, and/or provide services in a weekly group therapy session at a community-based EI program to ensure consistent care. Services may include the parent and child meeting with service providers in the community (eg, a caregiver and child meeting with a service provider at a playground), groups of families and their children meeting in one setting (eg, developmental therapy groups), and support groups for caregivers (eg, family members participating in a group to address common concerns).[3] The EI team needs to work collaboratively as it coordinates goals across settings and delivers services that best meet each family's individualized needs.

Although EI offers this rich array of child, parent, and family supports, professionals need to be mindful of families' individualized needs and perceptions of support for their children. In other words, practitioners must understand that parents' perceptions of and expectations for services can significantly impact intervention outcomes.[4] In one study of the transition from the neonatal intensive care unit (NICU) to home, mothers had varying perceptions of EI programs; those with high expressed needs benefited more from intervention, whereas those with low expressed needs showed fewer benefits.[4] When assessed at 6 months postdischarge, mothers with an increased expressed need for support benefited from EI programs; positive effects of the EI program included improvements in the mother's sense of competence, perceived control, mood, and responsiveness.[4] Benefits were proportionate for the mothers who needed the most support and those with infants with more severe disabilities. However, for mothers with low needs for support, participation in the EI program had negative effects on outcomes. Clearly, the EI team must be sensitive to each family's expressed need for information and services, recognizing cultural differences, family concerns, and family strengths for engaging with their children.

Interprofessional Screening Tools and Practices

Although many infants are identified for EI following discharge from the NICU, other infants have less obvious developmental problems, and parents may not recognize developmental delays. Professionals are often asked to provide screenings that serve as a safety net for families with limited access to health care. There is a referral process that is commonly used to ensure that families and children have

TABLE 7-1	
INTERPROFESSIONAL CARE BY PEDIATRIC THERAPISTS IN EARLY INTERVENTION	
DISCIPLINE	**ROLES AND RESPONSIBILITIES**
Shared knowledge	• Knows typical infant and child development and developmental risk factors • Understands common pediatric conditions (pathophysiology, clinical manifestations, and prognoses) • Appreciates the roles and responsibilities of team members in EI, including the family • Embraces the philosophy of family-centered care • Applies the International Classification of Functioning, Disability and Health (ICF) Model to examination and intervention • Understands the legal and philosophical underpinnings and implications of Individuals with Disabilities Education Act (IDEA) Part C of 2004 (Public Law 108-446) • Appreciates that EI should enhance the development of infants and toddlers, (including cognitive, physical, communication, social-emotional, and adaptive development) and enhance the capacity of families to meet the special needs of their children • Understands the Individualized Family Service Plan (IFSP) and its implementation • Embraces play-based therapy • Facilitates transition to and from EI • Values ethical practice
Interprofessional skills	• Communicates and collaborates interprofessionally and with others involved in the child's care • Determines optimal times for interactions (eg, screenings, examinations, interventions) based upon the child's tolerance and family routines • Screens for needed services (eg, physical therapy, occupational therapy, speech-language pathology) • Incorporates evidence-based literature in EI practice • Monitors and evaluates impact of recommended interventions • Instructs, consults, and communicates with family members, caregivers, team members, and community, as appropriate • Embraces family-centered care and cultural competency • Encourages interventions in the natural environments where families and their children live, learn, and play • Consults in areas of expertise and collaborates with health care professionals, families, policy makers, and community organizations to advocate for services to support families and their children • Helps families become self-advocates • Provides documentation that is objective, interpretive, thorough, and concise

(continued)

Table 7-1 (continued)

Interprofessional Care by Pediatric Therapists in Early Intervention

DISCIPLINE	ROLES AND RESPONSIBILITIES
Physical therapy	• Interviews the family for history and goals • Observes child's and family's routines related to the body structures' growth and development, functional and play activities, environmental factors (psychosocial and physical), personal factors (lifestyle behaviors), and participation • Examines and evaluates the child using standardized tests and measures that assess the various aspects outlined in the ICF Model (See Appendix A for a list of tests and measures used) • Develops and implements a plan to promote overall development, healthy growth, and the ability to move • Using clinical reasoning, designs, implements, and evaluates plans of care and therapeutic strategies appropriate to facilitate development • Monitors postural alignment, therapeutic positioning, skin integrity, equipment safety, pain, and vital signs, as needed • Develops and implements transition plans, including consultation with providers of specialized equipment or services in preparation for community-based care, and educates families, caregivers, and community members about potential risks and injuries related to toys (including motorized cars) and equipment (eg, seating devices, walkers, assistive devices, orthotics), risks for deformity, and risks for developmental delays
Adapted from American Physical Therapy Association. The role of physical therapy with infants, toddlers, and their families in early intervention. Academy of Pediatric Physical Therapy Web site. https://pediatricapta.org/special-interest-groups/early-intervention/pdfs/Role%20of%20PT%20in%20EI.pdf	
Occupational therapy	• Selects and administers formal and informal assessment procedures to identify developmental abilities, vulnerabilities, and limitations in daily life activities and occupations as they are influenced by medical status and neurobehavioral organization, sensory development and processing, motor function, pain, daily activity (eg, feeding), social-emotional development, physical environment, caregiving practices, positioning, and nurturance on the child's neurobehavioral organization, sensory, motor, and medical status • Formulates an individualized therapeutic intervention plan that supports the child's current level of function and facilitates optimal social-emotional, physical, cognitive, and sensory development of the child within the context of the family, home, and community • Modifies sensory aspects of the physical environment according to the child's sensory threshold • Participates with the child and caregivers in occupational therapy interventions that reinforce the role of the family as the constant in the life of the child and supports the child's medical and physiological status to enhance neurobehavioral organization; facilitate social participation; promote optimal neuromotor functioning and engagement in daily life activities; promote developmentally appropriate motor function and engagement in daily life activities through the use of biomechanical techniques, when appropriate; and facilitate well-organized behavior through adaptation of daily life activities
Adapted from American Occupational Therapy Association. Specialized knowledge and skills for occupational therapy practice in the neonatal intensive care unit. American Occupational Therapy Association Web site. http://www.aota.org/-/media/corporate/files/practice/children/browse/ei/official-docs/specialized%20ks%20nicu.pdf. Accessed March 24, 2017.	

(continued)

TABLE 7-1 (CONTINUED)	
INTERPROFESSIONAL CARE BY PEDIATRIC THERAPISTS IN EARLY INTERVENTION	
DISCIPLINE	**ROLES AND RESPONSIBILITIES**
Speech-language pathology	• Conducts clinical assessment of the child and family for communication, cognition, feeding, and swallowing problems • Conducts instrumental evaluation of the child for feeding and swallowing problems • Provides support and intervention/treatment for the child's communication, cognition, feeding, and swallowing problems (eg, facilitate nutritive sucking process in the development of feeding) • Establishes an intervention plan with the parent and caregiver training to facilitate the development of safe feeding and swallowing skills • Provides education, counseling, and support to families, other caregivers, and staff regarding preferred practices to support current and future communication, cognition, feeding, and swallowing skills

Adapted from American Speech-Language-Hearing Association. Knowledge and skills needed by speech-language pathologists providing services to infants and families in the NICU environment. American Speech-Language-Hearing Association Web site. http://www.asha.org/policy/KS2004-00080/. Accessed March 23, 2017.

access to EI services. Most typically, the referral source to EI is a physician or nurse practitioner, but it may also be parents who suspect that their infants have a developmental delay or disability. Once referred, a professional informs the family about how to sign up for an EI program. An EI case manager or officer informs the family of their rights, reviews the list of evaluators, obtains insurance/Medicaid information, and obtains other relevant information for setting up evaluations.

Screenings and formal evaluations must be conducted with the parents' consent. The EI team should be familiar with state guidelines and standardized evaluations that are used to determine eligibility for available services. (See Appendix B for a list of assessments that may be used in EI.) Evaluations should be written with an emphasis on family priorities, routines, and the child's unique needs. Reports by each professional are submitted prior to meeting to develop the IFSP.

Once children have entered the EI system, they have likely shown developmental delays in a number of areas, including motor, language, and/or cognition. Although an overview of comprehensive screening and evaluation for the purposes of obtaining EI services is beyond the scope of this section, there are many screening tools used by service providers once a child is receiving EI services. Most often, these screening tools can help identify infants needing additional services. In this section, we discuss how all members of the EI team can screen for the motor, visual, cognitive, social, and emotional development in young children. All pediatric screenings begin with close observations of infants because a great deal of information can be obtained from simply observing children's spontaneous behavior. Also, pediatric therapists are reminded that the infant's age should be based upon the extent of prematurity and should be adjusted accordingly. For example, an infant born 2 months prematurely would be tested at an age level that is 2 months less than her chronological age to adjust for the child's actual level of maturation.

Motor Screening

Observation is a critical skill for assessing young infants. In addition to recognizing delays in achieving developmental milestones, pediatric therapists should be aware of the following red flags for motor issues that can be easily identified by observing the infant's posture and movements[5]:

- Birth to 3 months: The infant has difficulty lifting head, has stiff legs with little or no movement, pushes back with head, keeps hands fisted, and lacks arm movement.

- At 6 months: The infant has a rounded back while sitting, is unable to lift head up while prone, has poor head control, has difficulty bringing arms forward to reach out, arches back and stiffens legs, holds arms held back, or has stiff legs.

- At 9 months: The infant predominately uses one hand, has a rounded back, has poor use of arms in sitting, has difficulty crawling, uses only one side of body to move, unable to straighten back, or cannot take weight on legs.

- At 12 months: The infant has difficulty getting to stand because of stiff legs and pointed toes; only uses arms to pull up to standing; sits with weight to one side; has strongly flexed or stiffly extended arms; needs to use hand to maintain sitting; does not babble, point, or make gestures.

The EI team should be alert to infantile myoclonic seizures, which are evidenced by a sudden contraction of the trunk flexor muscles, possibly accompanied by abrupt flexion of arms to the chest and thighs to the trunk.[6] In some instances, a sudden noise, some manipulation, or feeding precipitates an infantile myoclonic seizure; however, sometimes the seizures occur just before the onset of true sleep or immediately on waking. Apneic episodes (ie, suspension of breathing), episodic nystagmus (ie, eyes making repetitive, uncontrolled movements), episodic changes in tone and/ or color, and episodic sneezing may be seizure manifestations. Petit mal, minor motor, psychomotor, and grand mal seizures may all occur during infancy, but the minor motor type is most common. When the EI team is alert to these red flags, they can make additional examinations or referrals that might be appropriate for the infant.

Visual Screening

All members of the EI team must be aware of how vision impacts all other areas of development; therefore, each member is responsible for screening for any signs of visual impairment. Red flags for visual problems include[7] (1) appearance of any strabismus (cross-eyed) after 2 months of age; (2) wandering, uncoordinated eye movements; (3) nystagmus (dancing or jerky eyes); (4) holding items too close (within 6 inches) for visual inspection; (5) turning the head to the side habitually to look at items; (6) having to turn the head to focus on people or objects in their periphery, or (7) disregarding objects presented in the peripheral field. Red flags for blindness[7] include prolonged hand watching past developmental age of 5 months (shadowing), staring at lights in preference to people or objects, poking at eyes, rubbing eyes, rocking, spinning, head banging, smelling, sniffing, "rooting" to find objects, or prolonged mouthing of objects. For a full explanation of how to implement a vison screening for young children, refer to pages 17 to 23 in the Vision Screening Guidelines outlined at http://health.mo.gov/living/families/schoolhealth/pdf/VisionScreeningGuidelines.pdf.

Social-Emotional Screening

Social-emotional screening tools assess children's self-awareness, social awareness, and relationships with caregivers.[8] Also, autism-specific screening tools often target social-emotional components of child development and allow a service provider to assess a child's risk for autism symptoms. Specifically, autism-specific screening tools capture a child's social interaction and communication difficulties, as well as the presence of repetitive behavior, all of which are red flags

for a later diagnosis of an autism spectrum disorder. The interprofessional EI team can screen for children's social-emotional difficulties to guide treatment and involve family members in children's therapy services to the fullest extent possible. See Table 7-2 for screening tools appropriate for infants and toddlers.

Nutritional Screening

High-risk infants commonly have difficulties with eating and digestion, so parents and other caretakers oftentimes seek help with these problems. As part of an interprofessional team, it is helpful to screen for these issues because IDEA Part C provides nutrition services to address these concerns. If families have not had nutritional screenings, the team could either recommend one and/or ask if they have any concerns about the following[9]:

- Concerns about their child's weight or stature;
- Difficulties feeding (eg, how long it takes to feed; difficulty swallowing, chewing, or sucking; problems eating solids; delays in feeding skills);
- Problems with food intake (eg, food refusal, eating too little, poor appetite);
- Concerns about hydration, bottle feeding, or formulas;
- Questions about the use of nutritional supplements and medications;
- Gastrointestinal health concerns (eg, constipation, diarrhea, and/or vomiting);
- Food allergies and/or food intolerances;
- Problems with the use of a feeding tube;
- Pica (ie, eating non-food items); and/or
- Dental issues (eg, teething problems).

As part of a team who sees the family in the natural environment, many of these issues can be addressed with family education and referrals.

Individualized Family Service Plan

Eligibility for services is based upon state criteria. For example, Kansas outlines eligibility as:

...children with developmental delay (experiencing 25% or more between chronological age and developmental age, after correction for prematurity, and as measured by appropriate diagnostic instruments and procedures, in one of the following areas); or children under the age of three who are experiencing a discrepancy of 20% or more between chronological age and developmental age, after correction for prematurity, and as measured by appropriate diagnostic instruments and procedures, in two or more of the following areas: (1) physical development including health and nutritional status, vision,

TABLE 7-2				
SCREENING TOOLS FOR INFANTS AND TODDLERS				
TOOL	**AGE RANGE**	**AREAS OF DEVELOPMENT**	**COMPLETION TIME**	**SOURCE OF INFORMATION**
The Ages and Stages Questionnaires-3	1 month to 5½ years	Self-regulation, compliance, communication, adaptive function, autonomy, affect, social interaction	10 to 15 minutes	Parent, caregiver (readability: less than 6th grade)
The Brigance Infant and Toddler Screen	21 to 90 months	Fine motor, gross motor, language, daily living, social-emotional skills	10 to 15 minutes	Parent, caregiver (readability: not rated)
Brief Infant-Toddler Social and Emotional Assessment	12 to 36 months	Externalizing, internalizing, regulatory problems, maladaptive behaviors, 7 scales of competences	7 to 10 minutes	Parent, caregiver (readability: less than 6th grade)
Greenspan Social-Emotional Growth Chart	0 to 42 months	Growing self-regulation and interest in the world; engaging in relationships; using emotions in an interactive, purposeful manner; using interactive emotional signals to communicate and solve problems; using symbols to convey intentions or feelings and express more than basic needs; creating logical bridges between emotions and ideas	10 minutes (qualified examiner needed for scoring)	Parent, caregiver (readability: not rated)
Temperament & Atypical Behavior Scale	11 to 71 months	Temperament; attention and activity; attachment and social behavior; neurobehavioral state; sleeping; play; vocal and oral behavior; senses and movement; self-stimulatory behavior in infants, toddlers, and preschoolers	5 minutes	Parent, caretaker, teacher (readability: 3rd grade)
The Modified Checklist for Autism in Toddlers-Revised	24 to 36 months	Social interaction, communication, repetitive behavior	5 minutes (If the MCHAT-R indicates risk, a follow-up interview is necessary	Parent, caregiver
Communication and Symbolic Behavior Scales Developmental Profile-Infant Toddler Checklist	6 to 24 months	7 language indicators: emotion and use of eye gaze, use of communication, use of gestures, use of sounds, use of words, understanding of words, and use of objects	10 minutes	Parent, caregiver, teacher (readability: not rated)
Adapted from Henderson J, Strain PS. *Screening for Delays and Problem Behavior (Roadmap to Effective Intervention Practices)*. Tampa, FL: University of South Florida; 2009 and Wetherby A, Prizant B. *Communication and Symbolic Behavior Scales Developmental Profile-Preliminary Normed Edition*. Baltimore, MD: Paul H. Brookes Publishing Co; 2001.				

hearing, and motor, (2) cognitive development, (3) communication development, (4) social or emotional development, or (5) self-help/adaptive development. It also includes the professional judgment/informed clinical opinion of the multidisciplinary team to conclude a developmental delay significant enough for eligibility when appropriate tests are not available or when testing does not reflect the child's ability.[10]

New York State has similar criteria; however:

...to be eligible for the EIP [Early Intervention Program], the child must have a 12 month or 33% delay, or a score of at least 2 standard deviations below the mean, in an area of development (eg, communication development or social/emotional development or physical development, etc).[11]

For this reason, some families move to different states to optimize services for their children.

Once it has been determined that a child is eligible for services, the interprofessional team engages in an IFSP meeting. At this meeting, parents and professionals must work together to understand the child's strengths and needs, formulate family-centered goals, and discuss how to best serve the child and family. Based upon the important outcomes of this planning meeting, interprofessional competencies are essential. All must listen carefully to the outcomes desired by the family and be prepared to talk about options that meet both the child's and family's needs. During this meeting, EI services are specified, the plan is developed, and the family and representative for the state sign the IFSP. According to IDEA Part C,[3] each family must receive:

- A multidisciplinary assessment of the unique strengths and needs of the infant or toddler and the identification of services appropriate to meet such needs;

- Family-directed assessment of the resources, priorities, and concerns of the family and the identification of the supports and services necessary to enhance the family's capacity to meet the developmental needs of the infant or toddler; and

- A written individualized family service plan developed by a multidisciplinary team, including the parents, as required by subsection (e), including a description of the appropriate transition services for the infant or toddler.

- Periodic Review: the individualized family service plan shall be evaluated once a year and the family shall be provided a review of the plan at 6-month intervals (or more often where appropriate based on infant or toddler and family needs).

- Promptness After Assessment: the individualized family service plan shall be developed within a reasonable time after the assessment required by subsection (a)(1) is completed. With the parents' consent, EI services may commence prior to the completion of the assessment.

- Content of Plan: the individualized family service plan shall be in writing and contain:

  1. A statement of the infant's or toddler's present levels of physical development, cognitive development, communication development, social or emotional development, and adaptive development, based on objective criteria;

  2. A statement of the family's resources, priorities, and concerns relating to enhancing the development of the family's infant or toddler with a disability;

  3. A statement of the measurable results or outcomes expected to be achieved for the infant or toddler and the family, including pre-literacy and language skills, as developmentally appropriate for the child, and the criteria, procedures, and timelines used to determine the degree to which progress toward achieving the results or outcomes is being made and whether modifications or revisions of the results or outcomes or services are necessary;

  4. A statement of specific EI services based on peer-reviewed research, to the extent practicable, necessary to meet the unique needs of the infant or toddler and the family, including the frequency, intensity, and method of delivering services;

  5. A statement of the natural environments in which EI services will appropriately be provided, including a justification of the extent, if any, to which the services will not be provided in a natural environment;

  6. The projected dates for initiation of services and the anticipated length, duration, and frequency of the services;

  7. Identification of the service coordinator from the profession most immediately relevant to the infant's or toddler's or family's needs (or who is otherwise qualified to carry out all applicable responsibilities under this part) who will be responsible for the implementation of the plan and coordination with other agencies and persons, including transition services; and

  8. Steps to be taken to support the transition of the toddler with a disability to preschool or other appropriate services.[12]

- Parental Consent: the contents of the individualized family service plan shall be fully explained to the parents and informed written consent from the parents shall be obtained prior to the provision of EI services described in such plan. If the parents do not provide consent with respect to a particular EI service, then only the EI services to which consent is obtained shall be provided.

All of these aspects of EI are communicated in the IFSP process to ensure full participation of the family throughout the program.

WORKING WITH PARENTS AND CAREGIVERS IN EARLY INTERVENTION

Parent Advocacy in Early Intervention

Family-centered care in EI is grounded in the belief that parents are the experts on their own children; therefore, parents are integral in the creation and implementation of intervention goals. Service providers are a source of support and information for families; ultimately, the purpose of service providers in EI is to meet the needs of families. Families with children who receive EI services are often bombarded with information, appointments, and varying recommendations from doctors and therapists. Within this complex system, parents often find themselves acting as advocates for their children to receive particular services that match the needs of the family.

For families of children with special needs, *advocacy* is an empowerment and support process. The use of advocacy here is not necessarily meant to imply a parent's involvement in changing complex EI systems. Instead, advocacy is often a dynamic process in which parents strive to understand their rights and their child's rights and to gain as much information as possible about their child's diagnosis.[13] Through the advocacy process, families can express dissatisfaction and work with service providers within systems to create change.[13] Most parents are involved in advocating for their own children's therapeutic, educational, or other accommodation needs.[13]

Service providers can support advocacy efforts of parents of children with developmental conditions. A specific goal of IDEA legislation is to support the capacity of families to meet the special needs of the infants and toddlers.[1-3] When service providers enhance the capacity of families by preparing parents to be advocates for their children, therapists are meeting a key component of IDEA. EI programs and providers must promote parent advocacy and parent capacity by helping parents understand their rights, service options for their children, and options for action in the case that they feel appropriate services are not being provided for their children.[13]

Service providers in EI systems can promote parent advocacy skills by including parents in all aspects of therapy. When parents are aware and able to practice the strategies that service providers use, they feel more efficacious using such strategies in everyday activities. Through a coordinated effort, the EI team can educate parents on the child's health and/or developmental condition, provide information about parent support groups, and help caregivers locate and secure additional supports, such as respite care.

The Role of Parent Strain in Early Intervention

When very young children experience health and/or developmental difficulties, parents often experience psychological strain. When parents are faced with navigating the complexities of EI systems, they are often compelled to act as children's service coordinators and advocates. Extensive research has outlined the financial strain of having a young child with medical and/or developmental needs, as well as the time commitment of coordinating EI appointments that often occur outside of the home.[14] Mothers of children with disabilities have been found to decrease or leave employment to coordinate their children's care,[15] perpetuating financial difficulties. Parents of children with developmental conditions experience high levels of stress,[16] which is often magnified by social isolation.[17] Given the psychological strain that parents may experience, service providers are in a unique situation to support not only the development of children but also parent resilience. Research has extensively shown that the EI team can support parents to promote positive coping skills and responsive interactions with their children. As described in the interprofessional approaches to pediatric care, professionals working with families in EI should be mindful of the following principles of care:

- Service providers must build a *trusting relationship* with parents. By listening to parent concerns about any aspects of child development and taking time with new families to answer questions, professionals can create a space for parents to express both frustrations and accomplishments.

- EI providers must *value parents as the experts* of their own children. By showing that parents are valued in the process and involving parents in all aspects of care, service providers may help support parents to feel increasingly efficacious in their parenting role.

- The EI team must *construct goals with parents*; child goals can address development milestones as well as family routines. When families have effective everyday routines, parents are less stressed and children have more opportunities to practice skills to promote development. Parents should be made aware of this rationale for treatment.

- All members of the EI team should *accommodate families' schedules and roles*. For example, if a family has the goal of promoting a child's independent eating, service providers can offer to schedule a family visit during mealtime. When EI providers embed services in the daily-occurring routines of the family (eg, feeding, napping, driving in the car, changing diapers), they have a greater impact on child development and family routines.

- A parent may gain positive coping skills and decrease stress by attending a support group; a service provider may be able to *provide information about specific support groups* and respite to families of young children with medical and/or developmental conditions. The EI team can encourage parent education and advocacy by sharing resources.

The EI team should also be aware that children who are younger than 4 with intensive caring needs (eg, young children with health concerns, intellectual disabilities, mental health issues, and chronic physical conditions) are at increased risk for *adverse childhood events* (ACEs). ACEs are defined as negative and potentially traumatic events that can have detrimental effects on health and well-being.[18] These experiences range from physical, emotional, or sexual abuse to parental divorce or the incarceration of a parent or guardian. Parents and caregivers who are most likely to perpetrate abuse constituting ACEs are those who exhibit the following characteristics[19]:

- Lack of understanding of children's needs, child development, and parenting skills;
- History of child maltreatment in family of origin;
- Substance abuse and/or mental health issues, including depression in the family;
- Young age, low education, single parenthood, large number of dependent children, and low income;
- Nonbiological, transient caregivers in the home; and
- Thoughts and emotions that tend to support or justify maltreatment behaviors.

Children's risks are even greater if their families are socially isolated, disorganized, and stressed and have negative family interactions. Finally, ACEs are more common in communities prone to violence with concentrated neighborhood disadvantage (eg, high poverty, residential instability, high unemployment rates) and poor social connections.[20] The EI team must work collaboratively to address potential ACEs by developing a plan to address specific existing concerns and risk factors. As a team, they can advocate and provide evidence-based resources that are protective for child maltreatment, including connections with community-based groups, nurturing parenting skills, encouraging household rules and child monitoring, and facilitating access to needed health care and social services.

Parenting Styles

EI service providers must be mindful of how different types of parenting styles can influence a child's behavior.

Four different types of parenting styles include *authoritative, authoritarian, permissive*, and *uninvolved*.[21,22] Each style is differentiated by the extent to which a parent shows *demandingness* (how firm/domineering a parent is toward the child) and *responsiveness* (how sensitive/aware a parent is toward the child).

Research suggests that parenting styles fall along the continuum of demandingness and responsiveness.[21,22] Parents with an authoritative parenting style, featuring high demandingness/high responsiveness, provide children with firm direction and encourage freedom for child exploration. Children experiencing this type of parenting style tend to be more self-reliant, self-controlled, explorative, and self-contented. Parents who use an authoritarian parenting style, characterized by high demandingness/low responsiveness, expect child obedience and adhere to absolute values. Children of authoritarian parents tend to become more discontented, withdrawn, and distrustful. Authoritative or authoritarian styles have high expectations of their children (high demandingness) but respond differently to their children's abilities (differing degrees of responsiveness). Those with a permissive parenting style have limited demands, allow their children to regulate their own behavior (accepting whatever the child tends to do), and are very responsive. Children with permissive parents tend to become more self-reliant, self-controlled, explorative, and self-contented. Finally, the uninvolved parenting style is characterized by parents who demonstrate low expectations and decreased responsiveness. The uninvolved parenting style has been shown to contribute to poor child outcomes, such as child impulsivity, aggression, and decreased social skills.[21,22]

The EI team can help families build their parenting skills through realistic goals based on their children's strengths and current functioning. Parents that are overly focused on their children's deficits may not offer opportunities to practice skills that would build on their children's existing abilities and strengths. Given that infants need continual practice to develop their motor, language, and cognitive skills, the EI team can not only help parents set realistic goals but also show them how to monitor progress toward achieving their goals. For example, the typical attention span of a 1-year-old is only 3 to 5 minutes; a 2-year-old is only 4 to 10 minutes; and a 3-year-old is only 6 to 15 minutes. Parents should not expect their child to join them at the movie theater at such a young age but rather plan to watch a movie at home, providing short breaks to engage the infant in novel activities.

Pediatric therapists, using their knowledge of health conditions, developmental milestones, therapeutic approaches, prognostic indicators, and interprofessional collaboration, can help families and caretakers gauge their expectations for intervention outcomes and promote healthy infant-adult interactions.

Promoting Parent Responsiveness and Play

Play-based activities promote the infant's developmental skills and can be consistently provided by responsive parents. Pediatric therapists can help parents to incorporate playful ways of performing functional activities in the home and community, offering multiple opportunities to reinforce needed skills. As earlier stated, *parent responsiveness* is defined as how sensitive and aware parents are toward their children, and parents with different styles have varying levels of responsiveness toward their children.[23,24] When parents respond to their children's cues and interact warmly with their children, their children show better developmental outcomes over time.[25,26] For example, if a parent talks more to her child during daily routines, the child's language and communication are positively impacted. If a parent responds warmly to a child's cries, that child shows better social-emotional developmental over time. Service providers must work with parents to understand how to increase responsiveness to children during daily routines where interactions are most likely to occur.

There are a number of ways that the EI team can promote parent responsiveness. Service providers can help parents understand and interpret their children's cues.[25,26] For example, a young child with autism spectrum disorder (ASD) may appear disinterested in interacting with a parent; the child may avoid eye contact with the parent or turn his body away. Service providers can help the parent reframe her interpretation of this behavior. It may be that the young child does not understand how to interact with the parent or does not comprehend the words that the parent is using. Instead of thinking that the child does not want to interact, service providers can help educate the parent on what the child may be expressing when he turns away.

Another method the EI team can use to promote parent responsiveness is teaching parents specific strategies to engage their children; examples of such evidence-based strategies include using children's interests and promoting imitation.[27] When a parent follows the child's lead and/or uses a child's interest to engage him in an activity, the child is more engaged. Take the example of the young child with ASD. A parent is having difficulty engaging in play with the child, but the parent knows that the child loves trains. The parent may sit on the floor and play trains with the child. The parent can imitate the child's actions with the train, even if the actions seem repetitive, like spinning the wheels of the train. When the parent joins the child in his interest, the child is more likely to socially interact and engage with the parent. Imitation is a vital component of engaging in social interactions with young children; professionals and parents often expect that children should imitate their actions. When service providers model imitation for a child (eg, echoing the child's sounds no matter how functional,

imitating the child's motor actions even if repetitive), the child is more likely to then imitate an adult.

For young children, parent responsiveness is vital; when parents are more responsive, children show better language and cognitive outcomes. The EI team can become trained in specific practice models for promoting parent responsiveness, including, but not limited to, Responsive Teaching[24]; the Early Start Denver Model[25]; and Developmental, Individual-Difference, Relationship-Based (DIR)/Floortime.[26]

Supporting Families Transitioning From Early Intervention to School-Age Programs

The young child can transition out of EI services into a preschool program or be directed to other services to meet her needs before her third birthday. While beginning preschool poses challenges for all families, the transition between EI and preschool services is especially challenging for parents of children with special needs. EI teams should also be aware of common problems that families face, including (1) incompatible schedules, (2) conflicting philosophies between the IFSP and the Individualized Education Plan (IEP) that begins at age 3, (3) overlapping/duplicate forms, (4) lack of trust/respect for existing assessment information, (5) differing eligibility criteria, (6) unclear expectations/assumptions, (7) different cultures associated with different agencies/staffs, and (8) loss of funding (eg, waivers, insurance).[28]

The EI team should engage in ongoing collaboration to discern what the family needs, while advocating for necessary services. The EI team should also educate the family about the different regulations that impact services for infants younger than 3 as compared with those offered to children older than 3. Whereas IDEA Part C for EI is family focused and mandates family involvement, Part B for early childhood special education (ECSE) is child centered and focused on education, and the school assumes the responsibility for the child. Because IDEA requires a minimum of 6 months to prepare families for this transition, it is helpful to follow some simple guidelines to make the transition from EI to ECSE as easy as possible[29]:

- Allow time to address any questions the family may have about the transition from EI to ECSE.

- Help the family build a relationship with the ECSE program their child will attend. Part B of IDEA attempts to strengthen parental roles in the education process, encouraging patents to be involved in the IEP program and active in their children's education at school and at home.

- Help the family prepare for transition meetings by encouraging them to visit the preschool and meet with the preschool teachers and other staff prior to the transition meeting.

- Educate parents about the differences between IDEA Part C (EI) and Part B for ECSE. For example, Part C (EI) focuses on the *natural environment* as compared with Part B (preschool), which focuses on the *least restrictive environment*, enabling the child to participate with peers in the learning process as much as possible.
- Encourage families to discuss their expectations, family routines, and concerns about the transition from EI to ECSE.
- Increase parents' confidence in their children's ability to achieve goals in the new setting.
- Improve parents' self-confidence in their own ability to communicate with educational staff and to effectively influence the education system.
- Connect families with a parent support group, while considering child care, transportation, and other family barriers that might restrict participation.

As pediatric therapists, we can help parents make the difficult transition that all families face when their children enter school; in the case of children with special needs, we need to equip them with knowledge, emotional support, and confidence in their children's future success.

SUMMARY

Children younger than 3 who are at risk for developmental conditions and delays can benefit from EI services. As outlined in this section, IDEA is a federal mandate that ensures families and children have access to necessary services. Part C of IDEA is most relevant to EI; as part of this federal mandate, interprofessional teams of service providers serve families of young children with developmental concerns and conditions. Service providers implement developmental assessments and screening tools, and each family in EI has an IFSP. There are special considerations when working with families of young children with developmental conditions; in this section, we discussed parent advocacy, parent strain, parenting styles, ways to promote parent responsiveness, and supporting families from the transition between EI and ECSE. By providing services in natural environments and implementing evidence-based practices, interprofessional teams of EI therapists are in a unique position to support the daily lives of families of children with special needs.

INTERPROFESSIONAL ACTIVITY

Developing the Individualized Family Service Plan

As a team, develop an IFSP for one of the case studies below. Take turns having one person in your group play the role of the parent while others play the roles of professionals working with the family.

1. As a team, how would you describe your role in the EI program to this family?
2. Based upon criteria given in the case, is the child eligible for EI?
3. What concerns do you think the parent would have about the child?
4. How would you communicate with the family, given their situation?
5. As a team, how would you organize your screening of the child?
6. What types of recommendations would you make for the IFSP in terms of functional goals and parental involvement?

Case 7-1: A 1-month-old girl diagnosed as failure to thrive

Lilly was born at 30 weeks' gestational age. Following her premature birth, she was placed in the NICU, where she received treatment with oxygen, surfactant, and mechanical assistance to help her breathe. Lilly's birth weight was 1030 grams. She began feeding, receiving her mother's breast milk via a gavage tube. Lilly is able to grasp a finger. She can stay awake and alert for short periods. She is now 1 month old. Her height, weight, and head circumference continue to be below the 5th percentile, and her length is below the 10th percentile. Her mother, Margaret, is a waitress, recently divorced, who lives in a small, low-income apartment with a stairway entrance. Lilly has 2 older brothers, Jeremy (age 2) and Phillip (age 3). Margaret's ex-husband, Paul, a butcher, is seeking sole custody of his 2 sons, currently in Margaret's custody. Paul complains that Margaret spends too much time caring for Lilly. Margaret wants to prove that she is capable of caring for Lilly and both of her sons, so she is seeking support from the interprofessional team serving her in EI.

Case 7-2: A 2-month-old boy born with spina bifida

Jared was born at 35 weeks' gestational age with myelo-dysplasia (L2 with hydrocephalus and Arnold Chiari type II syndrome) by Cesarean section. Jared's diagnosis of a Chiari II malformation can be made prenatally through ultrasound. Jared had decompressive surgery involving removing the lamina of the first and second cervical vertebrae and part of the occipital bone of the skull to relieve pressure with shunt placement. He has been in the NICU since his birth, where he is receiving interprofessional care. Jared is allergic to latex and has difficulty maintaining his body temperature. He has difficulty with feeding, requiring more frequent feeds due to his problems with swallowing and breathing. Jared's mother, Sandra, and father, George, live with Alex, their 2-year-old son, in the basement of Sandra's mother's home. There are 10 steps into their basement apartment, which features linoleum floors, concrete walls, and poor lighting. They share a bathroom on the first floor of the house. Both parents work low-paying, full-time jobs, and Alex stays with his grandmother during the day. Flooding in their neighborhood (and in the basement) has led to reduced family income, limiting the family's resources to cover Jared's health care costs. Jared is now 3 months old and discharged from the NICU.

Case 7-3: A 9-month-old boy diagnosed with cerebral palsy

Solyna, age 42, and Sopheak, age 57, recently moved from Cambodia to a small town in the Midwest. Solyna had an uneventful pregnancy and gave premature birth to Narin, her only child. Given the unexpected early birth, the family was transferred to a large city for Narin's hospitalization. While the father continued working in the small town, his wife remained in the hospital with the newborn. Born at 32 weeks' gestational age, Narin spent his first 3 weeks in the NICU, where he was very quiet and did not cry much. As Narin became physiologically stable, he was discharged from the NICU and sent home to his rural hometown. Once at home, both parents became concerned when they noticed Narin's shaky movement pattern and his inability to hold his head up or roll by the time he was 6 months old. The family saw a pediatrician, who diagnosed Narin with cerebral palsy (mixed type with spasticity and athetosis) and suggested that the family seek out EI services for Narin. With the initiation of EI services, both parents were relieved and willing to do whatever was best for him. Although Sopheak is able to communicate in English, he is sometimes difficult to understand. Solyna has difficulty understanding and speaking English. Narin's aunt, Raksa (also from Cambodia), has since moved into the family's 2-story rental home to assist with Narin's care. Raksa does not understand or speak English. Narin's bedroom is on the second floor. Narin is now 9 months old and entering EI. His family is open to suggestions for ways to best manage Narin's delayed motor development; however, communication with the family during therapy sessions is challenging, especially when his father is not home. Narin continues to have difficulties with mobility, postural control, fine motor control, and language skill; however, he appears to be alert, engaged, and eager to learn.

Case 7-4: A 12-month-old girl born with Trisomy

Bo was born in Beijing, China, with Trisomy 21 (Down syndrome), diagnosed at birth. Born full-term, Bo exhibited generalized hypotonicity, muscle weakness, and hyperflexible joints. She also had an unrepaired atrioventricular malfunction and cervical instability.

Bo was adopted by her American parents and brought to the home when Bo was 10 months old. Bo did not receive any therapeutic interventions prior to entering the United States. Her parents also have 3 other adopted children, Susan (a 5-year-old daughter from Ecuador), Bill (a 7-year-old son from Guatemala), and Rachel (a 9-year-old daughter from Vietnam). Mary and Jake are her adoptive parents. Mary is a housewife who takes care of the children, and Jake runs his own business that frequently takes him out of town. Mary has sought EI services through the pediatrician who sees all the other children. Now that Bo is 1 year old, Mary is eager to learn about how to help Bo learn needed functional skills.

Case 7-5: A 1-year-old girl at risk for developmental delays

Carly was born at 26 weeks' gestation and spent the first 9 weeks of her life in the NICU. Carly was on a ventilator for 2 weeks while her lungs developed, and she had G-tube inserted for feeding for 6 weeks. Carly's mother, Grace, was homeless and became pregnant when she stayed in a homeless shelter during the winter. Grace was addicted to cocaine and was picked up by police a couple of times before Carly's birth. Grace did not receive any prenatal care during her pregnancy, but she went to the hospital to deliver her child in a warm environment where she could stay safely off the streets. Based upon her inability to care for the newborn, Grace immediately had to give Carly up for adoption. Carly was placed in foster care but did not receive immediate care for possible developmental delays. At 8 months, Carly was taken to the local general hospital for a developmental screening. Carly scored below the 25th percentile across all areas. Referred to pediatric therapists, Carly was further assessed using standardized tests and measures and continued to be below normal for motor activities. While in foster care, Carly received EI services with guidance given to her foster mother (Janice) and foster father (Bob). At 12 months old, Carly sits independently with support but is unable to belly crawl or creep. She is able to bring her hands to midline and transfer objects with a weak grasp. She can also respond to voices by babbling. Her mother has requested to have Carly returned to her, so the interprofessional team has been asked to make recommendations for a comprehensive EI program with sufficient supports to aid the mother in developing key parenting skills.

Developing a Plan of Care

1. Reflect on the frameworks of practice (Section 2), cultural competency (Section 3), typical development (Section 4), and management of care (Section 5).

2. Using interprofessional skills outlined in Section 1, discuss activities you would teach the family to encourage the infant's participation in each family's daily routine.

REFERENCES

1. US Department of Education. Thirty-five years of progress in educating children with disabilities through IDEA. US Department of Education Web site. https://www2.ed.gov/about/offices/list/osers/idea35/history/idea-35-history.pdf. Published November 2010. Accessed January 31, 2017.

2. US Department of Education. Part C–Infants and Toddlers with Disabilities. US Department of Education Web site. https://sites.ed.gov/idea/. Published 2017. Accessed December 5, 2017.

3. New York State Department of Health, Bureau of Early Intervention. Early Intervention Program: Group Developmental Intervention Services Standards. New York State Department of Health Web site. https://www.health.ny.gov/community/infants_children/early_intervention/docs/2013_11_grp_dev_inter_serv_standards.pdf. Published November 2013. Accessed January 27, 2017.

4. Affleck G, Tennen H, Rowe J, Roscher B, Walker L. Effects of formal support on mothers' adaptation to the hospital-to-home transition of high-risk infants: The benefits and costs of helping. *Child Dev.* 1989;60(2):488-501.

5. Pathways.org. Motor skills. Recognizing early motor delays (ages 0-6 months). Pathways Web site. https://pathways.org/topics-of-development/motor-skills-2/printouts/. Accessed February 13, 2017.

6. Kruer MC. Myoclonic epilepsy beginning in infancy or early childhood. Medscape Web site. http://emedicine.medscape.com/article/1176055-overview. Published March 14, 2016. Accessed February 13, 2017.

7. Missouri Department of Health and Senior Services. Guidelines for vision screening in Missouri schools. Missouri Department of Health and Senior Services Web site. http://health.mo.gov/living/families/schoolhealth/pdf/VisionScreeningGuidelines.pdf. Accessed February 13, 2017.

8. Robins RL, Casagrande K, Barton M, Chen CA, Dumont-Mathieu T, Fein D. Validation of the Modified Checklist for Autism in Toddlers, Revised with follow-up (M-CHAT-R/F). *Pediatrics.* 2014;133(1):37-45.

9. Washington Department of State Health. Nutrition screening for infants and children with special needs. Washington Department of State Health Web site. http://www.doh.wa.gov/Portals/1/Documents/Pubs/970-116_NutritionScreeningForInfantsAndYoungCSHCN.pdf. Published October 2008. Accessed January 26, 2017.

10. Kansas Infant-Toddler Services. At-Risk Infants or Toddlers. Kansas Department of Health and Environment Web site. http://www.ksits.org/download/part_c_manual/ELIGIBILITY.pdf. Published 2013. Accessed December 5, 2017.

11. New York State Department of Health. Eligibility requirements. New York State Department of Health Web site. https://www.health.ny.gov/community/infants_children/early_intervention/memoranda/2005-02/eligibility_criteria.htm. Accessed January 26, 2017.

12. Nachshen J, Jamieson J. Advocacy, stress and quality of life in parents of children with developmental difficulties. *Developmental Disabilities Bulletin.* 2000;28(1):39-55.

13. Bailey DB, Bruder MB, Hebbeler K, et al. Recommended outcomes for families of young children with disabilities. *Journal of Early Intervention.* 2006;28:227-251.

14. Seltzer MM, Greenberg JS, Floyd FJ, Pettee Y, Hong J. Life course impacts of parenting a child with a disability. *Am J Ment Retard.* 2001;106(3):265-286.

15. Parish SL, Seltzer MM, Greenberg JS, Floyd F. Economic implications of caregiving at midlife: Comparing parents with and without children who have developmental disabilities. *Ment Retard.* 2004;42(6):413-426.

16. Estes A, Munson J, Dawson G, Koehler E, Zhou XH, Abbott R. Parenting stress and psychological functioning among mothers of preschool children with autism and developmental delay. *Autism.* 2009;13(4):375-387.

17. Gupta VB. Comparison of parenting stress in different developmental disabilities. *J Dev Phys Disabil.* 2007;19(4):417-425.

18. Iowa ACEs 360. ACEs impact on brain development. Central Iowa ACEs 360 Coalition Web site. http://www.iowaaces360.org/aces-and-development.html. Accessed February 2, 2017.

19. Felitti VJ, Anda RF, Nordenberg D, et al. Relationship of childhood abuse and household dysfunction to many of the leading causes of death in adults: The Adverse Childhood Experiences (ACE) Study. *Am J Prev Med.* 1998;14(4):245-258.

20. Sacks S, Murphey D, Moore K. Adverse Childhood Experiences: National and state-level prevalence. Child trends Web site. http://www.childtrends.org/wp-content/uploads/2014/07/Brief-adverse-childhood-experiences_FINAL.pdf. Accessed January 27, 2017.

21. Baumrind D. Effects of authoritative parental control behavior on child behavior. *Child Dev.* 1966;37(4):887-907.

22. Baumrind D. Child care practices anteceding three patterns of preschool behavior. *Genet Psychol Monogr.* 1967;75(1):43-88.

23. Mahoney G, Perales, F. Wiggers, B, Herman B. Responsive teaching: Early intervention for children with Down syndrome and other disabilities. Down Syndrome Education Web site. https://www.down-syndrome.org/perspectives/311/. Published 2017. Accessed December 5, 2017.

24. Landry SH, Smith KE, Swank PR, Assel MA, Vellet S. Does early responsive parenting have a special importance for children's development or is consistency across early childhood necessary? *Dev Psychol.* 2001;37(3):387-403.

25. Rogers SJ, Dawson G. *Early Start Denver Model for Young Children With Autism: Promoting Language, Learning, and Engagement.* New York, NY: Guilford Press; 2010.

26. Greenspan SI, Wieder S. *Engaging Autism: Using the Floortime Approach to Help Children Relate, Communicate, and Think.* Boston, MA: Da Capo Press; 2009.

27. Zins JE, Elias MJ. Social and emotional learning: Promoting the development of all students. *J Educ Psychol Consult.* 2007;17(2-3):233-255.

28. IFSPweb. Planning for transitions. IFSPweb Web site. http://ifspweb.org/module3/transition-planning.php. Accessed January 27, 2017.

29. Johnson C. Supporting families in transition between early intervention and school age programs. Hands and Voices Web site. http://www.handsandvoices.org/articles/education/law/transition.html. Accessed January 27, 2017.

Section 8

Working With Families of Young Children With Special Needs

Ketti Johnson Coffelt, OTD, MS, OTR/L and Catherine Rush Thompson, PT, PhD, MS

OVERVIEW

This section provides an overview of how pediatric therapists work with families and other professionals to manage the special needs of young children. Once children reach the age of 3, they no longer qualify for early intervention (EI) services, as described in Section 7. For those children with ongoing special needs, this section outlines services available to preschool children aged 3 to 5 years. Federal and state laws dictate a different standard of care for children in the preschool setting from what was provided to families of children from birth to age 3. In addition to describing the changing focus of service provision from family-centered care in natural settings to providing supportive services for learning, this section describes risk factors, screening and assessment tools, and the roles of other professionals commonly encountered when working with this population. Finally, it differentiates the provision of educational vs medical services. Upon completion of this section, the learner will be able to (1) describe Individuals with Disabilities Education Act (IDEA) components relevant to therapists working with preschoolers, (2) discuss recommended interprofessional practices, (3) discuss family and developmental risk factors of young children, (4) identify age-appropriate standardized screening and assessment tools for young children and families, (5) describe the scope of practice of professionals young children in educational and other practice settings, (6) distinguish educational vs medical care for preschoolers, and (7) describe how to help families transition from EI to early childhood special education (ECSE).

EARLY INTERVENTION SERVICES FOR PRESCHOOLERS

Children aged 3 to 5 years who have special needs may qualify to receive free educational services to optimize their learning. Federal and state laws provide ECSE to those who qualify through Part B of IDEA.[1] IDEA Part B sets the standards for the achievement of educational goals and helps families and professionals work collaboratively to address the individual needs of these children with special needs. Children who generally qualify for special education services

Thompson CR. *Pediatric Therapy:*
An Interprofessional Framework for Practice (pp 115-132).
© 2018 SLACK Incorporated.

are those who received EI services and continue to have developmental delays. In addition, children with identified disabilities (eg, cognitive impairments; hearing impairments, including deafness; speech or language impairments; visual impairments, including blindness; emotional disturbance; orthopedic impairments; autism; traumatic brain injury; and other health impairments or specific learning disabilities) typically qualify.[1]

The Division for Early Childhood (DEC) of the Council for Exceptional Children has developed recommended practices to provide guidance to practitioners and families about the most effective ways to improve their children's learning outcomes. These outcomes include promoting the development of young children, birth through age 5, who have or are at risk for developmental delays or disabilities. The following recommendations relate to (1) assessment, (2) environment, (3) family, (4) instruction, (5) interaction, (6) teaming and collaboration, and (7) transition.[2] Many of these recommendations are highlighted in the previous section on EI, but several relate more directly to children who have transitioned from EI to ECSE and will be highlighted in this section.

In terms of *assessment practices*, recommendations include implementing *systematic ongoing assessment* to identify learning targets, plan activities, and monitor the child's progress to revise instruction as needed.[2] To achieve this end, assessments need to be sufficiently sensitive to detect each child's progress; ie, therapists must select tests that are not only valid and reliable but also particularly sensitive to small, incremental changes in measurable behavior. Equally important, practitioners need to report their results to others in a manner that is both understandable and meaningful for all, especially caregivers, developmental specialists, and teachers.

According to the DEC, *environmental practices* refer to the physical environment (eg, space, equipment, materials), the social environment (eg, interactions with peers, siblings, family members), and the temporal environment (eg, sequence and length of routines and activities).[2] Environmental practice recommendations address both *learning and safety* to promote each child's health and development. For ECSE, the DEC recommends providing service in inclusive, accessible environments during daily routines that promote each child's participation.[2] Using interprofessional collaboration, team members can modify and adapt the physical, social, and temporal environments to promote access to and participation in learning activities, incorporating assistive technology, as appropriate. In addition, environments should "provide ample opportunities for movement and regular physical activity to maintain or improve fitness, wellness, and development across domains."[2] This provision can be a challenge in some early childhood settings where space is limited. Through team collaboration, therapists can offer suggestions for incorporating active games as part of

the group's daily routines that further enhance participation and inclusion.

The concept of *family*, described as a family-centered framework and discussed in the sections on frameworks of practice and EI, continues to be emphasized in ECSE. For families who have had their children transition from EI to ECSE, opportunities for respectful team participation and advocacy skill building should have been ample and built upon. IDEA Part C (addressing families of children under age 3) and Part B (addressing children older than 3 years entering preschool) have different foci for care and instruction, so ECSE practitioners need to appreciate these differences, and parents need to be advised of realistic expectations. Differences in Part C and Part B are outlined in Table 8-1. Most notably, the shift in focus is from the child and family in a natural setting for IDEA Part C to the child solely in the preschool setting for IDEA Part B. Although parents are still actively involved in developing the child's Individualized Education Program (IEP) as part of the team, programs are incorporated into the daily routines in the preschool setting, as opposed to family routines in the child's natural settings, such as the home and community, as emphasized in EI.

Instructional practices are the foundation of ECSE, as the team (including physical therapists, occupational therapists, speech-language pathologists, teachers, and other services) work together to maximize learning and improve developmental and functional outcomes for young children who have or are at risk for developmental delays or disabilities. Interprofessional collaboration relies on a variety of intentional and systematic strategies to optimize learning outcomes; otherwise, the child and the family may be confused by a wide range of inconsistent and disparate information. Practices most relevant to ECSE include the following[2]:

1. *Identifying each child's strengths, preferences, and interests* to engage the child in active learning;

2. *Identifying skills to target for instruction* that help a child become adaptive, competent, socially connected, engaged, and well educated in inclusive environments;

3. *Gathering and using data to inform decisions* about individualized instruction;

4. *Planning for and providing the level of support, accommodations, and adaptations* needed for the child to access, participate, and learn within and across activities and routines;

5. *Embedding instruction* within and across routines, activities, and environments to provide contextually relevant learning opportunities;

6. Using *systematic instructional strategies with fidelity* to teach skills and to promote child engagement and learning;

7. Using *explicit feedback* and consequences to increase child engagement, play, and skills. Practitioners use

TABLE 8-1

DIFFERENCES BETWEEN THE INDIVIDUALIZED FAMILY SERVICE PLAN AND INDIVIDUALIZED EDUCATION PROGRAM		
FEDERAL LAW	**IDEA PART C**	**IDEA PART B**
Eligibility	Children with special needs from birth to age 3 years	Children with special needs aged 3 through 21 years
Focus	On the family's and caregivers' roles in supporting the child's health, learning, and development	On the child's learning and development
Program developed	Individualized Family Service Plan (IFSP)	Individualized Education Program (IEP)
Outcomes	The child and family	The child
Environment	The environment for learning is in the natural environment (often the home, child care, or the community)	Environments focus on the preschool (eg, classroom, playground, dining area), incorporating assistive technology, if needed; social interactions with other children are encouraged
Coordination	EI service manager or case worker coordinates services integrated by the IFSP; services may involve many agencies in providing services because of the child's age	Local school districts are authorized to coordinate and manage the child's services
Meeting with family	Offer information and resources and to define the various agencies' roles and financial responsibilities	Called to develop long-term and short-term goals for the child, accommodations and modifications, services, and child placement
Frequency of formal meetings	Typically every 6 months	Typically annually (those that involve the family)

Adapted from PACER Center. What is the difference between an IFSP and an IEP? PACER Center Web site. https://www.pacer.org/parent/php/PHP-c59.pdf. Pubished 2011. Accessed December 11, 2017.

peer-mediated interventions to teach skills and to promote child engagement and learning;

8. *Using functional assessment and related prevention, promotion, and intervention strategies* across environments to prevent and address challenging behavior

9. Implementing the *frequency, intensity, and duration of instruction* needed to address the child's learning needs;

10. *Using and adapting specific instructional strategies that are effective for dual language learners* when teaching English to children with disabilities; and

11. *Using coaching or consultation strategies* with others to facilitate positive adult-child interactions and instruction intentionally designed to promote child learning and development.

Additionally, recognizing the importance of cultural competency and the need to be sensitive and responsive, the

DEC also provides helpful recommendations for *interaction practices* that mirror those discussed in the section on cultural competency. The following DEC recommendations are designed to facilitate interactions that promote specific learning outcomes for each child[2]:

1. *Observing, interpreting, and responding contingently* to the range of the child's emotional expressions;

2. *Encouraging the child to initiate or sustain positive interactions with other children and adults* during routines and activities through modeling, teaching, feedback, or other types of guided support;

3. *Providing natural consequences for the child's verbal and nonverbal communication* and by using language to label and expand on the child's requests, needs, preferences, or interests.

4. *Observing, interpreting, and responding intentionally to the child's exploration, play, and social activity* by

joining in and expanding on the child's focus, actions, and intent; and

5. *Observing, interpreting, and "scaffolding" in response to the child's growing level of autonomy and self-regulation.* The idea of *scaffolding* is to provide assistance just slightly beyond the child's learning abilities, helping him build upon his existing abilities.[3] This is the primary strategy therapists can help teachers learn in respect to knowing the child's level of competence in performing motor, language, and cognitive skills.

A cornerstone of successful ECSE programs is using effective *teaming and collaboration practices*, as discussed in earlier sections. The DEC's recommendations for these practices are similar to those identified by organizations supporting interprofessional care; they recommend building relationships through respect, support, capacity enhancement, and cultural sensitivity. In addition to principles stated earlier in this book, it elaborates on assisting each other to discover and access community-based services and other informal and formal resources to meet family-identified child or family needs. Oftentimes, families and teachers seek out enrichment opportunities in the community, and therapists can provide appropriate options. With these practices in mind, pediatric therapists play an important role in anticipating family and developmental risk factors during these early childhood years (Table 8-2) .

FAMILY AND DEVELOPMENTAL RISK FACTORS

Any change to a family's routine can be stressful and pose unique risks. While prioritizing the educational and developmental needs of the child in the preschool, it is important to appreciate the family's culture, routines, and environment to ease the transition from EI to ECSE. In addition to the developmental risk factors described in Section 7, there are additional considerations for a child older than 3. What are the parents' desires for their child? What supports or limitations from the home setting may impact the child's skills and routines as they transition to a preschool classroom? This is an opportunity for team members to collaborate with each other as they gather information from the family pertinent to their perspective disciplines. While planning care, pediatric therapists need to be thoughtful and respectful of the parents' time by reducing redundancy in the types of questions asked about their child.

Risk factors for the child are likely to align with the nature and severity of the child's exceptionality. Is the child's condition progressive in nature? Is there an unusual demand for child caretaking? How dependent is the child upon others for her daily care, communication, and play exploration

of the environment? The family unit is at risk due to the unique demands placed upon them.

As the child enters preschool education, the family unit is vulnerable to a new set of professionals from the educational realm, who are ready to share their knowledge and expertise. Professionals must guard against overloading the family with "homework" that can be overtaxing. For example, expecting family members to therapeutically feed and position their child for every meal is not realistic and too demanding. Given that the overall goal is to support the learning and development of the child, practitioners need be nonjudgmental, allowing time for trust and relationships to develop to reassure vulnerable families.

All members of ECSE teams must pay close attention to how a child is learning, looking for potential signs of hearing, vision, and developmental problems. Common risk factors for all children aged 3 to 5 include developing ear and eye infections that impact their sensorimotor skills, play, social interactions, and knowledge development. Observations of children at play and while interacting with peers may provide valuable information for identifying those children who may be at risk. Carefully following a child's development across areas of preacademic skills, motor skills, sensory exploration, social/play interactions, communication skills, social behaviors, and self-care routines offers specific clues as to her need for further assessment by specific disciplines or the entire preschool educational team.

Specific communication, social interaction, and behavior problems may require observations of the child in a variety of contexts. These initial observations of her play skills, social skill development, and ability to follow daily routine tasks are the first steps in documenting the need for further evaluation for a child with suspected autism spectrum disorder (ASD).

- What is motivating to the child or of interest to her?
- What types of behaviors interfere with play and preacademic learning?
- How does the child play with toys?
- How does the child communicate with others?

The following questions can guide a practitioner to attend to behaviors for child who may have significant attention problems that many times are diagnosed as attention deficit hyperactivity disorder (ADHD)[4]:

- Does the child reportedly need constant attention and not play alone at home?
- Do parents report that the child has problems winding down at the end of the day, popping out of bed repeatedly?
- Is the child able to sustain attention (normal attention span for a 3-year-old is 7 to 9 minutes)?
- Is the child destructive with toys?

TABLE 8-2	
DEVELOPMENTAL OBSERVATIONS FOR CHILDREN AT RISK	
LEARNING AREAS	**COMMON OBSERVATIONS OR RISK FACTORS**
Preacademics	• Does the child initiate and complete task independently? • Is the child able to hold attention to complete task? • Is the child easily distracted? • Does the child play make-believe games? • Does the child remember parts of a story? • Is the child interested in knowing colors, ABCs, numbers? • Does the child use central or peripheral vision to perform tasks?
Motor skills	• Does the child sit using a slumped posture? • Is the child able to maintain head in erect position during play? • Does the child lean into furniture or consistently lay down during play? • Is the child able to maintain balance while using hands? • Does the child run easily? • Does the child climb on playground equipment? • Does the child only play on one piece of playground equipment (eg, only being pushed on a swing)? • Does the child use both hands together while manipulating items? • Does the child use one hand predominately, with the other by her side? • Is the child able to pick up small items? • Does the child drop items? • Does the child have hand strength to hold items?
Sensory exploration	• Does the child prefer solitary play? • Does the child prefer to be moving or active? • Does the child bump into furniture or others during play or transitions? • Is the child able to touch various textures during play (eg, water, paint, glue)? • Does the child have difficulty grading pressure while holding items (too much or too little)? • Does the child seek movement by rocking, spinning, or jumping? • Does the child repeat words or self-vocalize? • Does the child excessively look at, touch, mouth, or smell objects?
Social/play interactions	• Does the child separate from his parents? • Does the child play alone or in isolation? • Is the child interested in playing with others? • Is the child only interested in preferred toys? • Does the child play with others, or beside them? • Does the child move away from others during play? • Does the child take turns?

(continued)

TABLE 8-2 (CONTINUED)
DEVELOPMENTAL OBSERVATIONS FOR CHILDREN AT RISK

LEARNING AREAS	COMMON OBSERVATIONS OR RISK FACTORS
Communication skills	• Does the child make eye contact with others? • Does the child smile, laugh, express feelings? • Does the child communicate using words? • Does the child understand 2- to 3-step directions? • Does the child express wants and needs using words? • Will the child approach others?
Self-care routines	• Is the child independent in toileting? • Does the child need repeated prompts to finish a learned task? • Does the child use both hands to pull up and down pants? • Does the child manage clothing items, knowing which items belong to her? • Is the child able to manipulate fasteners? • Does the child use a spoon to scoop items?
Social behaviors	• Is the child able to organize behavior response to the situation? • Do specific tasks or environments calm or arouse the child? • Does the child pick up on social and environmental cues? • Does the child demonstrate restricted interests or repetitive behaviors?

- Does the child have difficulty playing with other children, with a higher incidence of biting, kicking others, or pushing peers? The child should be able to engage in cooperative play and display kindness and caring.

- Is the child overly active, appear clumsy, and have a higher incidence of falling or accidents?

- Does the child yell or overreact to everyday situations? By age 3 to 4 years, a child should be able to tolerate changes in routines.

Communication among the preschool team members is crucial because each discipline may have similarities and differences in terminology associated with ASD or ADHD during the initial phases of observation of children who may be at risk.

All children at this age typically become more mobile both inside and outside as they explore their expanding environment. As children explore and learn from the interactions with objects in the environment, they are at a potential risk for falls, burns, poisoning, getting hit by a car, accidental drowning, or accidental gunshot. All adult caregivers and providers of the child are responsible for their safety and teaching them basic safety rules.

All children at this age are at risk for suspected neglect or abuse from adults with whom they come into contact with due to their helplessness. The adults could be familial and/or provide care to the child or play a peripheral role within the child's social environment. Typical indicators of child neglect include lack of supervision, adequate clothing and hygiene, medical and dental care, adequate nutrition, and shelter. As practitioners, there is a sensitivity to identifying neglect based on family cultural values and expectations and differing child rearing practices. A family living with poverty is not an indicator of child neglect.

As mentioned in Section 7, types of child abuse include physical, sexual, and emotional trauma. Signs of physical abuse of a young child could include any or all of the following: bruises, burns, lacerations and abrasions, skeletal injuries, and head and internal injuries. A child experiencing emotional abuse may show signs of being overly compliant and passive. Conversely, the child could display extremely aggressive, demanding, and rage-like behaviors.

A child who has been abused most often will display a lag in development when compared with same-age peers, particularly in the area of self-care. The child may exhibit a lack of curiosity and enjoyment, display self-stimulating behaviors, and have a fear of physical contact from others. The child may revert to an earlier developmental state. For example, a 5-year-old who was previously toilet trained might begin to wet herself. Sometimes the child will act out sexual or abusive scenarios with toys or objects without ever vocalizing the signs of abuse. Certain parent groups are more susceptible and at risk for possible child neglect or abuse, specifically parents with disabilities themselves and adults with drug and alcohol addictions. Our role and responsibility is to find assistance and resources for these parental groups. We are required to respect family and cultural differences and provide alternatives and education for enhancing their parenting skills.

The law stipulates that any person (medical, educational, or otherwise) who has definite contact with the child and suspects abuse is a mandated reporter. If there is reasonable cause to suspect neglect and/or abuse of a child, practitioners are instructed by law to contact and report the issue to a state department of social services. To report any suspected child abuse, contact the Childhelp National Child Abuse Hotline at 1-800-4-A-CHILD (1-800-422-4453). To report child sexual abuse, call 1-888-PREVENT (1-888-773-8368).

SCREENING AND ASSESSMENT TOOLS

As stated by IDEA of 2004,[1,2] no single measure or assessment tool should be used as sole criteria for determining an IEP for a child. The evaluation should "use a variety of assessment tools and strategies to gather relevant functional, developmental, and academic data including information provided by parent."[6] Special education preschool teams are required to consider information from the multiple sources, including the family and medical and service provider reports, but are not bound by any recommendations or decisions offered by medical teams. This is true for children with the medical diagnosis of ASD or ADHD because there is no automatic eligibility guarantee for special education or related services under IDEA.

A referral for evaluation under IDEA Part B (covering preschoolers and school-aged children) must follow federal law and regulations and individual state regulations and comply with individual service provider practice acts. Informed written consent must be obtained from a parent before evaluations are conducted by the preschool educational team. Under IDEA Part B, a request for an initial evaluation may come from a parent, state agency, or local educational agency (LEA).

Oftentimes in the preschool environment, assessment information is gathered from adults in the child's environment, from the teaching staff, and from parents or caregivers. Self-report measures, interviews, and observations should be considered by service providers as providing information about how the child performs and communicates in the context of the task and situation.

Discipline-specific evaluation tools used by service providers are conducted to determine eligibility for special education instructional and related services. In most preschool cases, the evaluation process culminates in identification of

the child's strengths and needs, with an emphasis on the child's performance in preacademic and nonacademic skills and routines. Table 8-3 lists commonly used assessments for ECSE.

ECSE teams (including physical therapists, speech-language pathologists, and occupational therapists) involve bottom-up and top-down approaches, incorporating observations within preschool environments (eg, playground, classroom, hallway, gym, library, art room, bathroom), appropriate discipline-specific evaluation measures, data collection, and identification of student goals. Researchers have identified the following essential components for team members to consider when collaborating in the development and implementation of an integrated educational program[6]:

- Goals belong to the learner and not individual team members.

- Team members need to contribute needed information and skills to enhance achievement of all goals and objectives.

- Professionals provide unique perspectives through their respective disciplinary methods and skills.

- Interprofessional collaboration addresses the child's needs more successfully in a wider variety of contexts.

- Effective integration involves focusing on meaningful activities to the learner.

ECSE programs are designed to meet the individualized needs of each child and are generally available in most school districts. Parents who suspect their young child may have a developmental delay or disabling condition that may affect their child's learning can contact their local school district to make a referral for an ECSE evaluation. Children with mild, moderate, and severe deficits typically qualify for education-related services provided in local preschools.

In contrast, children needing *medical attention* must go to a clinic or hospital for an evaluation and/or treatment by a medical professional, which is oftentimes costly to the family in terms of time, energy, and money. Medical professionals perform discipline-specific, age-appropriate, standardized assessments, clinical examinations, and observations to select interventions to promote the best *health outcomes* for the child. In the medical model, parents are typically held responsible for locating and paying for the needed therapeutic services. Health insurance may assist with payment, but not always. Table 8-4 lists the distinctions between the educational vs the medical model of care commonly applied to young children and their families.

Some children with special needs may receive therapy in both educational and medical settings, depending upon their health condition, because educational goals may not fully address the medical needs of children with certain diagnoses. For example, a child with Down syndrome may be engaged in preschool learning activities to develop motor, language, and cognitive skills but may also be monitored in

TABLE 8-3
FORMAL AND INFORMAL TYPES OF EARLY CHILDHOOD ASSESSMENT (3 TO 5 YEARS)

FORMAL ASSESSMENTS	DESCRIPTION	EXAMPLES
Norm-referenced assessment	Compares child's performance to a normative group of pre-school children	• Peabody Developmental Motor Scales (Second Edition) • Miller Function & Participation Scale (M-FUN) • Bruininks-Oseretsky Test of Motor Proficiency (Second Edition) • Assessment of Motor and Process Skills (AMPS) • School Assessment of Motor and Process Skills (School AMPS) • Motor Free Visual Perception Test (Third Edition) • Beery-Buktenica Developmental Test of Motor Integration (Sixth Edition)
Criterion-referenced assessment	Indicates child's performance based on a set of criteria	• Hawaii Early Learning Profile (HELP) • School Function Assessment (SFA) K-6 • Gross Motor Function Measure (GMFM) • Knox Preschool Play Scale • Child Sensory Profile-2 • Developmental Assessment for Individuals with Severe Disabilities (DASH-3) • Wee-FIM II • Pediatric Evaluation of Disability Inventory (PEDI)
INFORMAL ASSESSMENTS	**DESCRIPTION**	**EXAMPLES**
Self-report measures	Questionnaires completed by parent or teacher using scales and checklists of behaviors and skills	• Pediatric Evaluation of Disability Inventory (PEDI)
Interview	Structured and semi-structured interview to gather and review pertinent information	• Clinical interview with parents and observation of child • Interviews with parent and teacher and observation of child in class or within school context
Observations/ semi-structured checklists	Authentic and ecologically based observations of child's skills and performance in context, activity, interaction	• Observations within classroom, bathroom, outside, snack time, arrival and dismissal • Preschool educational checklist • Self-care checklist • Reflex integration/righting and equilibrium reactions • Range of motion/strength/muscle tone/posture • Sensory system observations • Social-emotional observations • Cognitive/perceptual/body awareness observations
Review of medical records	Respond to initial referral by reviewing medical reports	Practitioners in medical setting discuss orders with other providers

	TABLE 8-4	
	EDUCATIONAL VERSUS MEDICAL MODELS	
CRITERIA	**EDUCATIONAL**	**MEDICAL**
Team	IEP team (including child, family, and educational staff)	Health care professionals
Payment	Federal and state funds support services	Insurance/Medicaid with payment by the family
Focus	Student learning and safety; adaptations and interventions to allow the student to participate, access special education and the school environment	Therapy addresses medical conditions and aims to improve health, fitness, and wellness
Location	School (classroom, hallways, lunchroom, playground); includes transportation and home-based education, if needed	Acute hospital, subacute hospital, and rehabilitation setting (inpatient clinic, outpatient clinic, homebound); home programs are commonly given to the family following the child's hospitalization
Eligibility	Determined by IDEA Part B criteria measured by the preschool team	Determined by health needs appraised by physician or other health professional
Delivery	Services may include inclusive direct, indirect, or consultative services, collaborating with the IEP team for program development and implementation	Services typically involve direct one-on-one interventions to achieve prescribed goals
Documentation	Jargon-free reports for use by family members, IEP team, and related school staff	Discipline-specific reports that meet professional standards and reimbursement criteria
Example: Child with a fractured femur	This is a temporary medical condition that is not covered by IDEA Part B or C. This child would not qualify for physical therapy services in a school setting as long as the child had access to a wheelchair and/or crutches to move between classes	This injury would get immediate attention in an acute care hospital. After the immediate repair and casting of the femur, the child would receive instruction in gait training and wheelchair mobility, followed by outpatient care to regain strength and endurance for walking

an outpatient clinic for leukemia. Ideally, professionals communicate across practice settings to coordinate information sharing with families and to optimize care for children with special needs.

Scope of Practice for Professionals Working With Children 3 to 5 Years

Preschool Setting

Preschool education programs provide the *social context for knowledge development* of preschool-aged children. The aim of preschool education is to deliver safe and quality care, preparing the child for the role of student. Therapists may play an important role in screening children in preschools to assess their developmental skills. Children with disabilities can receive unique and individualized educational programming from the preschool IEP team, as described early in this section. Collaborative relationships develop among the preschool team (typically comprising the parent, teacher, psychologist, principal, speech-language pathologist, occupational therapist, and physical therapist). These educational teams identify the strengths and needs of the child using dynamic evaluation approaches to develop appropriate educational goals and objectives for the child's learning and success in the preschool environment. Successful team interaction is essential for effective intervention services for the child with special needs.[7]

Medical Setting

A preschool-aged child may be referred to or seen within a medical setting for a multitude of reasons based on a medical illness or injury. The physical therapist, occupational therapist, and speech-language pathologist assess the child's needs from their respective scopes of practice and provide evidence-based interventions, along with home programming instructions for parents or caregivers. Family-centered care is widely accepted by hospital and pediatric rehabilitation teams for the child and family. Team meetings are quickly established for the care of the child and to ensure that the family becomes familiar with therapy services for contributions to team decision making. Each discipline brings its respective knowledge of age-appropriate developmental skills. Fostering the child's normalcy is a team goal in this environment, so therapists encourage the child to resume activity as soon as possible, performing their daily tasks and interacting with others. Promoting play and daily routines may help the child cope and manage his inpatient or outpatient experience.

Scope of Practice in Various Settings

The scope of therapeutic practice varies with practice setting because the focus of care is different. Table 8-5 gives examples of the scope of practice and types of service provided to children (3 to 5 years) by physical therapy, speech-language therapy, and occupational therapy in preschool vs other settings.

Interprofessional behaviors are key to success within and across practice settings. Collaboration and discussion among service providers and key stakeholders (eg, parents, teachers, caretakers, and other family members) promotes seamless care and achieves desired outcomes. Although each professional may provide separate services, the interprofessional team values frequent communication to coordinate services and best address the changing needs of the child, family, and teaching staff. Team model approaches offer comprehensive joint planning and decision making.

Becoming an effective team member takes effort through active listening and reflection in communication practices within and between the child's medical and educational team. As practitioners, it is important to know the role and responsibility for each scope of practice area and to appreciate the similarities and difference between service providers. Through this understanding and awareness, team members generate plans and actions contributing to the overall learning and development of the child. For example, a preschool team (comprising a teacher, physical therapist, occupational therapist, and speech-language pathologist) is presented with the situation of a preschool child with ASD who has limited interaction with playground equipment and peers during outdoor recess time. This limited interaction can negatively impact the child's psychosocial and physical development. Each team member can contribute to a team solution for this child's recess, using the knowledge and skills from her respective practice area (Table 8-6).

Often, physical therapists, occupational therapists, and speech-language pathologists working in educational settings travel to multiple building sites, delivering services to a wide range of school-aged children. Given that pediatric therapists may not be on site for daily consultation and program implementation, they must engage in frequent check-ins and facilitate the transfer of training and information between team members for continuity of care.

Referrals

When a young child demonstrates developmental, learning, or behavioral difficulties, the child is closely observed by the teacher, who documents the child's behavior. These issues are brought to the interprofessional team for discussion with the goal of developing and implementing strategies toward resolution of these difficulties. Although

TABLE 8-5		
PROFESSIONALS' THERAPEUTIC SCOPE OF PRACTICE IN EDUCATIONAL AND OTHER SETTINGS		
SERVICES	**FUNCTION OF PROVIDER IN PRESCHOOL SETTING**	**FUNCTION OF PROVIDER IN MEDICAL/COMMUNITY SETTING**
Focus	• Learning through play-based and educational activities	• Return to health through therapeutic and age-appropriate means, including play
Interprofessional	• Education to team and family • Assessment and management of learning activities impacted by disabilities	• Education to team and family • Evaluation and management of acute medical conditions
Physical therapy	• Assessing and addressing factors that impact learning and movement (eg, memory, attention, postural control, mobility, transfers, gross motor skills, pain, breathing, strength, speed, endurance, balance, coordination, functional skills, play activities, and interpersonal skills • Interventions include training and environmental adaptations (eg, equipment, assistive devices, wheelchair seating, safety, risk reduction)	• Assessing and addressing impairments that impact daily function, including postural control and movement (eg, musculoskeletal, cardiopulmonary, respiratory, integumentary, genitourinary, gastrointestinal, and other body systems) • Interventions include management of body systems (eg, pain and burn management) and training in functional skills
Speech-language therapy	• Articulation • Language • Social communication • Play • Augmentative communication • Oral motor and swallowing • Learning and cognition	• Augmentative and alternative communication • Play and social interaction • Communication • Feeding and swallowing • Learning and cognition
Occupational therapy	• Play and learning • Functional motor skills (eg, self-help, eating, managing personal items, toileting) • Preacademics (eg, hand skills, prewriting, visual perceptual skills) • Social participation • Sensorimotor skills • Behavior regulation skills • Feeding and oral motor skills • Adaptive equipment/positioning • Assistive devices	• Learning and behaviors • Functional daily tasks (eg, toileting, grooming, dressing, bathing, transfers) • Play and motor skills (fine and gross) • Feeding and swallowing • Assistive technology devices • Adaptations/modifications to task and environment

TABLE 8-6		
EXAMPLES OF SHARED PLANNING AND RECESS INTERVENTIONS FOR CHILD WITH AUTISM		
PRESCHOOL TEAM MEMBERS	UNIFIED TEAM INTERVENTIONS	DISCIPLINE SPECIFIC INTERVENTIONS
• Physical therapist • Speech-language pathologist • Occupational therapist • Early childhood special education teacher	• Use of group play skills to increase gross motor skills on playground equipment • Visual supports to increase social initiation and group play at recess • Use of social stories to improve social skills during recess • Adult support to assist with turn-taking and group play with playground equipment • Adult modeling and prompting during recess play	• Multisensory activities • Motor imitation training • Physical exercise routines or movement activities • Peer training with model with specific playground equipment • Social stories/narratives • Joint attention training • Natural behavioral interventions; occurs in context • Use of special interests/ personal motivation

interprofessional team members can develop appropriate plans for helping the child with these difficulties, some problems may fall outside of their scope of practice and require referral to other experts. Table 8-7 lists common referrals made for preschool children with special needs.

REIMBURSEMENT

Within the medical setting, inpatient and outpatient services are funded by various sources, including a combination of private insurance carriers, Medicaid, state-funded programs, and/or Medicare. Local insurance companies may have different requirements for therapeutic services, equipment, and assistive devices. Each state has Medicaid protocols and regulations related to funding of therapeutic services. Medicare guidelines are more widespread across the United States. Care for young children can be cost prohibitive, and team members should always be mindful of families' limited financial resources and regulations dictating reimbursement for care.

Coordination of care is essential for reducing confusion for families. Service providers need to share the various concerns of families, including, but not limited to, (1) services provided, including type, intensity, frequency, and duration; (2) cost of services; (3) expected outcomes; (4) short-term and long-term goals; (5) the family's role in care; and (6) plans for when the child is ready to transition to other settings. It is recommended that a case manager work with the

therapy service team and the family to ensure that all parties understand service options and projected costs to coordinate therapeutic care.

In terms of reimbursement, IDEA Part B funds the education of children with disabilities, offered as *free and appropriate public education* (FAPE). Pediatric therapists should become familiar with federal and individual state laws and regulations that define the standards that qualify a preschooler with a disability for these free services. According to IDEA Part B, speech-language services are considered part of special education services and are offered for children with problems with communication and language. Similarly, physical therapy and occupational therapy are offered to children with disabilities but are considered *related services*. Under IDEA 2004, ECSE eligibility is cross-categorical. This means that preschool children with disabilities can present with a wide range of functional and ability levels and receive educational and related services. Examples of ability levels could include a child who has developmental delays in one or more of the following areas: fine motor skills, gross motor skills, communication and language skills, social-emotional skills, and cognitive skills. A child could present with a more global developmental delay, such as ASD, or display mild to severe forms of neurological or musculoskeletal disorders. These children with disabilities all qualify for free educational services tailored to their needs by the interprofessional team and outlined in the IEP.

	TABLE 8-7	
EXAMPLES OF SHARED PLANNING AND RECESS INTERVENTIONS FOR CHILD WITH AUTISM		
PROFESSIONAL	**FORMAL EDUCATION/TRAINING**	**EXPERTISE**
Certified orthotist	Nationally board certified: formal education in biomechanics and material sciences	Designing custom devices, custom-fit orthosis (eg, supramalleolar orthosis, ankle-foot orthosis, knee-ankle-foot orthosis)
Ophthalmologist	Nationally board certified medical doctors: completed residency in ophthalmology	Diagnosing, managing, and treating medical conditions that cause visual impairments
Feeding and swallowing specialist	Advanced certified training: continuing education and training for competence in assessment and intervention of dysphagia	Managing eating and swallowing problems based upon their advanced knowledge of normal and abnormal oral reflexes, swallowing phases, and instrumental assessments (eg, video fluoroscopy and fiber optic endoscopy)
Optometrist	Nationally board certified: doctor of optometry	Providing primary eye care and diagnosing and treating medical conditions causing vision loss
Wheelchair seating specialist/assistive technology provider	Rehabilitation Engineering and Assistive Technology of North America (RESNA) Certification: completed training for customizing positioning equipment and/or assistive devices	Performing equipment evaluations and customizing and fabricating equipment based upon their knowledge of medical necessity

ADVOCACY

For successful programming, all service providers should be advocates for parents/caregivers and children with special needs. As discussed in earlier sections of this book, pediatric therapists working with young children must respect family differences and help families cope and develop effective parenting strategies. Furthermore, the interprofessional team can help families develop their advocacy skills by providing information about their children's physical and mental health conditions and learning needs and by offering suggestions for medical equipment, assistive technology, adaptive devices, and intervention programming to supplement services received during school. Therapists' responsibilities include finding appropriate local, regional, and national resources for the parent to become further informed.

In addition, it is important to recognize the valuable information that families can share with the interprofessional team. Families know their children best and can share valuable insights from their personal experiences, their unique knowledge, and their successes with their children.

The Children Action Network (CAN), as part of the DEC of the Council for Exceptional Children, works to shape policy by providing feedback on current and upcoming legislation, regulations, and funding.[8] Nationally, the DEC works with other organizations such as the National Association for the Education of Young Children (NAEYC) to promote developmentally appropriate practice and provide guidance on inclusion. According to CAN:

> Professionals working with young children with disabilities and children at risk for developmental delays hold a unique perspective. It is imperative that they share their experiences with policy makers…staying informed about key issues through newsletters and email alerts, building and maintaining relationships with policy makers, and sharing perspectives through phone calls, emails, personal visits with elected officials.[9]

Pediatricians, EI providers, special educators, and programs serving individuals with developmental disabilities can strengthen advocacy efforts by aligning efforts with partners such as Head Start and the Women, Infant,

Children (WIC) Program. Advocacy backed by research of evidence-based practice will help to educate those responsible for developing policy and providing needed support. The DEC supports ongoing research efforts related to the individual and unique needs of young children with and at risk for disabilities and their families in early childhood settings.

Transitioning From Early Childhood Special Education to Kindergarten Programs

Finally, the DEC recommends *transition practices* that facilitate the move from one setting to another. Just as infants transition into ECSE from EI, young children with special needs graduate from preschool to enter kindergarten or school-age programs. Not only do parents of children with significant disabilities share common concerns with other families for young children entering a new school, they also worry about losing their strong support systems and wonder how, when, where, and by whom their child's special services will be provided.[10] Thus, entrance into school for children with disabilities can be exceedingly complex and anxiety laden for families.[10] Prior to the transition to elementary school, the ECSE team must identify developmental and family risk factors to ensure that concerns are addressed in the child's educational programs, appropriate referrals, and consultation. Throughout the transition process, ECSE practitioners should support the adjustment of the child and family by exchanging information between settings before, during, and after transitions, as well as incorporating planned strategies to support the adjustment.[10] Table 8-8 lists helpful steps in the collaborative transition process.

Resources For Early Childhood Special Education

Many resources are available to help young children with disabilities. The Centers for Disease Control and Prevention (CDC) and the National Center on Birth Defects and Developmental Disabilities have produced a toolkit to help parents learn about the milestones in their children's growth from birth to age 5, as well as developmental delays and other disabilities. The *Learn the Signs. Act Early.* campaign and Toolkit for Parents on Early Development (www.cdc.gov/ncbddd/autism/actearly) are available in English and Spanish and are designed to help parents recognize any delays so that their children can be screened and receive early treatment, if necessary. The toolkit includes an informational card on developmental milestones, a growth chart, and a series of fact sheets on milestones and developmental and behavioral delays. These materials can be downloaded from the website or ordered in bulk.

Additional websites that can support healthy growth and development of young children include the following:

- BAM! Body and Mind (https://www.cdc.gov/bam/index.html). "This website, developed by the Centers for Disease Control, provides child- and youth-friendly information about disease, food and nutrition, physical activity, and safety as it relates to a young person's life and body."

- The National Dissemination Center for Children with Disabilities (NICHCY) (https://www.nidcd.nih.gov/directory/national-dissemination-center-children-disabilities-nichcy) provides information to parents, communities, educators and the general public on specific disabilities; programs and services for infants, children and youth; U.S. special education law; and effective educational practices. NICHCY also offers links to state agencies, parent groups and organizations around the country that offer assistance and information."

- Born Learning Campaign (www.bornlearning.org). "The United Way of America, partnering with the Ad Council and Civitas, created a website that helps parents, caregivers, and communities create high-quality early learning opportunities using everyday events for young children. The website provides comprehensive developmental information on children from birth to 5 years of age."

- Pacer Center: Parent Advocacy Coalition for Educational Rights (www.pacer.org). "The center was created by parents with children with disabilities to help other parents with similar experiences. The site offers a wealth of resources, including associated links, newsletters, and publications on issues related to special education and disability."

- AblePlay (www.ableplay.org). "Developed by the National Lekotek Center, AblePlay™ is a toy rating system and website that provides comprehensive information on toys for children with special needs, so parents, special educators, therapists, and others can make the best choices. Toys are categorized according to disability and age group."

- CanChild Centre for Childhood Disability Research (www.canchild.ca). "The focus of this organization is to support research on children and youth with disabilities within communities where they live. Links on the website for families and providers offer comprehensive summaries of research findings that relate to improved quality of life for families and children."

TABLE 8-8	
STEPS IN THE COLLABORATIVE TRANSITION PROCESS	
TIME OF YEAR	**TASK AND PERSON RESPONSIBLE**
November prior to transition into kindergarten	Individualized Education Program (IEP) team/preschool team: • Writes a kindergarten transition letter to the family of a child receiving special education services who will be eligible for kindergarten the following year • Asks the family for a response to the transition letter • Invites the family to become part of a collaborative decision-making team for the transition
December to April	Sending school staff, including physical therapist, occupational therapist, and speech-language pathologist: • Observes the receiving kindergarten and meet with kindergarten teachers, related services staff, and school principal
December to April	Family (at their convenience with IEP team or separately): • Observes the receiving kindergarten and meets with kindergarten teachers, related services staff, and school principal
December to April	IEP team and receiving school: • Hold an informal collaborative meeting to discuss the transition process
February to April	Receiving school: • Observes the child in the preschool classroom • Shares information related to child's preparation for entering kindergarten
April to June	Physical therapist, occupational therapist, and speech-language pathologist: • Share relevant progress records • Makes recommendations to the IEP team regarding goals, activities, and needed equipment/assistive technology
April to June	Parents, parent representatives, sending and receiving school staff, and district administrator: • Have the annual IEP review/initial school-age special education meeting to develop the IEP; all collaborating team members attend and participate
May to June prior year	IEP team, including family: • Participate in the annual IEP meeting • Discuss the child's progress • Develop an IEP for the upcoming year • Discuss changes to anticipate in kindergarten and encourage the family's involvement
April to August	Receiving school staff: • Orders needed materials and equipment
August/ September	Family and child: • Participate in orientation activities
September	Receiving school staff: • Ensures that the child is included in kindergarten with proper supports and services for success

SUMMARY

Educational services for young children with special needs older than 3 are specified in IDEA Part B. The DEC of the Council for Exceptional Children provides guidelines for implementing this law, offering interprofessional best practices for optimizing outcomes for these children. Pediatric therapists play key roles in identifying both family and developmental risk factors, selecting age-appropriate screening and assessment tools commonly used with this population, and recognizing the scope of practice for professionals working with 3- to 5-year-olds. As part of the team providing ECSE, therapists must shift their focus from family-centered EI to child-centered education, supporting the child's IEP for academic readiness to enter elementary school. Service for these young children and their families continues to build on advocacy for families' needs, educational services for their children, and community development for increased opportunities for inclusion.

INTERPROFESSIONAL ACTIVITY

Working With Young Children, Their Families, and Their Teachers

As you look at the following case studies, review the relevant information, reflect on the roles of all involved, and answer each of the following questions with your interprofes-sional team:

1. How would you describe your role in the ECSE program to this family?

2. Based upon criteria given in the case, is the child eligible for ECSE?

3. What concerns do you think a preschool teacher would have about the child?

4. How would you communicate with the family, given their situation?

5. As a team, how would you organize your assessment of the child?

6. What types of recommendations would you make in terms of functional goals, based upon IDEA Part B?

7. What information would you give the parents and teacher to promote advocacy?

8. How would you help this child and his/her family transition to elementary school?

Case 8-1: A 3-year-old girl at risk for developmental delay

Nicole was born at 36 weeks' gestation via Cesarean section with a 6-day stay in the neonatal intensive care unit (NICU) before going home. Her mother reports that Nicole did not smile until 4 months, sat independently at approximately 12 months, and started walking around 29 to 30 months. She reports that Nicole has received physical therapy, occupational therapy, and speech-language therapy since she was 12 months old. She was diagnosed with a developmental delay. Nicole is now integrated into a half-day preschool program 4 mornings a week. She is mobile in her environment but demonstrates poor balance and uses a wide base of support, her arms at shoulder height when walking. Nicole can kick a ball but falls once with 3 kicks. She ascends and descends stairs in marking time with both hands holding onto the rails. She is unable to walk heel to toe, stand on one foot, or jump. Nicole throws a ball with trunk rotation to assist in the throwing motion. She demonstrates palmar grip around all objects. Her mother states that Nicole mainly prefers to use her left hand, but she does not currently show any hand preference when coloring and will switch hand usage. Nicole uses her thumb and all 4 fingers to grasp smaller-sized objects and turn the pages of a thick book. She has limited social play skills and prefers to play by herself. Her attention span is limited, and she is distracted if the task is too hard for her to complete. She is unable to understand or follow simple tasks, requiring extra cues from adults. She has difficulty expressing her wants and needs to peers and adults. Her developmental screening continues to reveal functional skills at the developmental age of 15 to 20 months.

Case 8-2: A 4-year-old boy with cerebral palsy

Adam is a 4-year-old boy with spastic cerebral palsy presenting with intermittent hypertonicity of all extremities and hypotonicity of head, neck, and trunk. He has obligatory tonic reflexes for asymmetrical tonic neck reflex (ANTR) and symmetrical tonic neck reflex (STNR) and poor gross motor control. Adam has fair fine motor control of his left hand/fingers when provided postural support in a position chair with lap tray. When positioned properly, he is able to reach and grasp items asymmetrically with his left hand/arm. He has limited right arm and hand use and requires physical cues to place in midline for hold-and-do tasks.

When concentrating on throwing or maneuvering with his left hand/arm, his right hand is observed to present with palmar reflex as he clutches fingers together tightly. Although cognition appears to be on target, his speech is severely dysarthric, making communication a concern. It is often hard to hear Adam as he speaks due to limited breath control. He is unable to assume sitting or standing and cannot maintain sitting without support and physical assistance. He is dependent upon an adult for mobility in a manual wheelchair that he is currently outgrowing. Adam currently has a normal body mass index for his age. He likes to look at books and is developing reading skills. He watches and will interact with peers if they are within his proximity. Adam will be going to a new elementary school next fall, and the IEP team will be addressing his needs for adaptive equipment and devices to function in the kindergarten classroom. His mother would like recommendations for therapeutic positioning to prevent deformities, continued focus on Adam becoming toilet trained, and options for assistive technology to keep up with the kindergarten curriculum.

Case 8-3: A 3-year-old boy with cerebral palsy

Art is a 3 year 11 month old boy who was born prematurely (at 32 weeks' gestation) via emergency Cesarean section (C-section) due to fetal distress. He weighed 2250 grams at birth (low birth weight) and remained in NICU for 6 weeks with ventilation. Art's feeding was poor; he had a weak suck; and he had difficulty coordinating respiration. Motor milestones were delayed due to persistent primitive reflexes, variable muscle tone and intermittent clonus. Art was diagnosed with cerebral palsy, athetoid type prior to his first birthday. Art has been followed by physical therapy, occupational therapy, and speech-language pathology since birth and through a children's therapy center prior to transitioning to a LEA preschool program. Art currently attends preschool 5 mornings a week for special education and related services in addition to receiving weekly therapeutic services in the home.

Art displays irregular, involuntary movements of arms and legs. He can become quite excited when the other children are around him which increases his muscle tone and movements. His jerky movements make it extremely difficult to isolate movement of one part of his body. Accessibility for Art is a key focus of his IEP preschool team for social participation and functional control/coordination to assist with his play, gross motor, fine motor, and self-care tasks. He is dependent upon adults for postural control, functional mobility, hygiene (toilet care), and feeding. Prior to transitioning to preschool programming, Art received a customized wheelchair with tray and is currently being fitted for new ankle foot orthoses to provide postural support. When he is on a crowded bus, Art becomes excited and his arms get caught in the wheelchair during the bus ride to and from school. When Art is properly positioned, he is able to activate a switch for cause and effect toys using elbow motion to press down on the "big red button." The IEP preschool team is addressing positioning and communication needs during the day. Another area of importance is to create an area in the preschool room that can be modified to help reduce Art's tendency to become overstimulated by sensory input, allowing him to engage in functional and play tasks. The development of Art's oral motor skills is of importance to his family as they are fearful of recommended placement of a gastrostomy tube (G-tube) for his feeding and nutritional needs. Frequent discussion and contact between the school, family, and other professionals working with Art is essential.

Case 8-4: A 3-year-old boy with autism spectrum disorder

Caleb is a 3 year 6 month old boy with a diagnosis of ASD and developmental delay. He lives at home with his parents and older brother who is home-schooled. His mother reports that she had a normal pregnancy and that Caleb was delivered by C-section. His developmental milestones are delayed in the areas of communication and motor skills. There is a family history of ASD, seizures, and diabetes and heart problems.

Caleb has received educational services through First Steps (EI) and is currently attending ECSE and receiving physical therapy, occupational therapy, and speech-language pathology services. He requires one-on-one direction for preacademic and the majority of functional tasks. He consistently displays self-stimulatory behaviors when not engaged. Typical sensory behaviors for Caleb include arm/hand flapping, twirling a toy/object, flicking fingers at lights in room, and twirling his body in circles. He will run, but will put his arms out in a medium guard position. His balance and coordination are delayed for climbing stairs, throwing and catching balls, and jumping or standing on one foot. Caleb enjoys swinging, but becomes agitated if assisted to climb upon other playground equipment (eg, monkey bars, slide). He often gets upset when he has to be brought in from recess activities. He is able to imitate simple motor actions with practice. He avoids using classroom tools such as scissors, chalk, markers, and brushes. His attention to non-preferred tasks is limited. He is visually distracted by events occurring in the classroom and can become over stimulated from noise and will cover his ears. He will spend time looking at a computer screen and iPad if allowed. During snack time, Caleb eats only preferred items such as chips and crackers. He uses his fingers to eat and will not try fruit or vegetable items. He is able to drink from a straw but needs help to open milk carton. Caleb has limited speech and will repeat sing-song rhymes, or repeat simple greetings such as "Hi, hi," or "Goodbye, goodbye." He often walks out of his shoes, and is unaware of his coat or backpack and what he should do with these items.

Case 8-5: A 4-year-old girl with multiple disabilities

Monica is 4 years 7 months old with a diagnosis of 18q syndrome, ocular apraxia. This syndrome causes growth problems and developmental delays. She lives with her parents and younger brother and sister. Monica's family is involved with many medical needs and regularly communicates with preschool staff. She has received services since infancy and is being evaluated as she transitions into school-age programming next fall. She is currently in an ECSE classroom and receives physical therapy, occupational therapy, speech-language therapy, and special education programming. She is nonambulatory and has a wheelchair with customized tray. Monica is able to sit without support for longer periods of time (4 to 6 minutes) and demonstrates fair postural control while in sitting position with proper setup. She does not have protective responses to catch herself if she loses her balance in sitting. When pulled to sit, she is able to maintain her head in midline position. She presents with decreased muscle tone overall. She does have full range of motion for arms, hands, and legs. With positioning and lap tray, Monica is able to reach and grasp medium-sized objects with elbow extended, forearm pronated, and wrist flexed. She attempts to grab smaller objects using a raking motion with her fingers. She is able to poke or press a switch with either her right or left palm or index finger when positioned in a prone stander with tray.

Monica is dependent upon adults for feeding. She typically holds her mouth in an open position, with drooling observed. When food is introduced, she holds her head in extensor pattern. She is able to close her lips around a straw and suck for regular liquids, with some spillage as she releases the straw from her lips. Monica has minimal spillage when taking thickened or semisolid liquids from a nosey cup. She will not bite solid-type foods. Monica uses a munching/chewing pattern of her jaw and lips when food items are placed on her tongue. She has limited lateral, side-to-side movements of her tongue. When provided food items to the side of her mouth, Monica is beginning to move her tongue to the side to initiate a munching/chewing pattern. She grinds her teeth during nonfood activities. She is dependent in hygiene and dressing activities. She will quiet her arms while being dressed with a shirt or coat. She smiles and enjoys music and animated videos with her peers.

REFERENCES

1. Center for Parent Resources and Information. Part B of IDEA: Services for School-Aged Children. Center for Parent Resources and Information Web site. http://www.parentcenterhub.org/repository/partb/. Published September 24, 2010. Accessed January 24, 2017.
2. Division of Early Childhood. DEC recommended practices in early intervention/early childhood special education. Division of Early Childhood Web site. http://www.dec-sped.org/dec-recommended-practices. Published 2014. Accessed January 24, 2017.
3. Verenikina I. Scaffolding and learning: Its role in nurturing new learners. In: Kell P, Vialle W, Konza D, Vogl G, eds. *Learning and the Learner: Exploring Learning for New Times.* Wollongong, Australia: University of Wollongong; 2008:236.
4. Morin A. ADHD: What you're seeing in your preschooler. Understood Web site. https://www.understood.org/en/learning-attention-issues/child-learning-disabilities/add-adhd/adhd-what-youre-seeing-in-your-preschooler?gclid=Cj0KEQiAwrbEBRDqxqzMsrTGmogBEiQAeSE6ZQnNqaCl5cI2kglJs6JzrZ79Xjqb6sfAIOBph0hEOEQaAtXe8P8HAQ. Published 2014. Accessed January 27, 2017.
5. US Department of Education. Building the Legacy: IDEA 2004. US Department of Education Web site. http://idea.ed.gov/explore/view/p/,root,regs,300,D,300.304,.html. Published July, 2013. Accessed December 11, 2017.
6. Rainforth B. Analysis of physical therapy practice acts: implications for role release in educational environments. *Pediatric Physical Therapy.* 1997;9:54-61.
7. Bose P, Hinojosa J. Reported experiences from occupational therapist interacting with teachers in inclusive early childhood classroom. *Am J Occup Ther.* 2008;62:289-297.
8. DEC. Promoting the Health, Safety and Well-Being of Young Children with Disabilities and Developmental Delays. University of Kansas Web site. https://kskits.drupal.ku.edu/sites/kskits.drupal.ku.edu/files/docs/DEC_Promoting_the_Health_Safety_Well_Being.pdf. Published September, 2012. Accessed December 11, 2017.
9. Turnbull A, Turnbull R, Erwin E, Soodak L, Shogren KA. *Families, Professionals and Exceptionality: Positive Outcomes Through Partnership and Trust.* 6th ed. Upper Saddle River, NJ: Pearson; 2011.
10. Fenlon A. Paving the way to kindergarten for young children with disabilities. Reading Rockets Web site. http://www.readingrockets.org/article/paving-way-kindergarten-young-children-disabilities. Published 2005. Accessed January 24, 2017.

Section 9

Providing Support for Children 5 to 21 Years in the Educational Setting

Joan Delahunt, OTD, MS, OTR/L; Mildred Oligbo, PT, DPT; Pamela Hart, PhD, CCC-SLP; and Catherine Rush Thompson, PT, PhD, MS

OVERVIEW

This section builds on foundational interprofessional concepts, discussing how physical therapists, occupational therapists, and speech-language pathologists work collaboratively with others to support school-aged students in educational settings. While many children with congenital problems receive therapy services from birth through early intervention (EI) services and early childhood special education (ECSE), others begin receiving special education at age 5 or later. This section illustrates how the interprofessional team supports a child's education from 5 to 22 years of age, describing common risk factors, including bullying and cyberbullying, obesity, youth suicide, concussions, addiction to drugs, internet addiction, school violence, low socioeconomic level, and academic failure. It also provides a range of discipline-specific and interprofessional tests and measures commonly used in educational settings. In addition, it offers suggestions for evidence-based strategies that can be used for team management of pediatric conditions commonly seen in elementary, middle, and high schools, including long-term therapeutic support provided to children with chronic conditions. Finally, it offers suggestions of how to build a children's self-advocacy as they develop into adults. Upon completion of this section, the learner will be able to (1) describe common risk factors that are encountered in educational settings, (2) compare and contrast tests and measures used by team members, (3) describe evidence-based interprofessional strategies used in school settings, and (4) discuss how the interprofessional team can empower children and adolescents to advocate for themselves.

INTERPROFESSIONAL SCHOOL SERVICES

Occupational therapists, physical therapists, and speech-language pathologists play important roles in the educational programming for children with special needs. In school settings, therapists and educators work together to support children with special needs across academic, psychosocial, and sensorimotor areas of development. The overarching goal of these collaborative services is to support each child's ability to achieve her highest potential within the educational curriculum. As such, therapists and educators must

Thompson CR. *Pediatric Therapy:*
An Interprofessional Framework for Practice (pp 133-148).
© 2018 SLACK Incorporated.

have extensive knowledge of individualized assessment and intervention, the range of possible assistive technologies to provide children the opportunity to access learning materials, and an understanding of how classroom design may impact learning for specific children. All children, regardless of the severity of their disability, are entitled to a *free appropriate public education* (FAPE) in the *least restrictive environment* (LRE). It is the role of interprofessional special education teams to address learning challenges and barriers so that each child is able to reach her highest learning potential, as discussed in Section 8.

CONSIDERATION OF RISK AND PROTECTIVE FACTORS IN AN EDUCATIONAL SETTING

Within educational settings, children, adolescents and young adults may encounter risk factors that can affect learning and participation. In this context, a *risk factor* is defined as an individual or environmental characteristic, condition, or behavior that increases the chance that a negative outcome will occur.[1] Conversely, the presence of *protective factors*, including social support and unique individual or environmental characteristics, conditions, or behaviors, can reduce the negative impact of risk factors.[1] The presence or absence, as well as the various combinations of protective and risk factors, contributes to the overall health of children and youth.

Common risk factors facing students include bullying and cyberbullying,[2] obesity,[3] youth suicide,[4] concussions,[5] addiction to drugs,[6] internet addiction,[7] school violence,[8] low socioeconomic level,[9] and academic failure.[10] Students' protective factors include, but are not limited to, emotional self-regulation, active engagement with school, positive engagement with peers, and athletics.[1] Professionals working in educational settings can serve as protective factors through mentoring and providing clear expectations for behavior and physical/psychological safety.[1] All of these protective factors aid in counterbalancing the negative risk factors' effect on youth.[1] Children and youth with medical conditions and disabilities are at increased risk for many of these risk factors, particularly obesity and bullying.[4] Conditions associated with an increased risk of suicide include chronic pain, loss of mobility, disfigurement, cognitive styles that make problem solving a challenge, asthma, multiple sclerosis, and spinal cord injuries.[4] All school personnel, including pediatric therapists, can provide social support and help children develop the protective factors that can help prevent academic failure.

SCREENING AND EVALUATION

Assessment of an individual student involves a multitude of factors, including age of the student, type of educational setting, specific areas of concern for the student, availability of screening and evaluation tools, and which professional team members should contribute to this process. As a school team, each member is asked to (1) provide individual viewpoints on what areas should be assessed, (2) suggest particular tools for assessment, (3) complete the agreed-upon assessment(s), (4) document assessment results, and (5) provide recommendations based upon interprofessional clinical decision making. Interprofessional collaboration emphasizes the expectation of all team members working in concert to provide a comprehensive picture of each student's strengths and areas of concern.

Within educational settings, specific guidelines for the process of qualifying a student for special education services helps to guide the interdisciplinary team in determining the focus for the initial evaluation. As a team, each member shares her observations of the student, and collaboratively they develop an evaluation plan that can be set into motion. During this process, each practitioner must openly discuss her concerns and ideas for evaluating specific areas of need.

Physical therapists, occupational therapists, and speech-language pathologists have unique expertise and discipline-specific tests and measures that address categories outlined in the International Classification of Functioning, Disabilities, and Health (ICF) Model (Table 9-1).[11] Although discipline-specific tests are useful in isolated situations, most assessments designed for use within educational settings are interdisciplinary in nature. Thus, team members are encouraged to perform screening and/or evaluation assessments collaboratively within the same educational environment(s), such as the classroom, gymnasium, playground, cafeteria, hallway, bathroom, or school bus. This shared experience allows for rich dialogue among all professionals. Additionally, this collaboration ensures a comprehensive plan of care culminating in the Individualized Education Plan (IEP),[12] as detailed in Section 8. However, some situations exist where team-based assessments do not provide enough detailed information about a student's performance. Individual school professionals may decide to assess the student independently, using discipline-specific measures to provide detailed data. The decision to complete an interdisciplinary team evaluation or several discipline-specific evaluations depends upon key factors, including (1) the familiarity of the team members with one another, (2) the intended purpose of the evaluation data, (3) the severity and chronicity of the student's condition, (4) prior evaluation data from other sources, (5) the availability of assessment tools, (6) time available for evaluation, and (7) state regulations regarding accepted assessment tools.

TABLE 9-1
DISCIPLINE-SPECIFIC ROLES AND RESPONSIBILITIES IN SCHOOL SETTINGS

RELATED SERVICES	PRIMARY FUNCTION IN SCHOOL SETTINGS
Physical therapy	• *Mobility throughout the school*: Training the child to move as independently as possible through hallways, negotiate stairs, and move on the playground (this may involve the use of adaptive and assistive devices, such as customized motorized wheelchairs, walkers, crutches, and orthotics) • *Transfers at school*: Teaching the child how to perform safe and efficient transfers to/from therapeutic equipment, transportation, desk seat, and toilet • *Postural control*: Positioning the child to facilitate attention, comfort, and safety during learning activities while preventing secondary complications • *Motor skills*: Enabling the child to engage in school-related activities (eg, gym, adaptive physical education, field trips, playground activities) • *Cardiopulmonary rehabilitation*: Ensuring that children with decreased endurance have properly paced activities throughout the school day • *Neuromuscular training*: Providing resources to enhance motor control • *Education of stakeholders*: School team members, children with special needs, all children in the school setting, families, legislators, community members
Speech-language therapy	• Articulation • Language • Social communication • Play • Voice • Resonance • Fluency • Social Skills • Feeding and Swallowing • Cognition • Literacy • Augmentative communication • Oral motor and swallowing • Learning and cognition • Education to team and family
Occupational therapy	• Play and learning • Functional motor skills (self-help, eating, managing personal items, toileting) • Preacademics (hand skills, prewriting, visual perceptual skills) • Social participation • Sensorimotor skills • Behavior regulation skills • Feeding and oral motor skills • Adaptive equipment/positioning • Assistive devices • Education to team and family

Common areas of concern for students with special needs range from their issues related to mental health and physical performance to environmental factors impacting a child's ability to learn. Practitioners can work collaboratively to determine which assessments best detect risk factors and issues impacting each child's learning. Table 9-2 displays the broad areas of concern paired with, based upon categories in the ICF Model, examples of team-based assessments and suggested team members. Additional details about these tests and measures are listed in Appendix B.

SCHOOL-BASED INTERVENTIONS

The educational environment provides a setting where students with special needs are given supports to aid their learning and development into adulthood. Within this complex environment, multiple factors influence the success of each child's ability to benefit from his educational experience. After identifying risk factors impacting a child's education, school professionals work together to foster the student's protective factors while developing additional strategies to boost the child's resilience.

Throughout the country, school professionals typically gather together weekly to discuss students who display at-risk behaviors in the school setting. In this dialogue, each professional shares observations and suggestions to assist the student. Teams also review each student's protective factors, which may include a supportive family, close communication with a trusted teacher, and/or the student's level of motivation to achieve high grades. Together the team assesses all factors and provides a support plan for the particular student. This plan might incorporate the speech-language pathologist as a motivator for the student to participate in recess by developing a plan for using a peer buddy to facilitate playing on the playground equipment. Another example might be the school nurse, physical therapist, and occupational therapist working together to initiate a "healthy choices after school program" to target students with obesity. Physical therapists and occupational therapists may team with high school football coaches on concussion prevention and management programs. Through creative planning, school teams can work to address risk factors affecting students to facilitate improved educational outcomes. Table 9-3 lists common problems or risk factors encountered in the school setting, protective factors, and interprofessional strategies commonly used to manage these problems.

RESPONSE TO INTERVENTION

One collaborative process used to deliver services in educational settings is called *Response to Intervention* (RtI). RtI is a multitiered approach designed for the early identification and support of students with learning and behavior needs.[13,14] Within this methodical process, school professionals gather to follow the recommended guidelines implicit within each tier and outlined in this model. School professionals may be asked to assist general education teachers within this practice. The RtI process begins with high-quality instruction and universal screening of all children in the general education classroom.[13,14]

Common issues within the general education classroom include difficulties with handwriting, language, social interaction, sitting at a desk, following directions, and reading and math skills. General education teachers identify a student's specific challenges and initiate the 3-tiered RtI process. Tier 1 involves whole-class intervention strategies; Tier 2 focuses on small-group interventions; while Tier 3 is reserved for individualized, intensive interventions.[13] RtI addresses both the academic and behavioral health needs of all students, particularly those at risk. Figure 9-1 illustrates the tiered RtI model used to provide appropriate, inclusive services for children identified at-risk in the classroom.

Pediatric professionals can contribute to this tiered process through consultation and classroom support. Speech-language pathologists, occupational therapists, and physical therapists are most commonly involved in Tier 3 interventions but may be invited to assist at any tier. For example, within Tier 1, the teacher may invite the occupational therapist to suggest age-appropriate self-care and fine motor skills that enable children of all ability levels to succeed. Tier 2 interventions involve small groups, so the physical therapist may assist in adaptive physical education classes, aiding children needing additional physical prompts or supports. Tier 3 interventions are more intensive and specialized to individual students. At this tier, pediatric professionals work directly with the student on targeted skills to determine whether an IEP is needed. An example of Tier 3 interventions includes a speech-language pathologist working for a trial of 4 sessions with a first-grade student on producing developmentally appropriate sounds correctly in his speech. Following this structured intervention, the therapist may encourage a transdisciplinary approach for reinforcing this skill development. The speech-language pathologist would provide discipline-specific assessments and high-quality, evidence-based instructional methods and interventions; data collection and data-based decision making; and progress monitoring. Across all 3 tiers of RtI, pediatric professionals seek to find strategies to effectively integrate evidence-based interventions into the daily school routines of the student.[15,16]

TABLE 9-2			
INTERPROFESSIONAL ASSESSMENTS IN THE EDUCATIONAL SETTING			
CATEGORY	ASSESSMENT	DESCRIPTION	INTERPROFESSIONAL TEAM MEMBERS
Participation (including activities, environmental factors)	Scales of Independent Behavior-Revised (SIB-R) Ages: 3 months to over 90 years	Measures functional independence and adaptive functioning (motor skills, social interaction and communication skills, personal living skills, and community living skills) in school, home, employment, and community settings	School psychologist, physical therapist, occupational therapist, speech-language pathologist, general education teachers, special education teacher, behavior therapist, parents
	School Function Assessment (SFA) Ages: Elementary school students	Measures function in the school environment, including participation in school activity settings, task supports, and activity performance (physical and cognitive/behavioral tasks)	Physical therapist, occupational therapist, school counselor, general education teachers, special
Activities (including function in educational settings)	Assessment of Functional Living Skills (AFLS) Ages: 2 years and up	Provides a systematic way to evaluate, track, and teach functional, adaptive, and self-help skills	Behavior therapist, occupational therapist, general education teacher, special education teacher, school psychologist, speech-language pathologist
	Assessment of Motor and Process Skills (AMPS)	An observational assessment with 16 motor and 20 process skills items, including complex or instrumental and personal activities of daily living	Physical therapist, occupational therapist, speech-language pathologist, general education teacher, special education teacher
	Bruininks-Oseretsky Test of Motor Proficiency (BOTMP) Ages: 4½ to 14½ years	Assesses balance, strength, coordination, running speed and agility, upper limb coordination (ball skills), dexterity, fine motor control, visual-motor	Physical therapist, occupational therapist
	Developmental Assessment for Individuals with Severe Disabilities–Third Edition (DASH-3)	Criterion-referenced assessment with 5 scales to measure rate of developmental progress	Physical therapist, occupational therapist, general education teacher, special education teacher, school psychologist, speech-language pathologist
	Functional Independence Skills Handbook (FISH)	Determines a person's ability to perform certain functional activities from daily life. It was developed for special education teachers, paraeducators, and parents working with individuals with severe developmental disabilities.	Behavior therapist, occupational therapist, general education teacher, special education teacher, school psychologist, speech-language pathologist
			(continued)

TABLE 9-2 (CONTINUED)			
INTERPROFESSIONAL ASSESSMENTS IN THE EDUCATIONAL SETTING			
CATEGORY	**ASSESSMENT**	**DESCRIPTION**	**INTERPROFESSIONAL TEAM MEMBERS**
Activities (including function in educational settings)	Functional Assessment and Curriculum for Teaching Everyday Routines (FACTER)	Assesses and teaches students with moderate to severe developmental disabilities everyday routines	Occupational therapist, general education teacher, special education teacher, school psychologist, speech-language pathologist
	Pediatric Evaluation of Disability Inventory (PEDI) Ages: 6 months to 7 years, 6 months	Uses 271 items to assess self-care (eating, grooming, dressing, bathing, toileting), mobility (transfers, indoors and outdoors mobility), and social function (communication, social interaction, household and community tasks); includes scales for environmental modification and amount of caregiver assistance	Parent, general education teacher, special education teacher, physical therapist, occupational therapist, speech-language pathologist
	Vineland Adaptive Behavior Scales (VABS) Ages: Birth to 90 years	Measures adaptive behavior (motor, social interaction and communication, self-care skills and community skills)	School psychologist, physical therapist, occupational therapist, speech-language pathologist, general education teachers, special education teacher, behavior therapist, parents
Impairments (focus on mental health)[38,43]	Behavioral and Emotional Screening System Student Self-Report Form (BESS) Grades: 3 to 12	Uses a 30-item rating scale for child-reported risks for behavioral and emotional problems	School psychologist, counselor, occupational therapist, school nurse, general education teacher, special education teacher, behavior specialist, principal
	Patient Health Questionnaire-9 item Grades: 6 to 12	Screen for anxiety	School psychologist, school counselor, general education teacher, special education teacher, occupational therapist, school nurse, principal, physical therapist
	5-Item Screen for Child Anxiety-Related Emotional Disorders Grades: 6 to 12	Screen for anxiety	School psychologist, school counselor, general education teacher, special education teacher, occupational therapist, school nurse, principal, physical therapist

TABLE 9-3
RISK FACTORS AND INTERPROFESSIONAL MANAGEMENT

RISK FACTOR	PROTECTIVE FACTOR	STRATEGY DESCRIPTION	TEAM MEMBERS
Bullying[40] and cyberbullying[47]	• Social support • Opportunities for children to talk about problems • Be as obvious about discussing cyberbullying as bullying face-to-face[48]	• Create a community for adults and pupils to send a unified message against cyberbullying/ bullying • Install a cell phone monitoring app (eg, Pumpic)	• All team members and school
Obesity[44,46]	• Support group, including team members and at-risk youth	• "Healthy choices" after-school program[39] • Graded exercise programs	• Teacher, occupational therapist, physical therapist, school nurse, school nutritionist
Youth suicide[42] The most frequently cited risk factors for suicide are: • Major depression (feeling down in a way that impacts your daily life) or bipolar disorder (severe mood swings) • Problems with alcohol or drugs • Unusual thoughts and behavior or confusion about reality • Personality traits that create a pattern of intense, unstable relationships or trouble with the law • Impulsivity and aggression, especially along with a mental disorder • Previous suicide attempt or family history of a suicide attempt or mental disorder • Serious medical condition and/or pain	• A crisis intervention team • Receiving effective mental health care • Positive connections to family, peers, community, and social institutions such as marriage and religion that foster resilience • The skills and ability to solve problems	• Identify at-risk student through a risk assessment	• All team members and school staff
Concussion[49,50]	• Close coach-player relationship • Neck strength is a significant predictor for concussion[49]	• Concussion prevention program • Protective helmets and facial protective equipment[50]	• Teacher, physical therapist, occupational therapist, speech-language pathologist, football coach, school psychologist

(continued)

Table 9-3 (continued)

Risk Factors and Interprofessional Management

RISK FACTOR	PROTECTIVE FACTOR	STRATEGY DESCRIPTION	TEAM MEMBERS
Drug addiction and substance abuse[45]	• School domain protective factors[51] • Opportunities for youths who perceive more chances • Involvement in prosocial activities • Involvement in school • Rewards for prosocial youths	• Involve students with clubs at school • Provide teacher-student mentors • Educate students about drugs and drug abuse • Offer support groups to students and their parents who struggle with drug or substance abuse	• Teacher, coach, occupational therapist, school counselor, social worker
Internet addiction[52]	• Parent-child relationship[52] • Emotional regulation[52]	• Surround students with a supportive environment • Controlling the computer and internet use • Promoting book reading • Providing treatment to those with a psychological problem	• Teacher, social worker, school counselor, occupational therapist, speech-language pathologist
School violence[53]	• Intensive supervision[52] • Clear behavior rules[52] • Consistent negative reinforcement of aggression[52] • Engagement of parents and teachers[52]	• Strong connections with students and school professionals[52] • Commitment to school (an investment in school and in doing well at school)[52] • Close relationships with peer role models[52] • Membership in peer groups that do not promote antisocial behavior[52] • Involvement in prosocial activities[52]	• Teachers, school counselor, speech-language pathologist, occupational therapist, physical therapist, social worker, coach, building principal

(continued)

TABLE 9-3 (CONTINUED)

RISK FACTORS AND INTERPROFESSIONAL MANAGEMENT

RISK FACTOR	PROTECTIVE FACTOR	STRATEGY DESCRIPTION	TEAM MEMBERS
Academic failure[53]	• Strong relationship between school connectedness and educational outcomes[53] • School attendance[53] • Staying in school longer[53] • Higher grades and classroom test scores[53] • Students who do well academically are less likely to engage in risky behaviors[53]	• Perceived adult support • Relationships with strong peers • Dedication to school by both students and school personnel	• Teachers, school counselor, speech-language pathologist, occupational therapist, physical therapist, coach, building principal
Low socioeconomic status[54]	• Adult caring and support[56] • Opportunities for meaningful participation[56] • High expectations[56]	• Engage community partners to provide a range of services at the school that students and their families need, such as dental services, health screenings, child care, substance abuse treatment)[54,55] • Nurturing staff and positive role models[56] • Creative, supportive school leadership[56] • Peer support, cooperation, and mentoring[56] • Personal attention and interest from teachers[56] • Warm, responsive school climate[56] • Minimum mastery of basic skills[56] • Emphasis on higher-order academics[56] • Avoidance of negative labeling and tracking[56] • Leadership and decision-making by students[56] • Student participation in extracurricular activities[56] • Parent and community participation in instruction[56] • Culturally diverse curricula and experiences[56]	• Teachers, school counselor, speech-language pathologist, occupational therapist, physical therapist, coach, building principal

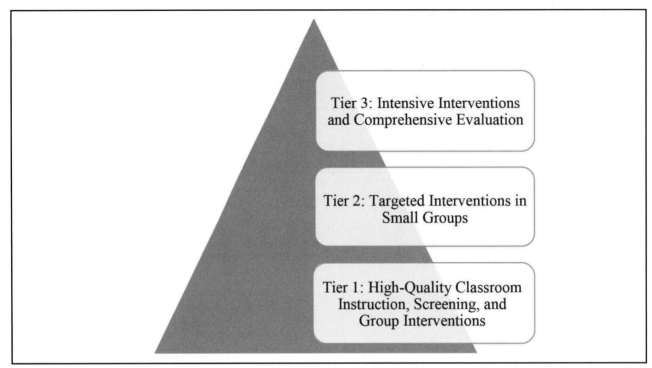

Figure 9-1. Response to intervention strategies used in school settings.

INTERPROFESSIONAL MANAGEMENT FOR COMMON CHRONIC CONDITIONS

Students with chronic conditions commonly qualify for special education services. *Chronic conditions* are defined as health issues that have persisted for 3 months or more, impacting a child's normal daily activities and typically involving extensive medical care.[17] Evidence reveals that the current prevalence of pediatric chronic conditions averages 26%.[18] Some examples of chronic conditions include, but are not limited to, asthma, diabetes, cerebral palsy, sickle cell anemia, cystic fibrosis, cancer, aids, epilepsy, spina bifida, obesity, and congenital heart defects.[19-22]

Chronic health conditions during childhood and adolescence impact physical, emotional, and/or mental functioning, leading to disruptions in school attendance and in completion of school work.[18] Due to their high number of required hospitalizations and ongoing medical appointments, students with chronic conditions do not enjoy the consistency of school participation compared with their peers. Therefore, school professionals must collaborate to create cohesive plans to support these particular students to maintain active engagement within the educational setting.[15,16] For children with complex medical conditions, physical therapists, occupational therapists, and speech-language pathologists serve as ongoing school-based health care resources for students, teachers, and parents.

A key variable present with children with chronic condition is stress.[21] *Stress* for children with chronic conditions can be described as a state of mental or emotional strain or tension resulting from adverse or very demanding circumstances.[21] Stresses in childhood differ from those experienced by adults. Table 9-4 provides a list of common stressors experienced by children and youth.

Recognizing potential stressors and students' emotional responses and identifying and reducing the stress triggers can effectively build trust among the student, the family, and the school team. Guided by the special education process, school professionals can incorporate data gathered from a variety of sources (eg, student observations within school settings, attendance records, results of previous and current assessments, interviews) to generate a comprehensive individualized plan that incorporates stress reduction. Details of this plan might include strategies for completing assigned work when the student is receiving extended medical treatment, scheduling in planned rest breaks at school, or creating a protocol to guide consistent care following a seizure at school.

Designing specific plans to support individual students living with chronic conditions requires clear communication among all school professionals, from the administrator to the paraprofessional aide. Additionally, time to meet and review current support plans is imperative. Many schools incorporate weekly school assistance team meetings into their calendar to ensure consistency with expectations and outcomes.

TABLE 9-4

STRESSORS AND STRESS MANAGEMENT FOR CHILDREN AND YOUTH

AGES	STRESSOR	SIGNS OF STRESS	SOLUTION
Across lifespan	• Inability to meet demands • Over-challenging situations (where the students' resources do not meet the demands) • Changes in schedules, changes in plans • Daily hassles • Major life events: pregnancy, moving • Minor losses (time, money, distant friends) • Major losses (money, friends, pets, parent[s] death or divorce, job, personal relationship) • Personal disability	• Changes in behavior: o Acting irritable or moody o Withdrawing from activities that used to give them pleasure o Routinely expressing worries o Complaining more than usual about school o Crying, displaying surprising fearful reactions o Clinging to others o Sleeping too much or too little o Eating too much or too little	• Refer to the school counselor or psychologist if behaviors persist: • Listen and observe closely • Mitigate losses • Help students develop strategies to reduce the impact of losses • Build self-confidence and coping skills • Maintain a routine • Give opportunities for choice and taking control • Respect the students' personal rights • Treat students fairly • Maintain a structured social schedule, allowing students to opt out • Encourage physical activity • Model healthy behaviors
6 yrs	• Meeting parent expectations • Full-time school schedule		
7 yrs	• Need for praise from family and peers • Being forced to leave a favorite activity		
8 yrs	• Physical appearance • Abilities compared with peers' • Need for positive feedback • Lack of choice		
9 yrs	• Fear of embarrassment		
10 to 12 yrs	• Puberty: developing at different rates • Over-extended schedules • Lack of freedom • Peer pressure		
13 to 18 yrs	• School pressures/deadlines • Involvement in too many activities • Physical appearance • Peer acceptance	• Significantly avoiding teachers • Long-term absences • Not completing schoolwork	

Adapted from American Psychological Association. Identifying signs of stress in your children and teens. American Psychological Association Web site. http://www.apa.org/helpcenter/stress-children.aspx. Accessed February 17, 2017; American Academy of Pediatrics. Helping children handle stress. HealthyChildren Web site. https://www.healthychildren.org/English/healthy-living/emotional-wellness/Pages/Helping-Children-Handle-Stress.aspx. Updated November 21, 2015. Accessed February 16, 2017; and National Association of School Psychologists. Stress in children and adolescents: Tips for parents. St. Mary's County Public Schools Web site. https://schools.smcps.org/fairlead/images/pdfs/Stress.pdf. Published 2008. Accessed February 17, 2017.

During these meetings, team members share their expertise with one another with the goal of creating a unified plan to meet each student's individual needs. For example, a physical therapist might meet with the special education teacher, occupational therapist, and paraprofessional aide to review mobility activities and therapeutic positioning for a child with spastic cerebral palsy. The occupational therapist might provide adaptations for taking notes during class, such as using a recorder (including the student's ability to operate it independently). Similarly, the speech-language pathologist may discuss a student's communication skills, elaborating on vocabulary that meets the unique social and emotional needs of the child. This educational training ensures that all members of the team receive the same information and understand scheduled activities, the frequency and duration of interventions, and who is responsible for their implementation. Documentation of team interaction is crucial to ensure consistency. Examples may include team meeting notes, a copy of the child's revised schedule, handouts for specific exercises, and/or positioning recommendations for eating in the cafeteria, on the school bus, or sitting at a desk.

LEGAL AND ETHICAL ISSUES IN SCHOOL SETTINGS

As described in Section 8, the Individuals with Disabilities Education Act (IDEA) Part B provides federal funding to assist school districts in providing necessary resources to educate students with disabilities.[22] Key to implementation of this law is the requirement for students to be educated in the LRE.[22] Education alongside healthy peers is considered the LRE, making it a priority to provide supportive services in the regular classroom to the greatest extent possible. Alternative settings are considered only if the severity of the disability renders this option impossible, even with supports. According to the US Department of Education, most children with severe disabilities who require multiple types of special education services are educated primarily in self-contained classrooms.[22] This finding indicates that school districts continue to struggle with providing adequate supports to educate children with multiple needs in inclusive settings.

Parents have reported educational issues as some of the most stressful aspects of raising a child with special needs.[23,24] Parents of children with special needs in segregated and integrated environments have reported positive and negative aspects of both.[25] In one study, 262 mothers of children placed in either inclusive or specialized placements were interviewed by researchers.[25] Mothers of children in inclusive settings felt certain that their children's social needs were being met but sometimes felt the educational program was not as tailored to their children's specific needs.

In contrast, mothers of children in specialized settings reported an understanding of the potential benefits of an inclusive placement for their children but were more comfortable with the services their children received in the specialized setting. Mothers of children in both types of settings reported fears that their children would be made fun of in regular classroom environments.[25]

The long-term impacts of initial educational placement decisions are substantial. Researchers have reported the critical need to maximize learning opportunities for children with severe disabilities during the school years because fewer changes in social, educational, and cognitive skills occur after children leave school settings. These initial decisions regarding educational placement tend to remain constant across a child's school career and eventually influence postsecondary placement decisions in the community.[26-28] One study found that graduated students with special needs who had been educated in regular classroom environments obtained jobs and other independent life skills to a much higher degree than those educated in special classroom placements.[29] Likewise, in a 5-state study of 40 students with special needs, those educated in inclusive settings demonstrated significantly higher skills in adaptive and social behaviors than children who received services in segregated environments.[30]

Specific to children with highly complex needs requiring multiple services, the best outcomes have been reported for individuals educated in regular classrooms.[31] Similarly, researchers reviewing the educational records of 13 students with complex needs overwhelmingly reported greater success for students engaged in inclusive settings.[32] However, the researchers pointed out that training and support for interprofessional teams must be provided during the process. From the perspectives of interprofessional teams who serve school-aged children with complex needs, it has also been reported that professionals believe these children can be successfully educated in inclusive settings with appropriate supports.[33]

ADVOCACY: EMPOWERING CHILDREN AND THEIR FAMILIES

All professionals have the desire to empower children and their families to become self-advocates.[34] As noted in the ICF Model, *participation* at home, in school, and in the community involves an awareness of the health conditions, both mental and physical, that play a role in an individual's ability to perform age-appropriate activities. Barriers to full participation are more easily addressed by support services provided in educational settings, but these are not necessarily available to students and their families as they leave educational settings. Developing advocacy skills in parents begins during EI and ECSE. Children's self-advocacy can be developed as early as elementary school. Ways that the interprofessional team can help students develop self-advocacy skills include the following[35]:

- Writing down students' ideas, questions, and concerns before the IEP meeting

- Helping students rehearse what they want to say in the IEP meeting

- Teaching students to introduce themselves properly

- Talking to students about their interests, strengths, and desires for the future

- Teaching students to explain their disability to classmates, teachers, and others

- Encouraging students to ask for explanations if they don't understand something

- Reviewing what the team has agreed to at the end of the meeting

With their unique training and knowledge, physical therapists, occupational therapists, and speech-language pathologists in the educational setting have the opportunity to work with the same children over extended periods of time, allowing more opportunities to help children develop these self-advocacy skills.[36] These efforts support a *student-centered education* that can lead to academic success and the development of skills needed in adulthood. The interprofessional team can also promote "Kids As Self Advocates (KASA), a national, grassroots project created by youth with disabilities for youth."[37] This group offers teens and young adults with disabilities a forum for speaking out and sharing information.

In addition, pediatric therapists can collaborate with the educational team to ensure that students have needed accommodations for inclusion and participation in school activities. Advocacy includes providing team members with information about current evidence-based interventions; making recommendations and referrals for needed services based upon the needs and goals of students, families, and educators; supporting the acquisition of assistive technology (AT) and durable medical equipment (DME); and communicating with other service providers in medical settings to ensure continuity of care.[34]

Professionals in educational settings must engage in ongoing advocacy to meet individual student's needs while simultaneously ensuring that federal and state laws and regulations continue to support inclusive services in schools and the community. Pediatric professionals, especially those aligned with professional and nonprofit organizations, are well positioned to advocate for programming, policies, and decisions that impact children with disabilities in the educational setting. As policies are being updated and new programming opportunities arise, pediatric therapists have the responsibility to work with the special education team and administrators to ensure that the needs of all are taken into consideration.

TRANSITION SERVICES

The National Association of Special Education Teachers (NASET) describes the transition from high school:

Depending on the nature and severity of the disability, special education professionals and parents may play more of an ongoing role in the child's life even after he or she leaves secondary education. Historically, parents and their children have spent years actively involved in Individual Educational Plan (IEP) development and meetings, transitional IEP (ITEP) development, and Committee on Special Education (CSE) meetings concerning educational and developmental welfare. Depending upon the mental competence (the capability to make reasoned decisions) of the child with disabilities, some parents may have to continue to make vital decisions affecting all aspects of their children's lives; they need not shy away, thinking that they are being too overprotective if they are involved in the child's life after the child leaves school. On the other hand, the parents of children not affected by diminished mental competence should use all their energies to encourage the child's steps toward independence.[38]

Postsecondary goals must take into account the student's interests, preferences, needs, and strengths. Options available post–high school may include postsecondary education, vocational education, integrated employment (including supported employment), continuing and adult education, adult services, independent living, or community participation, depending upon available resources.[39] School practitioners can aid during this transition process by compiling a list of available resources for families, such as grants, extracurricular activities, social services, respite care for the family, assistance with navigating the health care system, and available postsecondary options.

For those students who intend to go on to postsecondary education from high school, the US Department of Education offers a website that provides vital information for this transition: https://www2.ed.gov/about/offices/list/ocr/transitionguide.html#introduction.[40] In addition to offering guidance in terms of civil rights issues, the site answers common questions about the admissions process and postadmission considerations (eg, having documentation of disability). "Students with disabilities possess unique knowledge of their individual disabilities and should be prepared to discuss the functional challenges they face and, if applicable, what has or has not worked for them in the past."[40] Keys to student success include strong self-advocacy skills, a solid preparatory curriculum for postsecondary education, a good understanding of the student's own disability, self-responsibility, strong computer and self-management skills, and gaining familiarity with the educational setting and learning expectations (eg, college visits and participation in orientation). The educational team should help students with disabilities develop these key abilities linked to success, facilitating their transitions from high school to postsecondary education.

The educational opportunities for growth and development during childhood and youth are tremendous; however, they may be overlooked if the educational team lacks the long-range perspective needed to help students successfully transition from childhood to adulthood. The interprofessional team must share discipline-specific knowledge and resources to optimize students' educations and, ultimately, their transitions to adulthood.

INTERPROFESSIONAL ACTIVITY

Interprofessional Care in Elementary School

After reviewing Case 9-1, answer the following questions as an interprofessional team:

1. Discuss interprofessional and discipline-specific assessments you would recommend for this child.
2. Discuss possible SMART goals that you share with the teachers and family in an IEP meeting. (SMART = Specific [simple, sensible, significant], Measurable [meaningful, motivating], Achievable [agreed, attainable], Relevant [reasonable, realistic and resourced, results-based], and Time bound [time based, time limited, time/cost limited, timely, time-sensitive].)
3. Describe age-appropriate therapeutic activities you would recommend for this educational setting.
4. Discuss appropriate supports for the child's IEP, including assistive technology such as adaptive devices to promote functional independence.

Case 9-1: A 6-year-old boy with cerebral palsy and spastic athetosis

This new kindergartner qualifies for special education services at a rural elementary school. The occupational therapist, speech-language pathologist, and physical therapist are all contract service providers who are assigned to this school 2 days per week. The new kindergartner is Narin,

born prematurely and diagnosed with cerebral palsy at 2 years old. He was briefly enrolled in EI, then he transitioned to ECSE in a different state. Standardized assessment at age 4½ indicated that Narin's fine motor and gross motor skills were more than 2 standard deviations below normal when he was enrolled in kindergarten. Narin's parents are originally from Cambodia and are involved parents. His father is able to communicate in English but is sometimes difficult to understand. His mother speaks and understands a little bit of English. Narin's aunt also lives with them to assist with his care and does not understand or speak English. His family still believes Narin will "recover" and will be a "normal" child and therefore do not see a need to invest in new adaptive equipment. Narin is an only child.

The following is a summary from Narin's ECSE team:

- *Strengths*: Narin is eager to come to school and is very well liked by his classmates at preschool. He is very talkative, but his speech is difficult to understand. He enjoys coming to preschool and is eager to participate in therapy sessions. He invites his classmates to be part of the group play during therapy.
- *Needs*: Narin has had difficulty engaging in play with his classmates, circle time, and class activities. He has difficulty with attention due to his limited postural control and motor skills to engage in learning activities. He is able to say a few words but is difficult to understand. He lacks postural control in sitting and is dependent in mobility (he is pushed in a child stroller). He is unable to transition from one position to another.
- *Preschool supports*: Narin currently has no technological support because his parents do not see the need for investing resources in any adaptive equipment or assistive technology. He requires 1:1 assistance throughout his day (eg, feeding, taking off coat, mobility, toileting, transfers, fine motor skills for learning activities).

He has benefited from a supportive preschool staff, including good follow-through with recommendations and encouraging Narin's participation in all activities as much as he is able. Narin has received occupational therapy, speech-language therapy, and assistive technology services. His elementary school is 2 stories, and the school made certain that all of Narin's classes were on the first floor.

Interprofessional Care in High School

Consider the recommendations you would have made for Narin across his elementary school years. He has since graduated from the local elementary school and must transition directly to the local high school because there are no middle schools in this small town.

1. Discuss interprofessional and discipline-specific assessments you would recommend for Narin.
2. Discuss possible SMART goals[41] that you share with the teachers and family in an IEP meeting.

3. Describe age-appropriate therapeutic activities you would recommend for this educational setting.

4. Discuss appropriate supports for Narin's IEP, including assistive technology and adaptive devices to promote functional independence.

5. Describe how you would help Narin develop self-advocacy and prepare for transitioning out of high school into the adult world.

Modifications in Care Based Upon a Health Condition

As a team, discuss modifications you would recommend for Narin's school schedule and therapeutic interventions based upon his new health condition.

Case 9-2: A 16-year-old boy with a new diagnosis of leukemia

Narin is now 16, and he was diagnosed with leukemia in the past month. His parents report having difficulty understanding the health care system in regard to all the services he receives outside of school, their health insurance, and working with durable medical equipment (DME) companies. Narin's parents are also deeply disappointed that he is still not able to walk. A conversation was held with the family offering education about Narin's medical condition. They are also worried about the leukemia and state that they do not understand the doctor's explanation about the diagnosis and his prognosis. Narin has expressed being worried about his leukemia diagnosis. They are also worried about Narin's future, especially as they are getting older. (His mother is 60 and his father is 68.) Recommendations for social work involvement and family counseling were made this summer.

The following is Narin's current level of function:

- *Strengths*: Narin is a friendly young man who enjoys watching wrestling and playing video games with his friends. He enjoys having his friends over. Narin effectively uses an augmentative communication device for classroom work and for talking with his friends. He also uses a modified computer for in-class quizzes. With postural support in his adapted wheelchair, Narin can attend to classroom activities for up to 20 minutes. Using a rollator walker, Narin is able to walk 20 feet in 3 minutes on level surfaces.

- *Needs*: Narin is dependent in all motor activities in the school setting, requiring supervision when using his motorized wheelchair for classroom mobility and hallway transitions. He requires adult assistance during adaptive physical education class; when transferring to playground equipment; and for eating, position changes, and transfers.

REFERENCES

1. US Department of Health and Human Services, Substance Abuse and Mental Health Services Administration. Risk and protective factors for mental, emotional, and behavioral disorders across the life cycle. http://dhss.alaska.gov/dbh/Documents/Prevention/programs/spfsig/pdfs/IOM_Matrix_8%205x11_FINAL.pdf. Published 2009. Accessed February 16, 2017.

2. Kowalski RM, Giumetti GW, Schroeder AN, Lattanner MR. Bullying in the digital age: A critical review and meta-analysis of cyberbullying research among youth. *Psychol Bull.* 2014;140(4):1073-1137.

3. Birbilis M, Moschonis G, Mougios V, Manios Y; Healthy Growth Study group. Obesity in adolescence is associated with perinatal risk factors, parental BMI and sociodemographic characteristics. *Eur J Clin Nutr.* 2013;67(1):115-121.

4. Sheftall AH, Asti L, Horowitz LM, et al. Suicide in elementary school-aged children and early adolescents. *Pediatrics.* 2016;138(4):e20160436

5. Chrisman SP, Rivara FP, Schiff MA, Zhou C, Comstock RD. Risk factors for concussive symptoms 1 week or longer in high school athletes. *Brain Inj.* 2013;27(1):1-9.

6. Degenhardt L, Coffey C, Romaniuk H, et al. The persistence of the association between adolescent cannabis use and common mental disorders into young adulthood. *Addiction.* 2013;108(1):124-133.

7. Kuss DJ, Van Rooij AJ, Shorter GW, Griffiths MD, van de Mheen D. Internet addiction in adolescents: Prevalence and risk factors. *Computers in Human Behavior.* 2013;29(5):1987-1996.

8. Niolon PH, Vivolo-Kantor AM, Latzman NE, et al. Prevalence of teen dating violence and co-occurring risk factors among middle school youth in high-risk urban communities. *J Adolesc Health.* 2015;56(2):S5-S13.

9. Brody GH, Yu T, Chen YF, Kogan SM, et al. Cumulative socioeconomic status risk, allostatic load, and adjustment: a prospective latent profile analysis with contextual and genetic protective factors. *Dev Psychol.* 2013;49(5):913-927.

10. Needham BL, Crosnoe R, Muller C. Academic failure in secondary school: The inter-related role of health problems and educational context. *Soc Probl.* 2004;51(4):569-586.

11. World Health Organization. International Classification of Functioning, Disability and Health. World Health Organization. Web site. http://www.who.int/classifications/icf/en/. Updated January 27, 2017. Accessed February 16, 2017.

12. Special Education Guide. The IEP process explained. Special Education Guide Web site. http://www.specialeducationguide.com/pre-k-12/individualized-education-programs-iep/the-iep-process-explained/. Accessed February 16, 2017.

13. Morin A. At a glance: 3 tiers of RTI support. Understood Web site. https://www.understood.org/en/school-learning/special-services/rti/at-a-glance-3-tiers-of-rti-support. Published 2014. Accessed February 16, 2017.

14. RTI Action Network. What is RTI? RTI Action Network Web site. http://www.rtinetwork.org/learn/what/whatisrti. Accessed February 16, 2017.

15. Peranich L, Reynolds KB, O'Brien SP, Bosch J, Cranfill T. The roles of occupational therapy, physical therapy, and speech/language pathology in primary care. Encompass Web site. http://encompass.eku.edu/ot_fsresearch/1. Published 2010. Accessed February 16, 2017.

16. Goldstein DN, Cohn E, Coster W. Enhancing participation for children with disabilities: application of the ICF enablement framework to pediatric physical therapist practice. *Pediatr Phys Ther.* 2014;16:114-120.

17. van der Lee JH, Mokkink LB, Grootenhuis MA, Heymans HS, Offringa M. Definitions and measurement of chronic health conditions in childhood. *JAMA.* 2007;297:2741-2751.

18. Van Cleave J, Gortmaker SL, Perrin JM. Dynamics of obesity and chronic health conditions among children and youth. *JAMA.* 2010;303(7):623-630.

19. Torpy JM, Campbell A, Glass RM. JAMA patient page. Chronic diseases of children. *JAMA.* 2010;303(7):682.

20. Boyse K, Boujaoude L, Laundy J. Children with chronic conditions. University of Michican Web site. http://www.med.umich.edu/yourchild/topics/chronic.htm. Published November 2012. Accessed February 16, 2017.

21. Robison LL, Armstrong GT, Boice JD, et al. The Childhood Cancer Survivor Study: A National Cancer Institute-supported resource for outcome and intervention research. *J Clin Oncol.* 2009;27:2308-2318.

22. US Department of Education. OSEP policy documents regarding the education of infants, toddlers, children and youth with disabilities. US Department of Education Web site. https://www2.ed.gov/policy/speced/guid/idea/letters/revpolicy/tplre.html. Accessed February 17, 2017.

23. Kurth JA, Morningstar ME, Kozleski EB. The persistence of highly restrictive special education placements for students with low-incidence disabilities. *Res Prac Persons Severe Disabl.* 2014;39(3):227-239.

24. Brown J, Rodger S. Children with disabilities: Problems faced by foster parents. *Children and Youth Services Review.* 2009;31(1):40-46.

25. Leyser Y, Heinze A, Kapperman G. Stress and adaptation in families of children with visual disabilities. *Families in Society: The Journal of Contemporary Social Services.* 1996;77(4):240-249.

26. Guralnick MJ, Connor RT, Hammond M. Parent perspectives of peer relationships and friendships in integrated and specialized programs. *Am J Ment Retard.* 1995;99(5):457-475.

27. Beadle-Brown J, Murphy G, Wing L. The Camberwell cohort 25 years on: Characteristics and changes in skills over time. *J Appl Res Intellect Disabl.* 2006;19(4):317-329.

28. Hendrickson JM, Smith CR, Frank AR, Merical C. Decision making factors associated with placement of students with emotional and behavioral disorders in restrictive educational settings. *Education and Treatment of Children.* 1998;21:275-302.

29. Smart M. Transition planning and the needs of young people and their carers: the alumni project. *British Journal of Special Education.* 2004;31(3):128-137.

30. Myklebust JO, Båtevik FO. Earning a living for former students with special educational needs. Does class placement matter? *European Journal of Special Needs Education.* 2009;24(2):203-212.

31. Fisher M, Meyer LH. Development and social competence after two years for students enrolled in inclusive and self-contained educational programs. *Res Prac Persons Severe Disabl.* 2002;27(3):165-174.

32. Camargo SP, Rispoli M, Ganz J, Hong ER, Davis H, Mason R. A review of the quality of behaviorally-based intervention research to improve social interaction skills of children with ASD in inclusive settings. *J Autism Dev Disord.* 2014;44(9):2096-2116.

33. Hunt-Berg M. The Bridge School: Educational inclusion outcomes over 15 years. *Augment Altern Commun.* 2005;21(2):116-131.

34. Soto G, Müller E, Hunt P, Goetz L. Critical issues in the inclusion of students who use augmentative and alternative communication: An educational team perspective. *Augment Altern Commun.* 2001;17(2):62-72.

35. Pacer Center. How you can help your child learn to be a good self-advocate. Pacer Center Web site. http://www.pacer.org/parent/php/PHP-c95.pdf. Accessed February 16, 2017.

36. American Physical Therapy Association. Vision statement for the physical therapy profession and guiding principles to achieve the vision. American Physical Therapy Association Web site. http://www.apta.org/Vision/. Updated September 9, 2015. Accessed December 12, 2017.

37. Kids as Self-Advocates. http://fvkasa.org/index.php. Accessed February 17, 2017.

38. Allison VL, Nativio DG, Mitchell AM, Ren D, Yuhasz J. Identifying symptoms of depression and anxiety in students in the school setting. *The Journal of School Nursing.* 2014;30(3):165-172.

39. Centers for Disease Control. Make a difference at your school. Centers for Disease Control Web site. https://www.cdc.gov/healthyyouth/keystrategies/pdf/make-a-difference.pdf Published January 2008. Accessed February 18, 2017.

40. Copeland WE, Wolke D, Angold A, Costello EJ. Adult psychiatric outcomes of bullying and being bullied by peers in childhood and adolescence. *JAMA Psychiatry.* 2013;70(4):419-426.

41. Darney D, Reinke WM, Herman KC, Stormont M, Ialongo NS. Children with co-occurring academic and behavior problems in first grade: Distal outcomes in twelfth grade. *J Sch Psychol.* 2013;51(1):117-128.

42. Davidson L, Linnoila M, eds. *Risk factors for youth suicide.* New York, NY: Taylor & Francis; 2013.

43. Dowdy E, Furlong M, Raines TC, Bovery B, Kauffman B, Kamphaus RW, Murdock J. Enhancing school-based mental health services with a preventive and promotive approach to universal screening for complete mental health. *Journal of Educational and Psychological Consultation.* 2015;25(2-3):178-197.

44. Malik VS, Willett WC, Hu FB. Global obesity: trends, risk factors and policy implications. *Nature Reviews Endocrinology.* 2013;9(1):13-27.

45. National Research Council (US) and Institute of Medicine (US) Committee on the Prevention of Mental Disorders and Substance Abuse Among Children, Youth, and Young Adults: Research Advances and Promising Interventions. *Preventing Mental, Emotional, and Behavioral Disorders among Young People: Progress and Possibilities.* Washington, DC: National Academies Press; 2009. https://www.ncbi.nlm.nih.gov/books/NBK32775

46. Ogden CL, Carroll MD, Curtin LR, Lamb MM, Flegal KM. Prevalence of high body mass index in US children and adolescents, 2007–2008. *JAMA.* 2010;303:242-249.

47. Snakenborg J, Van Acker R, Gable RA. Cyberbullying: Prevention and intervention to protect our children and youth. *Preventing School Failure: Alternative Education for Children and Youth.* 2011;55(2):88-95.

48. Tangen D, Campbell M. Cyberbullying Prevention: One Primary School's Approach. *Australian Journal of Guidance and Counselling.* 2010;20(02):225-234.

49. Collins CL, Fletcher EN, Fields SK, et al. Neck strength: a protective factor reducing risk for concussion in high school sports. *J Prim Prev.* 2014;35(5):309-319.

50. Navarro RR. Protective equipment and the prevention of concussion-what is the evidence? *Curr Sports Med Rep.* 2011;10(1):27-31.

51. Arthur MW, Hawkins JD, Pollard JA, Catalano RF, Baglioni Jr AJ. Measuring risk and protective factors for use, delinquency, and other adolescent problem behaviors: The Communities That Care Youth Survey. *Eval Rev.* 2002;26(6):575-601.

52. Koo HJ, Kwon JH. Risk and protective factors of Internet addiction: a meta-analysis of empirical studies in Korea. *Yonsei Med J.* 2014;55(6):1691-1711.

53. Centers for Disease Control and Prevention. School Violence: Risk and Protective Factors. Centers for Disease Control and Prevention Web site. https://www.cdc.gov/violenceprevention/youthviolence/schoolviolence/risk.html. Published February 10, 2015. Accessed February 19, 2017.

54. Centers for Disease Control and Prevention. School Connectedness: Strategies for Increasing Protective Factors among Youth. Centers for Disease Control and Prevention Web site. https://www.cdc.gov/healthyyouth/protective/pdf/connectedness.pdf. Published 2009. Accessed February 20, 2017.

55. Gambone MA, Klem AM, Summers JA, Akey TM, Sipe CL. Turning the Tide: The Achievements of the First Things First Education Reform in the Kansas City, Kansas Public School District. Philadelphia, PA: Youth Development Strategies, Inc; 2004.

56. Florida Department of Education. Section 2: Identification of Risk and Protective Factors. Florida Department of Education Web site. http://www.fldoe.org/core/fileparse.php/7771/urlt/0084829-sec2.pdf. Accessed February 20, 2017

Section 10

Providing Interprofessional Medical Care for Children and Adolescents

Brandi Dorton, DPT; Stephanie Orr, PT, DPT, PCS; Joan Delahunt, OTD, MS, OTR/L;
Lynn Drazinski, MA, CCC-SLP; and Catherine Rush Thompson, PT, PhD, MS

OVERVIEW

In the health care setting, pediatric therapists play an integral role in the management of children and adolescents with *acute and chronic medical conditions.* Although many children with medical conditions are eligible for early intervention (EI) and school-based programs discussed earlier in this book, the focus of interprofessional care differs based on practice setting. For programs offered through the Individuals with Disabilities Education Act (IDEA) Parts B and C (as described in Sections 7, 8, and 9), the interprofessional focus of care is on child-centered and family-centered interventions to enhance parenting skills and increase participation in daily life activities in the home and community, as well as providing needed supports to help children with special needs learn in the least restrictive educational (LRE) settings. Within the medical setting, pediatric therapists are clinicians who work in partnership to create a collaborative plan of care for each child (including a discharge plan) based upon health outcomes rather than educational outcomes.

Clinicians in health care settings work collaboratively to manage a wide variety of conditions affecting developmental,

behavioral, and motor milestones, emphasizing the child's return to daily activities. Examples of conditions seen in both educational and health care settings include Down syndrome, cerebral palsy, autism spectrum disorder (ASD), attention deficit hyperactivity disorder (ADHD), muscular dystrophy, and spinal muscular atrophy, among others. However, children with pathologies needing medical diagnoses and acute interprofessional care are typically managed best in a clinic, hospital, or rehabilitation setting where the focus is on stabilizing the health condition, recovering function, and building the needed skills and endurance to resume regular activity.[1-3] For example, physical therapists, occupational therapists, and speech-language pathologists work with children and adolescents with acute traumatic brain injuries and traumatic spinal cord injuries until they are ready to return home and engage in their daily routines at school, leisure and/or work, and home.

Pediatric therapists in health care settings also serve a wide range of medical needs related to: (1) surgical management of conditions (eg, pre- and post-procedure care for posterior spinal fusions and postoperative care for bone fractures); (2) management of complications from congenital

Thompson CR. *Pediatric Therapy:*
An Interprofessional Framework for Practice (pp 149-163).
© 2018 SLACK Incorporated.

diagnoses (eg, bronchopulmonary dysplasia and congenital heart defects); (3) reducing conditions related to prolonged hospitalization; (4) providing intensive care during the onset of new conditions, such as stroke, conversion disorder, or chronic pain; (5) discharging patients from medical care; and (6) supporting the child and family during terminal illness.[1-3]

Physical therapists, occupational therapists, and speech-language pathologists are responsible for screening, evaluation, and developing a plan of care to assist children in restoring their prior level of function, reaching their full potential with new deficits, or preventing further decline in function. Using a collaborative team approach, pediatric therapists work together to determine the needs of a patient, equipment or adaptations required for optimal function and mobility at home and integration in the community, and the appropriate discharge plan for services after an inpatient stay.[1-3]

AGE-SPECIFIC RISK FACTORS

Therapists each contribute to the screening process for risk factors and ensure that they are addressed quickly during an inpatient hospitalization. Risk factors are managed by evidence-based intervention (eg, therapeutic positioning to protect skin integrity, preventing contractures or loss of range of motion, avoiding abnormal postures that may develop after a neurological insult, and encouraging engagement in healthy behaviors). Being cognizant of an individual's communication style is also vitally important for understanding a patient's wants and needs during her care.

It is crucial to be aware of age-specific risk factors in the acute care setting to best serve the needs of children and their families. Whereas some children may have risk factors addressed in EI and educational settings, children entering medical care without prior special education needs may not have had prior medical attention to these issues. Health screenings in all settings can help prevent future disability. Understanding typical human growth and development (Section 4) will also help provide a framework for typical behaviors to expect in terms of developmental milestones for each age group. Table 10-1 lists recommendations for pediatric health and wellness in medical settings.

Pediatric patients who are immobile due to new or pre-existing conditions, regardless of their age, are at high risk for loss of skin integrity, loss of range of motion/contractures, dislocations, and respiratory complications due to prolonged positioning.[4]

SCREENING AND EVALUATION

In medical settings, physicians will oftentimes refer their pediatric patients to physical therapists, occupational therapists, and speech-language pathologists to determine if their specialized services are warranted. After receiving a referral, each therapist will begin a screening and evaluation process to determine the level of need and corresponding plan of care. Therapists in the health care setting perform a thorough chart review of the patient's medical history and an interview with the pediatric patient (if appropriate) and family as part of the assessment of the child's current skills, developmental history, home setting, interests and activities, and specific health concerns. With this foundational information, pediatric therapists have the ability to collaborate during the evaluation process, providing more coordinated services and an integrated plan of care.

Often the initial screening or evaluation will occur with multiple disciplines present, as in other practice settings. Multidisciplinary evaluations are commonly used to determine plans of care for various types of pediatric care, such as burn care, pain management, and management of feeding disorders.[5,6] During the initial assessment, disciplines work together to ask questions to understand the patient's prior level of function in all areas. This information assists the team in determining the most appropriate plan of care, including the expected duration of treatment to regain these prior skills.[7,8] A child's communication style and cognitive status are important to all team members, as these factors critically impact how all disciplines will engage the pediatric patient most effectively.

Although some areas of assessment overlap, it is essential that pediatric therapists recognize and trust each other's expertise and communicate thoroughly to ensure that referrals are appropriate and sufficiently comprehensive. Effective interprofessional collaboration between pediatric therapists can increase efficiency and reduce costs of care.[9] As outlined in Section 1, interprofessional care relies on role clarification, child-/family-/school-centered care, interprofessional communication, conflict resolution, team functioning, and collaborative leadership.

Listed in Table 10-2 are examples of common areas that all disciplines may evaluate together during the initial interaction with the pediatric patient (eg, attention, arousal, cognition, sensorimotor function, pain, and cardiopulmonary function). This areas of evaluation are augmented by discipline-specific tests and measures deemed necessary by the clinicians to complete a comprehensive plan of care that addresses the pediatric patient's specific needs. Although not

TABLE 10-1

RECOMMENDATIONS FOR PEDIATRIC HEALTH AND WELLNESS

AGE	RECOMMENDATIONS FOR PEDIATRIC HEALTH AND WELLNESS
Neonate and infant (birth to 1 year)	• Monitoring growth and development • Assessing anthropometrics: length/height and weight, head circumference, weight for length, and body mass index (making a referral if the child is at risk for failure to thrive) • Assessing/reviewing vital signs, including cardiorespiratory function • Assessing neurodevelopmental skills, including screening for autism • Assessing behavior of infant and mother (related to postpartum depression) • Assessing sensory systems: vision and hearing • Instructing families in health promotion • Introducing the Back to Sleep Program and Prone to Play Program • Educating about appropriate sensory stimulation and decreasing noxious stimulation • Educating about parental/caregiver bonding opportunities • Suggesting therapeutic positioning throughout day (eg, to prevent torticollis) • Progressing feeding by breast or bottle to finger food
Toddler (1 year to 3 years)	• Monitoring growth and development • Instructing families in health promotion • Ensuring safety in sleep and play environments • Monitoring developmental skills to discern decline or lack of progression • Addressing decreased or absent play exploration with toys and books • Addressing delays with language development • Noting attachment to family members or interactions with peers • Addressing delays with self-care skill development (dressing, toileting, feeding, bathing, and grooming)
Child (3 to 10 years)	• Monitoring growth and development • Screening for mental health concerns, such as depression or the need for professional psychological support • Monitoring for safety awareness during learned mobility • Preventing muscle atrophy from prolonged bed rest • Preventing loss of range of motion • Decreasing dependence on adult for self-care needs (dressing, eating, grooming, bathing) • Addressing low interest in social opportunities • Monitoring decreased participation with leisure opportunities • Noting a decline or lack of progression in academic skills
Adolescent (11 to 21 years)	• Monitoring growth and development, as needed • Watching for signs of drug use and abuse (eg, sudden change in behavior, mood swings, irritable and grumpy and then suddenly happy and bright, withdrawal from family members, careless about personal grooming, loss of interest in hobbies, sports and other favorite activities, changed sleeping pattern; up at night and sleeping during the day, red or glassy eyes, sniffling or runny nose) • Education about sexually transmitted diseases, if appropriate • See recommendations for Child

Adapted from American Academy of Pediatrics. AAP Schedule of Well-Child Visits. HealthyChildren Web site. https://www.healthychildren.org/English/family-life/health-management/Pages/Well-Child-Care-A-Check-Up-for-Success.aspx. Published June 27, 2017. Accessed December 11, 2017 and American Academy of Pediatrics. Recommendations for Preventive Pediatric Health Care. American Academy of Pediatrics Web site. https://www.aap.org/en-us/documents/periodicity_schedule.pdf. Published February, 2017. Accessed on December 11, 2017.

TABLE 10-2
EXAMPLES OF INTERPROFESSIONAL AREAS OF EVALUATION

CATEGORY	DESCRIPTION OF INTERPROFESSIONAL ASSESSMENTS
Body systems	*Neurological structures and functions are assessed* (eg, cognition, cranial and peripheral nerve function, reflexes, and motor control for functional skills). Cognition abilities, including attention and arousal, are assessed subjectively during patient/therapist interaction. The child's ability to understand is important for communication during instruction and education in therapy. As the fifth vital sign (in addition to temperature, blood pressure, pulse rate, and respiration rate), pain should be monitored each visit. Pain at rest and with activity is important to note to determine how the patient will tolerate future therapy sessions.
	Cardiopulmonary structures and functions are assessed (eg, skin color, breathing patterns, heart rate, respiratory rate, oxygen saturation, and edema) at rest, during therapy sessions, and following activities.
	Integumentary structures and functions are assessed (eg, skin appearance, presence of wounds, bruising, rashes, and/or callus formation), especially related to the use of splints, orthotics, or other external pressures.
	Musculoskeletal structures and functions are assessed (eg, strength, range of motion, and endurance for performing functional motor functions).
	Other body structures and functions (eg, gastrointestinal, genitourinary, limbic, endocrine) are monitored to insure the child's safety, comfort, and health.
Activities: developmental skills and play activities	Developmental skills (gross motor, fine motor, communication, feeding, emotional, psychosocial skills) and play activities are observed, assessed, and integrated into therapeutic activities that prepare the child for functional independence after discharge.
Environmental and personal factors	Interprofessional teams assess and recommend appropriate adaptations, assistive devices, and environmental modifications to enhance function, as needed. Personal factors, including motivation, adherence to recommendations, and lifestyle living habits, are used for personalizing care.
Disability	Goals are designed toward restoration of function, reducing disability and promoting improved quality of life following hospital discharge.

Adapted from American Academy of Pediatrics. HealthyChildren Web site. https://www.healthychildren.org/English/Pages/default. aspx; American Academy of Pediatrics. AAP Schedule of Well-Child Care Visits. HealthyChildren Web site. https://www.healthychildren. org/English/family-life/health-management/Pages/Well-Child-Care-A-Check-Up-for-Success.aspx; and American Academy of Pediatrics. Recommendations for Preventive Pediatric Health Care. American Academy of Pediatrics Web site. https://www.aap.org/en-us/documents/periodicity_schedule.pdf.

exhaustive, Table 10-3 provides examples of discipline-specific tests used to further examine common areas of concern.

The subjective interview is typically the most convenient time for eliciting each patient's and family's goals. The team may assist the patient and family in determining these goals based on information related to the home environment, school environment, and the child's prior level of function. Once goals have been established, the interdisciplinary team works together to ensure progress is made toward the goals vital to the pediatric patient and family.

EVIDENCE-BASED STRATEGIES FOR PREVENTATIVE CARE

Patients and their families may encounter pediatric therapists for needs other than gaining new skills and function. For example, clinicians play a critical role in implementing support for patients and their families, preventing secondary complications, and easing challenges with daily care through family education.

TABLE 10-3		
EXAMPLES OF DISCIPLINE-SPECIFIC TESTING USED IN HOSPITAL-BASED SETTINGS		
DISCIPLINE	**AREA OF EXPERTISE**	**EXAMPLES OF DISCIPLINE-SPECIFIC TESTS**
Speech-language pathology	Language delay/disorder	Clinical Evaluation of Language Fundamentals (CELF)
	Speech sound disorder	Goldman Fristoe Test of Articulation
	Feeding disorder	Modified Barium Swallow
	Cognition	Woodcock-Johnson Test of Cognitive Abilities
	Literacy delay/disorder	Phonological Awareness Test
Physical therapy	Structural integrity	Anterior/posterior drawer test
	Respiratory function	Incentive spirometry
	Fitness	Fitness Gram
	Gait	Dynamic Gait Index
	Balance	Pediatric Balance Scale
	Endurance	6-minute walk test
Occupational therapy	Handwriting	Evaluation Tool of Children's Handwriting
	Play and leisure	Knox Preschool Play Scale
	Self-care	Assessment of Motor and Process Skills (AMPS)
	Sensory processing	Sensory Integration and Praxis Test
	Visual perceptual	Motor-Free Visual Perception Test
See Appendix B for a more comprehensive list of pediatric tests and measures with references.		

Developmental/Behavioral Screenings

Typically, families provide preventive care for their children through routine medical checkups. For patients with medical diagnoses, preventative care typically includes periodic developmental or behavioral screenings to detect potential developmental delays and/or clinical manifestations of newly developing health problems. These screenings can include standardized tests or observational assessments by pediatric therapists. Early screening of infants, children, and adolescents can lead to more timely referrals and expedite the process of the patient receiving quality of care in the appropriate settings.[10,11]

Patient and Caregiver Education

Medical conditions, new or existing, may present the need for a caregivers' attention to a variety of issues to promote the child's health outcomes and prevent secondary complications for their children with chronic conditions. Secondary complications are clinical manifestations that develop in the course of a primary diagnosis, either as a

result of that medical condition or from unrelated causes. Pediatric therapists provide patient and family education to prevent secondary complications, including, but not limited to, the following:

- Maintenance of range of motion to avoid joint contractures leading to pain, impaired mobility, and/or difficulties with positioning in equipment;
- Weight bearing and positioning for bone health and to promote proper joint development and alignment;
- Therapeutic positioning recommendations for skin integrity, prevention of abnormal posture, tone management, vestibular system input, and vital body functions (including digestion and lung/cardiac health) to prevent secondary complications in children/adolescents with chronic diagnoses;
- Environmental modifications, such as visual schedules to promote increased participation in daily activities of self-care;
- Adaptive equipment for feeding, dressing, bathing, and toileting; and

- Adaptations for activities to promote language, cognitive, social, and academic development.

There is no one-size-fits-all prescription for children and youth, so the interprofessional team must work collaboratively with the family to determine the interventions and strategies most likely to yield successful outcomes. Professionals must be good listeners to capture what the family members value and provide a strong rationale for each intervention to gain patient and family endorsement.

Promotion of Health and Wellness

Health and wellness is important to every child, with or without disability. In addition to screening for age-related risk factors discussed earlier in this book, pediatric therapists need to consider additional potential risk factors associated with specific medical diagnoses. These risk factors, if addressed early, can prevent associated secondary complications. For this reason, pediatric therapists should recommend appropriate health promotion strategies as soon as possible. For example, children who have developmental disabilities often have limited physical activity and are at an increased risk for obesity. Health promotion strategies for this population may include increasing physical activity through adaptive sports, participation in Special Olympics, weight management to prevent difficulty with mobility, and lifestyle habits (including diet) to reduce additional risks of disability and chronic disease. The American Physical Therapy Association's Pediatrics Fact Sheet entitled *The Role and Scope of Pediatric Physical Therapy in Fitness, Wellness, Health Promotion, and Prevention* provides exercise considerations addressing both strength and aerobic activities for children with and without disability.[12] Similarly, speech-language pathologists promote the development and maintenance of effective personal and professional communication in individuals both with and without a communication disorder. The American Speech-Language-Hearing Association (ASHA) provides resources and activities related to communication wellness and the prevention of communication disorders.[13] The American Occupational Therapy Association (AOTA) emphasizes health promotion through the inclusion of health and wellness as one of the 7 identified areas of practice for occupational therapists.[14] Occupational therapists can create health-promoting play activities for children to enhance physical well-being while in medical care. Using evidence-based health promotion strategies increases the likelihood of accomplishing health outcomes that are sustainable across the child's lifespan.

EVIDENCE-BASED STRATEGIES FOR MANAGEMENT OF COMMON ACUTE CONDITIONS

The management of *acute medical conditions* of pediatric patients often includes interventions provided by occupational therapists, physical therapists, and speech-language pathologists. These services are usually provided in the inpatient setting throughout the duration of care. A pediatric patient may receive a combination of individual and cotreatment sessions to achieve goals set by the team and family. Treatments by the interdisciplinary team address the increased physical, social, and emotional needs of the patient, while conserving the child's energy for participation throughout the day.[15,16] Regardless of diagnosis, the interdisciplinary team will work together prior to discharge to determine the equipment needed for home, recommendations for continued therapies, and family training/education needs. Examples of acute medical conditions that require interprofessional care include traumatic brain injury, spinal cord injury, and deconditioning secondary to some acute medical conditions involving prolonged hospitalization and immobilization. Listed in Table 10-4 are common acute conditions typically addressed by the interdisciplinary team. The interprofessional team works together to ensure that appropriate preventive care is implemented consistently as part of the patient's overall management.

EVIDENCE-BASED STRATEGIES FOR MANAGEMENT OF COMMON CHRONIC CONDITIONS

A relationship with a team of pediatric therapists (whether short- or long-term) begins once an infant, child, or adolescent is diagnosed with a chronic condition. This team of dedicated therapists will play a significant role in the management of each patient's condition. Intervention may occur intermittently, addressing changes in the individual's medical status, growth, or development from the time of onset of the chronic condition until management becomes part of the child's daily routines in life. Although the condition may initially require therapy in an acute care setting, management will oftentimes continue through outpatient care in a hospital clinic or outpatient setting. Pediatric therapists provide interdisciplinary treatment for a wide range of chronic conditions, including developmental or behavioral

TABLE 10-4

EXAMPLES OF ACUTE CONDITIONS INVOLVING INTERPROFESSIONAL COLLABORATION

ACUTE CONDITION	INTERVENTION	PURPOSE
Brain injuries	Therapeutic positioning	Prevent skin breakdown, manage tone, encourage cardiovascular function through antigravity postures (while ensuring spinal precautions are followed)
	Joint mobility	Maintain range of motion and prepare for active movement; using pressure-relief ankle-foot orthoses and splints to maintain safe joint positioning
	Sensory stimulation	Orient a patient to her environment, activate increased motor responses using olfactory, vestibular, tactile, proprioceptive, and auditory stimulation
	Feeding	Increase tolerance of food texture and amount of intake, monitor for safety of suck/chew/swallow, position for safety, and advance independence
	Improved strength and motor control	Insure adequate head, trunk, and extremity motor control (postural control) and endurance for functional activities.
	Progressive mobility	Encourage movement, beginning with bed mobility, supported sitting, transfers and walking, using assistance, body weight support, treadmill training, aquatic therapy and/or functional electrical stimulation
	Adaptive equipment	Facilitate functional activities, using customized adaptive devices, as needed
	Patient and family education	Assist with home care at the patient's level at discharge
Spinal cord injury (acute phase)	Therapeutic positioning	Promote skin integrity, manage muscle tone, and provide breath support; progressive upright positioning in wheelchair or tilt table; use of abdominal binder, lower extremity compression garments
	Joint mobility	Maintain range through passive exercises, positioning or use of splints; obtain spinal precautions from the physician
	Communication	Develop functional communication (possibly needing augmentative or alternative communication) through promoting breath support and providing strategies for voice production and improved intelligibility
	Patient and family education	Reduce the risk of secondary complications (eg, pressure sores, orthostatic hypotension, autonomic dysreflexia, and temperature dysregulation) through providing pressure relief strategies, instructing in safe transfers, managing bowel and bladder, and carefully monitoring vitals
Spinal cord injury (rehabilitation phase)	Mobility	Promote mobility, including mat/bed mobility, transfers, wheelchair mobility, advanced wheelchair skills, and gait training using body weight support treadmill training, aquatic therapy, and functional electrical stimulation, as needed
	Balance training	Encourage development of balance during activities of daily living; ring and short sitting
	Feeding	Progress feeding/eating skills for increased independence
	Self-care	Advance skills in independent grooming, dressing, bathing, and management of bowel/bladder
	Communication	Provide strategies for improved intelligibility
	Patient and family education	Prepare family for assisting with home care at patient's level at time of discharge

(continued)

TABLE 10-4 (CONTINUED)		
EXAMPLES OF ACUTE CONDITIONS INVOLVING INTERPROFESSIONAL COLLABORATION		
ACUTE CONDITION	**INTERVENTION**	**PURPOSE**
Deconditioned patient from prolonged hospitalization	Functional mobility	Encourage functional mobility (as possible), taking into account (1) current developmental level, (2) functional mobility, (3) prior level of function, (4) range of motion, (5) tolerance to activity, (6) endurance, (7) vital signs, and lines/tubes (chest tubes, extracorporeal membrane oxygenation catheters, intravenous access, peripherally inserted central catheter lines) during assessment and intervention
	Self-care	Facilitate self-care participation through use of adaptive equipment for feeding, bathing, grooming, dressing, and toileting
	Communication	Support communication to advocate for individual needs; determine the need for augmentative or alternative communication, as needed
Orthopedic conditions, injuries, and surgeries	Functional mobility	Encourage mobility (eg, bed mobility, transfers, gait, stair management), taking into account restrictions on movement and weight bearing, through exercises to prevent loss of strength/endurance and gait training and stair management with appropriate assistive device(s) or modifications, as needed
	Self-care	Facilitate increased independence with dressing, bathing, toileting, and grooming, using modifications for activities of daily living, including adaptive equipment (eg, a reacher, grab bar, or bath chair) depending on the child's unique need
	Patient and family education	Promote family knowledge about the level of assistance required, modifications to home, and strategies for function in the community through education and demonstration, as needed

Adapted from Strenk M. Early physical therapy/occupational therapy intervention for traumatic spinal cord injury. Cincinnati Children's Web site. http://www.cincinnatichildrens.org/svc/alpha/h/health-policy/best.htm. Published September 5, 2014. Accessed December 28, 2017; International Brain Injury Association. Evaluation and treatment planning in children with TBI. International Brain Injury Association Web site. http://www.internationalbrain.org/articles/evaluation-and-treatment-planning-in-children-with-tbi/. Published December 10, 2012. Accessed February 12, 2017; University of Rochester Medical Center. The Pediatrics Orthopedic Team. University of Rochester Medical Center Web site. https://www.urmc.rochester.edu/encyclopedia/content.aspx?contenttypeid=90&contentid=P02775. Accessed February 12, 2017; and Wieczorek B, Burke C, Al-Harbi A, Kudchadkar SR. Early mobilization in the pediatric intensive care unit: a systematic review. *J Pediatr Intensive Care.* 2015;2015:129-170.

diagnoses, torticollis, scoliosis, chronic pain, cerebral palsy, congenital heart conditions, oncological diagnoses, muscular dystrophy, cystic fibrosis, and sickle cell anemia, among others. Table 10-5 lists common chronic medical conditions and examples of interprofessional therapeutic interventions.

LEGAL AND ETHICAL ISSUES

The same ethical and legal issues described in earlier sections of the book apply to care for children and their families in medical settings. In addition, providing medical services to pediatric patients under the legal age of medical consent presents legal and ethical issues for pediatric clinicians. "Parental permission and childhood assent is an active process that engages patients, both adults and children, in their health care."[17] While a free appropriate public education (FAPE) in school settings requires consent through the Individualized Education Program (IEP) process, medical care requires specific consent for medical management of pediatric conditions. Again, family-centered care is a cornerstone of pediatric therapy across practice setting, as discussed in earlier sections. Other legal and ethical issues related to medical care include providing prognostic information, maintaining patient confidentiality related to a child's medical condition and management, and providing end-of-life care.

TABLE 10-5
EXAMPLES OF CHRONIC CONDITIONS INVOLVING INTERPROFESSIONAL COLLABORATION

CHRONIC CONDITION	EXAMPLES OF TREATMENTS	PURPOSE
Developmental or behavioral diagnoses	Assessment and intervention	Facilitate development of functional skills (fine and gross motor, self-care, communication, play and leisure, visual motor and visual perceptual, sensory and social-emotional) using individual or small-group intervention targeting specific needs and shaping behavior
Torticollis	Range of motion	Promote head and neck movement and function related to active/passive range of motion and postural, facial, and cranial asymmetries through stretching, movement, and positioning
	Therapeutic positioning	Facilitate developmental milestones through active head/neck movements in prone and side-lying
	Parent education	Educate parents on positioning and stretches to increase neck range of motion for participation in play and sleep
Scoliosis	Stretching	Promote postural alignment and flexibility through stretching
	Bracing	Align posture externally using postural supports (eg, a thoracolumbosacral support), with ongoing monitoring and education about orthotic use
	Self-care	Engage in self-care in daily activities (dressing, bathing, toileting, and grooming) through increased use of arms and adaptive equipment, as needed
	Parent education	Educate family on energy conservation and orthotic use and maintenance
Chronic pain	Assessment	Determine possible causes of chronic pain, including range of motion, strength, balance, endurance, and functional limitations
	Physical conditioning	Increase physical conditioning through aerobic activity, including therapeutic exercise/activity and aquatic therapy
	Self-care	Promote self-care by addressing limitations in activities of daily living that are restricted by pain
Cerebral palsy	Range of motion	Maintain range of motion and joint mobility through passive and active range of motion, strengthening, casting/splinting, orthotics, and constraint-induced movement therapy
	Functional mobility	Encourage mobility through gait training, body weight–supported treadmill training, neurodevelopmental therapy, and aquatic therapy; ensure rehabilitation post-orthopedic surgeries (eg, crouch gait surgery or dorsal rhizotomy)
	Self-care	Promote independence in self-care (dressing, bathing, toileting, and grooming) through modifications, as needed
	Feeding	Promote independent feeding and healthy growth through feeding strategies

(continued)

TABLE 10-5 (CONTINUED)		
EXAMPLES OF CHRONIC CONDITIONS INVOLVING INTERPROFESSIONAL COLLABORATION		
CHRONIC CONDITION	**EXAMPLES OF TREATMENTS**	**PURPOSE**
Congenital heart conditions	Assessment and intervention	Promote developmental skills, increasing endurance and functional mobility (as tolerated with impairments associated with heart condition)
	Physical conditioning and mobility	Promote physical conditioning and mobility through aerobic activity to progress toward prior level/function or progression in developmental skill level, monitoring vital signs throughout interventions and modifying activity (as necessary) for energy conservation
	Feeding	Monitor feeding skills as related to intake and nutritional status
Oncological diagnoses	Assessment and intervention	Encourage participation in daily activity, addressing strength, balance, coordination, aerobic endurance, and motor skills while reducing infection risk
	Range of motion	Monitor and manage ankle strength due to risk for impairment from vincristine neurotoxicity
Muscular dystrophy	Functional mobility	Promote mobility and prevent disuse atrophy through submaximal levels of aerobic exercise, coordination and balance activities, aquatic therapy, and wheelchair use (including wheelchair prescription and management), avoiding overwork, strengthening regimes, repetitive eccentric movements, high load, or progressive resistive activities; prevent fractures and falls; maximize function of upper extremities
	Therapeutic positioning	Promote alignment and comfort in prone-lying, wheelchair positioning, and stander
	Stretching	Preventing contractures/scoliosis through stretching program and casting, orthotics and splints, knee immobilizers
	Family and patient education	Educate about energy conservation, muscle conservation, transfers/body mechanics, and proper equipment use

(continued)

Providing Prognostic Information

Providing prognostic information to families and others about therapeutic outcomes can be challenging. Developing a prognosis is aided by current evidence-based research and interprofessional collaboration. Each prognosis, based upon the unique characteristics of each pediatric patient and his given situation, requires sharing insights and engaging in collaborative clinical decision making. The work of occupational therapists, physical therapists, and speech-language pathologists is guided by each profession's code of ethics, which address the issue of providing prognostic information carefully and truthfully. Physical therapists "shall provide truthful, accurate and relevant information and shall not make misleading representations"[18]; occupational therapists should "fully disclose the benefits, risks, and potential outcomes of any intervention"[19]; and speech-language

pathologists "make a reasonable statement of prognosis, but they shall not guarantee—directly or by implication—the results of any treatment or procedure."[20] These guiding standards are particularly applicable in the medical setting, where conditions may have a sudden onset and may not be well understood by parents or guardians. Family education about the likely outcomes of therapeutic interventions can help families cope with the many stresses of medical care.[21] Furthermore, it can help the family and the patient make informed decisions about future plans and the child's return to function. Proactive care may be enhanced by the interprofessional team asking the following questions[21]:

1. Which aspects of the child's health and life are likely to get better or worse?

2. What acute illnesses is the child likely to experience?

	TABLE 10-5 (CONTINUED)	
EXAMPLES OF CHRONIC CONDITIONS INVOLVING INTERPROFESSIONAL COLLABORATION		
CHRONIC CONDITION	**EXAMPLES OF TREATMENTS**	**PURPOSE**
Cystic fibrosis	Stretching and strengthening	Maintain postural alignment through strengthening and maintaining joint mobility and joint health; focus on maintaining erect posture and preventing tightness in anterior musculature
	Physical conditioning	Promote lung and cardiac health and airway clearance techniques, which are used in conjunction with respiratory therapy
Sickle cell disease	Pain management	Manage pain through use of whirlpool sessions and transcutaneous electrical nerve stimulation
	Exercise therapy	Promote general health and development post-crisis
	Self-care	Promote independence in self-care (dressing, bathing, toileting, and grooming) through modifications, as needed
	Communication	Monitor communication indicating signs of a possible stroke and ensure effective modes of communication
	Patient and family education	Educate all patients to recognize signs of infection, increasing anemia, and organ failure; provide information on energy conservation techniques to manage daily life activities

Adapted from Aarts PB, van Hartingsveldt M, Anderson PG, van den Tillaar I, van der Burg J, Geurts AC. The Pirate group intervention protocol: Description and a case report of a modified constraint-induced movement therapy combined with bimanual training for young children with unilateral spastic cerebral palsy. *Occup Ther Int.* 2012;19(2):76-87; Audu O, Daly C. Standing activity intervention and motor function in a young child with cerebral palsy: A case report. *Physiother Theory Prac.* 2017;33(2):162-172; Bushby K, Finkel R, Birnkrant DJ, et al. Diagnosis and management of Duchenne muscular dystrophy, part 2: Implementation of multidisciplinary care. *Lancet Neurol.* 2010;9(2):177-189; Christensen C, Landsettle A, Antoszewski S, Ballard BB, Carey H, Pax Lowes L. Conservative management of congenital muscular torticollis: An evidence-based algorithm and preliminary treatment parameter recommendations. *Phys Occup Ther Pediatr.* 2013;33(4):453-466; Dong VA, Fong KN, Chen YF, Tseng SS, Wong LM. 'Remind-to-move' treatment versus constraint-induced movement therapy for children with hemiplegic cerebral palsy: A randomized controlled trial. *Dev Med Child Neurol.* 2017;59(2):160-167; Kozlowska K, English M, Savage B, Chudleigh C. Multimodal rehabilitation: A mind-body, family-based intervention for children and adolescents impaired by medically unexplained symptoms. Part 1: The program. *Am J Fam Ther.* 2012;40(5):399-419; Maakaron JE. Sickle cell anemia treatment & management. Medscape Web site. http://emedicine.medscape.com/article/205926-treatment. Updated July 27, 2017. Accessed March 30, 2017; Rigo M, Reiter CH, Weiss HR. Effect of conservative management on the prevalence of surgery in patients with adolescent idiopathic scoliosis. *Pediatr Rehabil.* 2003;6(3/4):209-214; Sharma GD. Cystic fibrosis treatment & management. Medscape Web site. http://emedicine.medscape.com/article/1001602-treatment. Updated July 31, 2017. Accessed March 30, 2017; and Ward R, Leitão S, Strauss G. An evaluation of the effectiveness of PROMPT therapy in improving speech production accuracy in six children with cerebral palsy. *Int J Speech Lang Pathol.* 2014;16(4):355-371.

3. What exacerbations of the existing chronic conditions is the child likely to experience?

4. What new comorbid conditions is this child likely to develop?

5. How can comorbid conditions be avoided?

6. If unavoidable, then how can one mitigate their severity should they occur?

7. What major medical needs (eg, medications, subspecialty consultation, equipment) is the child likely to need in the future to help treat the illnesses and conditions?

8. What decisions about major medical interventions (eg, major surgery) are the child and family likely to face?

9. What is the likely impact on the family (eg, marriage, employment)?

10. What will life be like for this child in 1, 5, 10, or more years?

Managing Patient and Family Confidentiality

The Health Insurance Portability and Accountability Act of 1996 (HIPAA) is a federal law providing patients with specific rights concerning the use and disclosure of their private health information.[22] According to this law, pediatric therapists are required to provide every patient with a Notice of Privacy Practices at the start of treatment. Although the therapist is not required to obtain the patient's signature on the notice, she must make a good faith effort to obtain the patient's written acknowledgment of receiving it. Within the medical setting, a pediatric therapist is likely to receive a variety of requests to disclose confidential information about particular patients. Examples may include a phone call from a foster parent, social worker, or attorney asking the therapist to discuss the patient's treatment plan or a request from a child's parent to have a copy of the child's record of therapy. Because each scenario is unique, the course of action that a therapist may follow in a given situation depends upon the specific facts and circumstances of the request and the applicable legal and ethical standards. Keeping this in mind, it is helpful to coordinate care between therapy settings, especially when children return to the educational setting. Appropriate release of information forms should be obtained prior to sharing any information.

End-of-Life Care

Pediatric therapists can play an important role in the medical management of children and adolescents with terminal medical diagnoses. Recommendations made by therapists at earlier points in a patient's history may be modified at this point to emphasize enhancing the quality of life. Regular monitoring of the patient's status can help to facilitate this goal.[23] This care, referred to as *palliative care*, is:

> an approach that improves the quality of life of patients and their families facing the problems associated with life-threatening illness, through the prevention and relief of suffering by means of early identification and impeccable assessment and treatment of pain and other problems, physical, psychosocial and spiritual.[19]

Functional communication should be monitored to assure the patient's ability to communicate for basic needs, including physical, psychosocial, and spiritual needs. Feeding skills should also be monitored, and earlier recommendations may be adjusted considering the patient's preferences for food and drink in the context of quality of life. Positioning for comfort and sleep must be considered individually for each patient. Discussing ideas for relaxation strategies and coping methods will be essential in facilitating healthy expression of the various emotions present in palliative care.

Creating a calming sensory environment within the medical setting allows the pediatric patient and family to spend quality time together by turning off the sound of monitors, lowering the lights, and reducing the number of intravenous lines and other tubes. Together with nursing, and under the direction of doctors, therapists can facilitate a calm environment for the child with limited medical equipment in the patient's room using soft lighting and music, gentle range of motion, and positioning for comfort.[24]

ADVOCACY

As part of the interprofessional team, pediatric therapists must serve as family advocates during stressful periods of medical care. Advocating for the patient's medical needs may be necessary when the roles and responsibilities of team members are not clearly understood by others involved in the management of complex medical conditions. For example, a doctor specializing in oncology may not recognize the supports that pediatric therapists can offer (see Table 10-5). Therapists can help the entire medical team appreciate their unique services through education and collaboration, potentially enhancing the overall quality of care for pediatric patients served in their setting.

Advocacy is especially critical during discharge, when the family may need referrals to community resources and programs for support and ongoing therapy. Furthermore, collaboration between the medical team and family members can ease the child's transition back to life outside the medical setting. Discharge planning should include resources for family education and social support, information related to the purchase of needed equipment and services, and resources that will best enable the child to resume daily activities and participation in her roles at home, at school, and in the community.

SUMMARY

In the health care setting, pediatric therapists play an integral role in the management of children and adolescents with both acute and chronic medical conditions. Clinicians work together to create a collaborative plan of care for each child (including a discharge plan) based upon the patient's health outcomes. Whereas therapy provided in medical settings may be discipline-specific for certain aspects of care, the interprofessional focus of medical care is on stabilizing the health condition and on building the child's needed skills and endurance to resume regular activity. During episodes of care, the interprofessional team educates the family about the child's interventions and the prognosis for reaching desired outcomes. Finally, pediatric therapists facilitate the end of medical care, whether it results in discharge or palliative care. In all cases, the interprofessional team members abide by their ethical codes and honor patient privacy, as outlined in HIPAA.

INTERPROFESSIONAL ACTIVITY

Prognosis for Therapeutic Interventions

1. Reflect on your professional roles as they relate to discipline-specific and interprofessional care in a medical setting.

2. Read Case 10-1 and consider how this patient's diagnosis would impact your interprofessional team's interactions with the child and family members.

3. Find evidence-based research to support your plan of care and your prognosis for this patient.

4. Answer the following questions:

    a. What is the prognosis for this patient's ability to resume prior activities?

    b. How would you share prognostic information with this child and family members?

    c. What should the team consider before discharging this child from services?

    d. How could the team provide family education regarding postoperative treatment?

    e. What are the legal and/or ethical issues that are involved in dealing with this case?

Case 10-1: A 7-year-old boy diagnosed with neuroblastoma (stage 4)

By family report, Tyler was a happy, healthy first grader until very recently. His family took an extended summer vacation through several national parks, enjoying outdoor activities such as camping, hiking, swimming, and fishing. Tyler's condition was first noted when he increasingly became easily fatigued and he bruised easily when hiking with his family. Tyler also began to refuse food, complaining of feeling full. He also reported problems urinating and having bowel movements. His most recent complaints include diarrhea, fever, high blood pressure (causing irritability), rapid heartbeat, reddening (flushing) of the skin, and sweating. Tyler was admitted to the children's hospital, and medical testing ensued.

The parents were stricken by grief when tests finally revealed that he had neuroblastoma and was also diagnosed with opsoclonus-myoclonus-ataxia syndrome or *dancing eyes, dancing feet*. Surgery was scheduled for later in the week. Tyler's family wanted to explore all possible options to ensure Tyler's recovery, so the medical team suggested that

they meet with the therapists to help them understand the rehabilitation process.

Interprofessional Management of a Youth With a Spinal Cord Injury

1. Consider your knowledge and skills working with patients with spinal cord injuries.

2. Look at current evidence-based management of adolescents with spinal cord injuries.

3. Reflect on skills that are discipline-specific vs interprofessional skills.

4. Consider the risk factors facing a youth returning to school postinjury.

5. Review Case 10-2 as you consider the best approach for managing this patient.

6. Answer the following questions:

    a. How would the interprofessional team approach evaluation and treatment?

    b. What factors would affect this patient's outcome?

    c. How could the team work together to ensure that this patient is discharged safely, including given needed supports (given this patient's limited support system) and services to optimize his long-term outcomes?

Case 10-2: A 15-year-old boy in a motor vehicle accident

Brendan was hospitalized after his involvement in a high-speed motor vehicle crash. He was diagnosed with traumatic complete spinal cord injury at the level of T11, right humerus fracture, concussion/closed head injury, and right pulmonary contusion. He underwent open reduction and spinal cord decompression and posterior spinal fusion with instrumentation from the levels of T10-L2 due to his injury. He did not receive any treatment surgically for his right humerus fracture and was placed in a splint with nonweight-bearing restrictions on the right upper extremity for the first 4 weeks of his inpatient stay. He presented with complete loss of motor and sensory function below T11 and was nonweight bearing on the right upper extremity, which made transfers and progression of mobility difficult. His verbal interactions were atypical and suggestive of cognitive deficits.

Brendan had a complex social situation with little support and visitors throughout his hospitalization. At discharge, it was apparent that his caregivers' ability to assist him at home would be very limited. He lived with his father in an apartment on the second level, and his father owned a large truck. Brendan was seen by the interdisciplinary rehabilitation team from his acute state through his discharge from inpatient rehab.

Using Interprofessional Collaboration to Assist in a Patient's Diagnosis

1. Reflect on the typical growth and development of an adolescent, including the various psychosocial stressors facing students in the high school settings.

2. Review Case 10-3 regarding a 16-year-old student who had a bicycle accident.

3. After reading the case and using evidence-based resources, answer the following questions:

   a. How should the interprofessional team approach this patient's evaluation and treatment?

   b. What is the team's plan for patient/family education related to understanding the possible causes of this patient's signs and symptoms?

   c. What types of referrals or follow-up would the team recommend, if any?

   d. What factors would most likely impact Amanda's discharge from medical care?

   e. How should the interprofessional team communicate with the high school about why Amanda was missing school?

Case 10-3: A 16-year-old girl diagnosed with general anxiety disorder

Amanda's history was normal with no evidence of any mental or physical health problems until the age of 16. On her 16th birthday, she was involved in a bicycle accident on her way home from school. She reportedly fell hard on her left side, but she did not remember if she hit her head. She was reportedly wearing a helmet at the time of her accident. She had a couple of minor scrapes on her left leg from the pavement.

Because she reported dizziness, she was tested for concussion at the time of injury at the local rural hospital, and results were negative. Since the injury 5 days ago, Amanda reports that her dizziness has converted to double vision, she has difficulty swallowing "like there is a lump in my throat," and she has noticed occasional slurred words. Amanda continues to have difficulty walking and a loss of balance since the accident. Prior to the hospital visit, Amanda was attending a charter high school, where she participated in sports (basketball and soccer) and served as president of the school's Student Council. She was a straight A student and she enjoyed socializing with friends. Amanda currently lives with her stepmother and father.

Earlier this week, Amanda's visited a large urban hospital for the first time to manage her problems. Upon receiving doctor's orders for physical therapy, occupational therapy, and speech therapy, each therapist read about Amanda's medical history in the online medical chart. The therapists met interprofessionally to discuss a potential schedule for Amanda's evaluation, keeping in mind her prior reports of agitation and exhaustion from her present medical condition and the demands of an extensive evaluation by all team members. To reduce stress, the interprofessional team decided to have the occupational therapist conduct the initial evaluation to begin the process of determining Amanda's needs.

Before the occupational therapist went to Amanda's room for the evaluation, Amanda's nurse told her that many members of Amanda's family had been visiting for quite some time and she felt that it was time for them to leave. As the occupational therapist entered Amanda's room, she saw many adults and children in the room talking, while Amanda lay in bed crying. After introducing herself, the occupational therapist described her role on the rehabilitation team. Then she calmly directed the family members to leave Amanda's room to give Amanda some time to rest.

When all the extra family members had left, the occupational therapist interviewed both Amanda and her mother. Her mother reported that Amanda experienced anxiety prior to her traumatic head injury and was on medication to control her anxiety. Her mother stated that Amanda's anxiety had become much worse since she fell and that the anxiety was making it much more difficult for her to do anything. As the conversation continued, the occupational therapist made the following observations of Amanda and her room: (1) she used her right hand to hold her cell phone (which she kept close to her on her bed), (2) her window blinds were open and bright sunlight was streaming into her room, (3) her television volume was very loud, (4) she was able to move her right arm and leg fairly well, (5) she moved her left arm and leg a little more slowly while in bed, and (6) she closed her eyes often when she spoke. When asked about her vision, Amanda reported that she saw double and it made her dizzy. The occupational therapist confirmed that closing eyes is a good strategy to manage double vision.

When asked about goals for therapy, Amanda's mother shared that she wanted Amanda to return home and back to school to finish her year, including having her as independent as possible with walking, dressing, showering, driving, and being a student able to continue earning A's in school. Amanda was not able to clearly state what she wanted to work on as goals. She kept her eyes closed and moaned because of reported pain in her left leg. The occupational therapist then briefly explained the rehabilitation process to Amanda and her mother, describing her daily schedule with the physical therapist, speech-language pathologist, and occupational therapist. Amanda and her mother said they understood the proposed therapy schedule.

After the description of Amanda's plan of care and schedule, her mother asked when she could go home. She expressed that she was concerned that Amanda would fall behind in her classes and that her grades would suffer. She also worried that Amanda would lose her starting position on the soccer team. The occupational therapist responded that the decision for discharge would be discussed by many team members along with Amanda and her parents on the basis that goals were met and Amanda's medical status had improved.

REFERENCES

1. Greenwood K, Stewart E, Milton E, Hake M, Mitchell L, Sanders B. Core competencies for entry-level practice in acute care physical therapy. www.acutept.org/resource/resmgr/Core_Competencies_of_Entry-L.pdf. Published 2015. Accessed March 30, 2017.

2. American Occupational Therapy Association. Occupational therapy in acute care. American Occupational Therapy Association Web site. http://www.aota.org/About-Occupational-Therapy/Professionals/RDP/AcuteCare.aspx. Updated 2017. Accessed March 30, 2017.

3. Lockwood S. Speech language therapy in a freestanding acute care hospital. *National Student Speech Language Hearing Association Journal*. 1992;19:5-10.

4. Agency for Healthcare Research and Quality. Measure: Initial risk assessment for immobility-related pressure ulcer within 24 hours of pediatric intensive care unit (PICU) admission. Agency for Healthcare Research and Quality Web site. https://www.ahrq.gov/sites/default/files/wysiwyg/policymakers/chipra/factsheets/chipra-16-p002-1-ef.pdf. Published May 2016. Accessed March 31, 2017.

5. Odell S, Logan DE. Pediatric pain management: the multidisciplinary approach. *J Pain Res*. 2013;6:785-790.

6. Jung JS, Chang HJ, Kwon JY. Overall profile of a pediatric multidisciplinary feeding clinic. *Ann Rehabil Med*. 2016;40(4):692-701.

7. Pollack MM, Holubkov R, Glass P, et al. Functional Status Score: A new pediatric outcome measure. *Pediatrics*. 2009;124(1):e18-e28.

8. National Center for Medical Home Implementation. Pediatric care plan. National Center for Medical Home Implementation Web site. https://medicalhomes.aap.org/Documents/PediatricCarePlan.pdf. Accessed March 30, 2017.

9. Sachdeva RC, Jain S. Making the case to improve quality and reduce costs in pediatric health care. *Pediatr Clin North Am*. 2009;56(4):731-743.

10. Majnemer A. Benefits of early intervention for children with developmental disabilities. *Semin Pediatr Neurol*. 1998;5(1):62-69.

11. Ahn S, Smith ML, Altpeter M, Post L, Ory MG. Healthcare cost savings estimator tool for chronic disease self-management program: a new tool for program administrators and decision makers. *Front Public Health*. 2015;3:42.

12. American Physical Therapy Association Section on Pediatrics. Fact sheet: Role and scope of pediatric physical therapy in fitness, wellness, health promotion, and prevention. Academy of Pediatric Physical Therapy Web site. https://pediatricapta.org/includes/fact-sheets/pdfs/12%20Role%20and%20Scope%20in%20Fitness%20Health%20Promo.pdf. Published 2012. Accessed March 20, 2017.

13. American Speech-Language-Hearing Association. Position statement: Prevention of communication disorders. American Speech-Language-Hearing Association Web site. http://www.asha.org/policy/PS1988-00228/. Published 1988. Accessed March 20, 2017.

14. American Occupational Therapy Association. Occupational therapy practice framework: Domain and process (3rd edition). *Am J Occup Ther*. 2014;68(Suppl 1):S1-S48.

15. Kumar SP, Jim A. Physical therapy in palliative care: From symptom control to quality of life: A critical review. *Indian J Palliat Care*. 2010;16(3):138-146.

16. Rushton C, Reder E, Hall B, Comello K. Interdisciplinary interventions to improve pediatric palliative care and reduce health care professional suffering. *J Palliat Med*. 2006;8(4):922-933.

17. Katz A, Webb S. Committee on Bioethics. Informed consent in decision-making in pediatric practice. *Pediatrics*. 2016;138(2).

18. American Physical Therapy Association. Criteria for Standards of Practice for Physical Therapy. American Physical Therapy Association Web site. https://www.apta.org/uploadedFiles/APTAorg/About_Us/Policies/HOD/Ethics/CodeofEthics.pdf. Published 2016. Accessed March 30, 2017.

19. American Journal of Occupational Therapy. Standards of practice for occupational therapy. *Am J Occup Ther*. 2005;59:663-665.

20. American Speech-Language-Hearing Association. Code of Ethics. American Speech-Language-Hearing Association Web site. http://www.asha.org/Code-of-Ethics/. Published March 2016. Accessed March 30, 2017.

21. Lucile Packard Foundation for Children's Health. What children with medical complexity, their families, and healthcare providers deserve from an ideal healthcare system. Lucile Packard Foundation for Children's Health Web site. http://www.lpfch.org/publication/what-children-medical-complexity-their-families-and-healthcare-providers-deserve-ideal. Published December 1, 2015. Accessed March 30, 2017.

22. US Department of Health and Human Services. Summary of the HIPAA privacy rule. Department of Health and Human Service Web site. https://www.hhs.gov/hipaa/for-professionals/privacy/laws-regulations/index.html. Accessed March 30, 2017.

23. World Health Organization. WHO definition of palliative care. World Health Organization Web site. http://www.who.int/cancer/palliative/definition/en/. Accessed March 20, 2017.

24. Michelson KN, Steinhorn DM. Pediatric end-of-life issues and palliative care. *Clin Pediatr Emerg Med*. 2007;8(3):212-219.

Appendix A

Interprofessional Engagement With Children
Testing Developmental Reflexes

Catherine Rush Thompson, PT, PhD, MS

Pediatric therapists share a common knowledge of neuromotor development and appreciate reflexes commonly demonstrated by infants and children. Engaging learners in a pediatric lab experience featuring developmental reflex testing offers an opportunity for interprofessional observation, discussion, and documentation of behaviors observed during the testing session.

PREPARATION FOR TESTING

Examiner(s): Prior to Testing

- Review all the developmental reflex tests. Consider which reflexes will be performed on the infant or child.
- Make a copy of the developmental reflexes instructions and a form to document findings.
- Plan to observe the infant's/child's spontaneous behaviors before structured testing.
- Decide who will conduct the various developmental reflex tests.
- Inform the family about how to prepare for the testing session.

- Dress appropriately. (Consider various positions the learner must assume during testing—allow for flexibility and modesty.)
- Wear professional attire including a nametag.
- Remove jewelry, scarves, or perfume.
- Plan the space and equipment needed for testing:
  - Area should be clean (wiped with sterile wipes) and free of clutter (use a freshly cleaned sheet for young infants).
  - Equipment appropriate for the ages tested should be available (eg, tilt board for tilting reactions).
- Sterilize hands immediately before testing.

FAMILY

- Prepare the infant/child for testing:
  - Ensure that the infant or child is well-rested and comfortable. Typically, infants younger than 6 months are tested in diapers, whereas children older than 1 year can wear comfortable clothing (preferably shorts and a short-sleeved T-shirt).

Thompson CR. *Pediatric Therapy:*
An Interprofessional Framework for Practice (pp 165-172).
© 2018 SLACK Incorporated.

◦ Share information about the child (eg, likes, dis-likes, medical history, developmental history).

- Bring the child's favorite blanket, toys, books, etc, for comfort during testing, as needed.
- Allow about 60 minutes for the entire test and discussion with the interprofessional team after testing.
- Ask the caretaker if she has any concerns and questions.

INSTRUCTIONS

Many of these reflexes can be observed spontaneously during interactions with a young child; however, specific stimuli commonly elicit predictable responses. If the typical or normal responses are not observed during the typical time frame, there could be factors limiting the child's response. The following procedures describe the stimulus and typical response for developmental reflexes commonly observed.[1-7]

Early Reflexes

These early reflexes are commonly observed in a newborn or young infant.

Rooting Reflex

(Performed on a hungry infant.)
- Procedure: The cheek or lips are brushed by a clean finger, pacifier, or facecloth.
- Response: The lips and tongue will tend to follow in that direction. Stimulation at corners of mouth elicits head turning toward stimulus.
- Evaluation
  ◦ *Normal*: This reflex is present from 28 weeks' gestation up to 4 months, although the reflex may persist up to 7 to 8 months depending upon the infant's state of hunger and awake-sleep cycle.
  ◦ *Abnormal*: Persisting beyond 8 months. Also note that excessive salivation, difficulty breathing, froth-ing, or structural facial anomalies should be noted. Asymmetry may indicate insult to one side of the brain or facial injury. Absent in babies depressed by barbiturates.
- Significance: This early reflex may contribute to typical breast feeding and survival.

Sucking-Swallowing Reflex

- Procedure: Place a finger or nipple in the infant's mouth.
- Response: Rhythmic sucking movements.

- Evaluation:
  ◦ *Normal*: This reflex is present from 28 weeks' gesta-tion and integrated by 2 to 5 months.
  ◦ *Abnormal*: Persistence beyond 3 months or lack of response suggests neuromuscular problems. Persistence may inhibit development of voluntary sucking movements and oral sensory stimulation. Sucking is often less intense and less regular during first few days of life.
- Significance: Failure to develop interferes with nourish-ment. Slower rate is seen in nutritive sucking, which may be needed to coordinate with respiration and swal-lowing in the feeding process.

The Moro Reflex

This reflex demonstrates the acquisition of adequate strength against gravity. The development of motor skills will suppress the expression of the Moro movement pattern.
- Procedure: Place child supine with head in the midline and arms on chest. Supporting the infant's head and shoulders, allow the infant's head to drop back suddenly 20 to 30 degrees with respect to trunk.
- Response: When the head is dropped, the infant typi-cally extends and abducts the arms, then the extremities are brought to midline. Lower extremity movement is generally less obvious, but the same pattern of hip abduction and extension is normally followed by flex-ion. This reflex is normally present at 8 weeks postna-tally and may be present until 5 to 6 months of age.
- Evaluation:
  ◦ *Normal*: This reflex is present at 28 weeks' gestation and is integrated by 5 to 6 months.
  ◦ *Abnormal*: Persistence of this reflex suggests neuropathology.

Note: This reflex differs from startle reaction, which can be elicited by a loud noise or sudden light and consists of a flexor movement only.

Traction Response

- Procedure: Place child supine with head in the midline. Grasp child's forearms and pull to sitting position, stretching the shoulder adductors and arm flexors.
- Response: Flexion of the shoulders, elbows, wrists, and fingers. Increased muscle tension in the shoulder mus-cles can be felt and observed even if head lag is present.
- Evaluation:
  ◦ *Normal*: This reflex is present at 28 weeks' gestation and is integrated by 5 to 6 months.

○ *Abnormal*: Lack of response or persistence suggests neuromuscular pathology.

• Significance: Persistence may inhibit voluntary reach and grasp.

Palmar Grasp

This reflex allows the infant to hold a rattle when placed in her hand.

• Procedure: Place infant supine with head in the midline and hands free. Place index finger in infant's palm from the ulnar side and gently press against the palmar surface.

• Response: Infant's fingers will flex around the examiner's finger.

• Evaluation:
  ○ *Normal*: This reflex is present at 28 weeks' gestation and is integrated by 5 to 6 months. Infants show differential responses to hard and soft objects.
  ○ *Abnormal*: Lack of response or persistence suggests neuromuscular pathology.

• Significance: Persistence may inhibit development of volitional grasp and release.

Plantar Grasp

Suppression may occur through experience standing at a support, cruising, and walking with and without assistance because these activities promote more functional postures for the toes.

• Procedure: Place child in supine with head in midline and legs relaxed. Exert pressure against the soles of infant's foot, directly below toes. This reflex can also be tested in standing.

• Response: Flexion of toes.

• Evaluation:
  ○ *Normal*: This reflex is present at 28 weeks' gestation and is integrated by 9 months. Infants show differential responses to hard and soft objects.
  ○ *Abnormal*: Lack of response or persistence suggests neuromuscular pathology.

• Significance: Persistence may inhibit development of volitional grasp and release.

Neonatal Neck-Righting Reaction

This is an immature rolling pattern that lacks trunk rotation and trunk segmentation.

• Procedure: Place child supine with head in midline and extremities extended. Rotate head to one side actively or passively.

• Response: The child will follow the direction of the head turn and roll toward that side without segmental rotation (this is a "log-roll").

• Evaluation:
  ○ *Normal*: This reflex is present at 34 weeks' gestation and is generally integrated by 4 to 5 months.
  ○ *Abnormal*: Persistence beyond 5 months. By 10 months, an infant will typically roll independently using this reflex to assist in voluntary movement. If it is much stronger in one direction than another, this is a red flag for possible neuromuscular impairment.

• Significance: This reflex allows child to roll supine to side and side to supine. Persistence may interfere with the development of segmental rolling. The individual may have difficulties with other movement patterns that require rotational components or may fail to develop a variety of movement patterns and thus be limited to more stereotypical responses.

Neck-Righting Acting on the Body

• Procedure: Place child supine with head in midline and extremities extended. Turn the child's head to one side and hold in this position with jaw over shoulder.

• Response: The child rolls segmentally in direction of head turning.

• Evaluation:
  ○ *Normal*: This reflex is seen at 4 to 6 months.
  ○ *Abnormal*: This reflex is typically integrated at 5 years (when child can get to standing without rotation).

• Significance: This reflex allows the child to roll supine to prone and prone to supine. This reflex is indicative of the development of rotation around the body axis (intra-axial rotation) and allows for rotational patterns necessary for rolling, attaining sitting, sitting, and standing.

Neonatal Body Righting

• Procedure: Place child supine with head in midline. Flex one leg up toward the chest, and rotate the child's leg across the body, rolling the baby over.

• Response: The child's thorax, chest, and head will follow the direction of the pelvis, and the body will roll toward that side without segmental rotation (log roll).

• Evaluation:
  ○ *Normal*: This reflex is typically seen at 34 weeks' gestation and is integrated at 4 to 5 months.
  ○ *Abnormal*: This reflex is abnormal if it persists beyond 5 months.

- Significance: This reflex allows child to roll supine to side and side to supine. Asymmetry is not normal. Persistence interferes with the development of segmental rolling and acquisition of other developmental milestones that require rotation (see neck on body righting reflex).

Body-Righting Reaction Acting on the Body

- Procedure: Place child in supine with head in midline and extremities extended. Flex one leg and rotate it across the pelvis to the opposite side.
- Response: Child will roll segmentally to prone (ie, first the trunk, then the pectoral girdle, and finally the head).
- Evaluation:
  - *Normal*: This reflex typically begins at 4 to 6 months and is integrated by 5 years (when child can get to standing without rotation).
  - *Abnormal*: Persistent and obligatory responses beyond 5 years.
- Significance: This reflex allows child to roll supine to prone and prone to supine. It is indicative of the development of rotation around the body axis (intra-axial rotation) and allows for rotational patterns necessary for rolling, attaining sitting, sitting, and standing.

Flexor Withdrawal

Do this test last because it can be noxious to the infant and can cause crying.

- Procedure: Place child supine with head in midline and legs relaxed and semiflexed. Apply a noxious stimulus, such as pin prick, to sole of one foot.
- Response: Brisk flexion of stimulated limb, withdrawing from the stimulus; includes toe extension, dorsiflexion, and hip/knee flexion.
- Evaluation:
  - *Normal*: This reflex typically begins at 28 weeks' gestation and is integrated by 1 to 2 months or when independent walking occurs.
  - *Abnormal*: Persistence of this reflex when walking occurs.
- Significance: Persistence may indicate a delay in postural maturation.

Note: This is a protective response that is never completely inhibited although it loses dominance.

Crossed Extension

- Procedure: Place child supine with head in midline. Hold one lower extremity extended at the knee and apply firm pressure or noxious stimulus to sole of the foot.

- Response: Flexion, adduction, and then extension of the opposite lower extremity as if to push the examiner away. If the stimulated extremity is not fixed, the stimulated leg will withdraw, and the opposite extremity will extend.
- Evaluation:
  - *Normal*: The onset of this reflex is 28 weeks' gestation, with integration at 4 months.
  - *Abnormal*: The absence of this reflex in the young infant or its persistence beyond 4 months is suspect.
- Significance: Failure to obtain or late persistence may indicate general depression of the central nervous system or sensorimotor dysfunction. Persistence may prevent typical reciprocal kicking and subsequent walking.

Proprioceptive Placing (Upper or Lower Extremity) (Placing Reaction)

- Procedure: Hold the child in a vertical position with examiner's hands under the arms and around the chest. Move the child so that the dorsum of one hand or foot presses lightly against the edge of the table.
- Response: Infant will flex arm or leg respectively and place hand or foot on the table.
- Evaluation:
  - *Onset*: The upper extremity placing reaction begins at birth in the full-term infant.
  - *Abnormal*: Absence in early infancy or persistence are suspect.
- Significance: Correlates with spontaneous stepping (stepping reflex). May be obtained at any age if traction is exerted against the ankle or the wrist to the point of discomfort.

Visual Placing

- Procedure: Hold the child vertically under the arms and around the chest. Advance the child toward a supporting surface such as a table top.
- Response: Child will lift hand, extend it, and place it on the support with fingers extended and abducted or will immediately orient and place foot on top of supporting surface.
- Evaluation:
  - *Normal*: This reflex begins at 3 to 5 months and persists throughout life.
  - *Abnormal*: Absent or delayed response.
- Significance: This reflex requires visual input, relied on for both postural control and guidance for locomotor progression. This reflex is associated with independent walking and is important for weight bearing.

Neonatal Positive Support

- Procedure: Hold infant in the vertical position with examiner's hands under the arms and around the chest. Allow feet to make firm contact with the tabletop or other flat surface.
- Response: Simultaneous contraction of flexors and extensors in lower extremities so as to bear weight on the lower extremities. The child supports only minimal amount of body weight, characterized by partial flexion of the hips and knees.
- Evaluation:
  - *Normal*: This reflex begins at 35 weeks' gestation and is generally integrated by 1 to 2 months.
  - *Abnormal*: Absence or persistence of this reflex.
- Significance: This is a prerequisite for spontaneous stepping reflex. A typical response is needed for erect standing and bipedal locomotion.

Positive Support Reaction (Lower Extremity)

- Procedure: Support infant in the vertical position with examiner's hands under the arms and around the chest. Allow feet to make firm contact with the tabletop or other flat surface.
- Response: Simultaneous contraction of the lower extremity flexors and extensors for full weight bearing on the lower extremities with hips and knees extended.
- Evaluation:
  - *Normal*: The onset is 6 to 9 months and persists throughout life.
  - *Abnormal*: Absence or delayed response.
- Significance: Neonatal positive support gradually merges into active standing. The infant may show periods of nonweight bearing (astasia).

Positive Support Reaction (Upper Extremity)

- Procedure: Place child prone on floor or lower child to surface to allow contact.
- Response: Simultaneous contraction of flexors and extensors in upper extremity for full weight bearing with shoulder flexion and elbow/wrist extension. An exaggerated or atypical response involves extensor muscles dominating flexors (ie, shoulders are internally rotated and adducted, elbows extended, wrists flexed, and ulnarly deviated with hands fisted).
- Evaluation:
  - *Normal*: The onset is 3 to 6 months and persists throughout life.
  - *Abnormal*: Absence or delayed response.

- Significance: This reflex allows for creeping, attaining sitting, and standing positions; allows for development of shoulder stabilization and protective reactions; and prevents total effectiveness of protective reactions if absent.

Spontaneous Stepping (Stepping Reflex or Automatic Walking)

- Procedure: Support the infant in the vertical position with examiner's hands under the arms and around the chest with the child's feet touching the table surface. Incline the child forward and gently move the child forward to accompany any stepping.
- Response: Child will make alternating, rhythmical, and coordinated stepping movements.
- Evaluation: The standing posture includes some flexion of the hip and knee. Automatic stepping may also be observed when the newborn is inclined forward while being supported in this position. During the first 4 months of life, the crouching position gradually diminishes; this is followed by increase in support, so that typical infants will usually support a substantial proportion of their weight by 10 months. Scissoring or standing on the toes are red flags for neuromuscular impairment. The feet may be examined for structural anomalies such as clubfoot.
  - *Normal*: The onset is 37 weeks' gestation and is integrated by 2 months.
  - *Abnormal*: Absence or persistence.
- Significance: Identical to kicking but different from early true walking. May show nonstepping phase (abasia). Stepping reaction is integrated in parallel with neonatal positive supporting. Disappearance may be result of dramatic increase in the mass of the legs, which can no longer be raised against gravity.

Attitudinal Postural Reflexes

Attitudinal reflexes are those that are associated with emerging muscle tone.

Asymmetrical Tonic Neck Reflex

- Procedure: Place child supine with head in midline (can also test in sitting, quadruped, or standing, depending on child's age). Turn child's head to one side either passively or actively (have child follow an object from one side to the other).
- Response: The infant tends to assume a fencing position, with his face toward the extended arm, while the other arm flexes at the elbow. The lower limbs respond

in a similar manner. The arm and leg on the face side extend; arm and leg on skull side flex OR increase in extensor tone noted in face limbs and flexor tone in skull limbs.

- Evaluation:
  - *Normal*: Onset as early as 28 to 38 weeks (lower extremities before upper extremities), commonly seen at 2 to 4 months, and integrated by 6 months. Response is never totally obligatory in a typical infant; usually seen more as a posture (ie, fencer's position).
  - *Abnormal*: Absence or persistence. Its presence after 7 months suggests neurological impairment and the need for a medical referral.
- Significance: In full-term infants, upper extremities participate more strongly than lower extremities. Persistence may interfere with development of typical rolling pattern, hand-to-mouth and hand-to-body exploration, visually directed reaching, midline hand activity, and symmetrical head lifting. Persistence may lead to scoliosis or hip subluxation.

Symmetrical Tonic Neck Reflex

- Procedure: Place the child in quadruped position or prone over the examiner's knee. Passively flex and then extend the child's head.
- Response: Flexion of the head produces flexion of the upper extremities and extension of the lower extremities. Extension of the head produces extension of the upper extremities and flexion of the lower extremities. There is no reciprocal movement.
- Evaluation:
  - *Normal*: Onset at 4 to 6 months and integration at 8 to 12 months.
  - *Abnormal*: Absence of muscle tone.
- Significance: Integration of this reflex coincides with crawling in 4-point position. Persistence may inhibit development of reciprocal creeping; the child will bunny-hop instead. Persistence may inhibit development of typical sitting posture.

Tonic Labyrinthine Reflex

- Procedure: Place child prone or supine with head in midline. Observe the child's tone and posture or try to passively move the head and limbs.
- Response: In prone, flexor tone dominates; child will not lift head or support weight on arms. In supine, extensor tone dominates; child will not flex in pull to sit.

- Evaluation:
  - *Normal*: The onset of this reflex can be as early as 38 weeks' gestation and integration at 6 months.
  - *Abnormal*: Absence in early infancy and/or persistence beyond 6 months is abnormal.
- Significance: Persistent obligatory response may prevent development of head lifting prone and/or supine, development of prone on elbows, rising to sitting, rolling, bringing hands to midline, and hand-to-mouth and hand-to-body exploration. Persistence may interfere with all activities requiring a controlled balance between flexors and extensors.

Galant Reflex (Incurvatum of the Trunk)

- Procedure: Place infant in prone in typical alignment. Gently stimulate with fingernail along paravertebral line about 3 cm from midline from shoulder to buttocks.
- Response: Lateral flexion of the trunk toward the side of the stimulus.
- Evaluation:
  - *Normal*: Onset begins at 32 weeks' gestation and integration by 2 months.
  - *Abnormal*: No response.
- Significance: This is one of the most common reflexes in typically developing newborns. Persistent response may lead to scoliosis.

Landau Reflex

- Procedure: Hold the infant in the air horizontally in the prone position. Be certain to offer full body support under the infant's abdomen, allowing the upper trunk and legs to move freely against gravity.
- Response: Extension of the neck and trunk with possible extension of the lower extremities against gravity.
- Evaluation:
  - *Normal*: Onset at 3 months and integration between 12 to 24 months.
  - *Abnormal*: Lack of extension of the neck and trunk or an exaggerated response with stiff extension of the entire body.
- Significance: This reflex indicates the infant's ability to move the body against gravity. An inability to move against gravity suggests low muscle tone and/or muscle weakness. An exaggerated response suggests increased muscle tone.

Righting Reactions

Optical Righting Reflex

- Procedure: Examiner holds the child in space prone, supine, or vertical and tilts the child in the vertical position; prone and supine position itself is stimulus.
- Response: Child rights head against gravity.
- Evaluation:
  - *Normal*: Onset at 2 months and persists throughout life.
  - *Abnormal*: Lack of response.
- Significance: Allows child to lift head in prone or supine and secures position of head in space.

Labyrinthine Head-Righting Reaction

The stimulus is the same procedure as above; however, you perform the test with the child's eyes closed or covered. A small bandana can be used to cover the eyes, but this is generally not tolerated for very long.

Landau Reflex (Sagittal Plane Righting Reflex)

- Procedure: Holding the infant in vertical suspension with the head, spine, and legs extended, the examiner passively flexes the head forward.
- Response: Total body flexion with neck flexion is seen as early as 3 months. At 6 months, vertical suspension elicits extension of the head, neck, and trunk.
- Evaluation:
  - *Normal*: Onset at 3 to 4 months, peaks at 5 to 6 months, and integration at 12 to 24 months.
  - *Abnormal*: Absence associated with muscle weakness or decreased extensor activity.
- Significance: Not an isolated reaction; produced by labyrinthine righting, optical righting, body-righting acting on the body, body-righting acting on the head, and neck righting. This reflex coincides with ability to assume pivot-prone or Superman posture.

Equilibrium Reactions

Protective Extension Forward (Upper Extremity) (Parachute Reaction)

- Procedure: Support infant in inverted vertical position in space with hands around the infant's body. Carefully plunge child downward toward a table or other flat surface.
- Response: Upper extremities will extend and abduct; fingers will extend and abduct as if to break the fall.

- Evaluation:
  - *Normal*: Onset at 6 to 9 months and persists throughout life.
  - *Abnormal*: Absence or delayed response.
- Significance: Coincides with ability to bring extended upper extremities forward for reaching out and bearing weight.

Protective Extension Sideward (Upper Extremity) (Propping Reaction)

- Procedure: Place child in sitting with legs out in front. Push child on one shoulder with enough force to displace center of gravity and cause child to lose balance.
- Response: Child will abduct arm with extension of elbow, wrist, and fingers on the side opposite of force and take weight on an open hand.
- Evaluation:
  - *Normal*: Onset at 7 months and persists throughout life.
  - *Abnormal*: Absence or delayed responses.
- Significance: Followed by positive supporting reaction as soon as contact is made with the surface.

Protective Extension Backward (Upper Extremity) (Propping Reaction)

- Procedure: Place child in sitting with legs out in front. Push child backward with enough force to displace center of gravity and cause child to lose balance.
- Response: Child will extend arms backward; full reaction involves backward extension of both arms. Frequently, an element of trunk rotation is seen and only one arm extends.
- Evaluation:
  - *Normal*: Onset is 9 to 10 months and persists throughout life.
  - *Abnormal*: Absence or delayed responses.
- Significance: Onset overlaps with other protective reactions of the upper extremities.

Protective Extension Downward (Lower Extremity) (Downward Parachute Reaction)

- Procedure: Hold child in vertical suspension and plunge child downward toward surface.
- Response: Lower extremities externally rotate and abduct and feet dorsiflex in preparation for standing.
- Evaluation:
  - *Normal*: Onset at 4 months and persists throughout life.

○ *Abnormal*: Absence or delayed response.

• Significance: Breaks a fall by extension of the knee joint.

Protective Staggering (Lower Extremity)

• Procedure: With child standing on solid surface, push child in all directions (forward, backward, and sideways).

• Response: Child will make corrective movements with limbs to restore center of gravity (eg, take steps forward or back, cross one foot over the other).

• Evaluation:
  ○ *Normal*: Onset at 15 to 18 months and persists throughout life.
  ○ *Abnormal*: Absence or delayed response.

• Significance: Keeps the body oriented in space when displaced by an external horizontal force. This reflex is needed for safe and independent ambulation.

Tilting Reactions

Tilting Reactions Dependent Upon Postures Tested

• Procedure: For each test, the therapist positions the child in the appropriate position (eg, prone, supine, sitting, quadruped, kneeling, or standing on a tilt board).

• Responses (dependent upon position tested):
  ○ Prone and supine: Child's trunk is curved away from the tilt, with the concavity of the spine upward; slight abduction of the upper arm and leg may be seen.
  ○ Sitting: To lateral tilt, body is laterally flexed away from the tilt, concavity of the spine upward, arm and leg on upper side abducted; to anterior tilt—spine extends and limbs retract; to posterior tilt—spine flexes and limbs advance.
  ○ Quadruped: To lateral tilt, body is laterally flexed away from the tilt with concavity of the spine upward; the head is slightly rotated so that the face turns toward the upper side; the arm and the leg on the upper side flex and the arm and leg on the lower side extend and abduct.
  ○ Standing: To lateral tilt, body is laterally flexed away from the tilt with the concavity of the spine upward; upper leg is flexed and upper arm abducted; lower leg is extended and strongly braced; to anterior tilt —spine extends, displacing the body backward, legs

extend, arms extend and are retracted; to posterior tilt—spine flexes, displacing the body forward, legs extend, shoulders are flexed and elbows extended

• Evaluation:
  ○ *Normal*: Typical onset for this reflex varies with postures used in testing: prone, 5 months; supine, 7 months; sitting, 7 to 8 months; quadruped, 9 months; standing, 12 to 21 months. Integration—persists throughout life.

• Significance: Adults rely most heavily on proprioceptive input, whereas children rely on visual input for postural orientation. These reflexes are necessary for maintenance of balance in all postures.

VIDEO RESOURCE

PediNeuroLogic Exam. http://library.med.utah.edu/pedineurologicexam/html/newborn_n.html. Updated August 2016. Accessed March 30, 2017.

The "Pediatric Neurologic Exam: A Neurodevelopmental Approach" uses over 145 video demonstrations and narrative descriptions in an online tutorial. It presents the neurological examination of the pediatric patient as couched within the context of neurodevelopmental milestones for newborns, 3-month-olds, 6-month-olds, 12-month-olds, 18-month-olds, and 2-and-a-half-year-olds.

REFERENCES

1. Meyers RK. Reflex testing methods for evaluating CNS development. Pediatrics. 1964;33(1).
2. New York State Department of Health. Motor disorders: Assessment and intervention for young children (age 03 years). https://www.health.ny.gov/publications/4961.pdf. Published 2011. Accessed March 30, 2017.
3. O'Dell N. The symmetric tonic neck reflex (STNR). http://www.ndc-brain.com/articles/SymmetricTonicNeckReflex.pdf. Accessed March 10, 2017.
4. Schott JM, Rossor MN. The grasp and other primitive reflexes. *J Neurol Neurosurg Psychiatr.* 2003;74(5):558-560.
5. Sohn M, Ahn L, Lee S. Assessment of primitive reflexes in high-risk newborns. *J Clin Med Res.* 2011;3(6):285-290.
6. Stanford Children's Health. Newborn reflexes. http://www.stanfordchildrens.org/en/topic/default?id=newborn-reflexes-90-P02630. Accessed March 30, 2017.
7. Mitchell RG. The Landau reaction (reflex). *Dev Med Child Neurol.* 1962;4(1):65-70.

Appendix B

Interprofessional Communication
Selecting Tests and Measures

Catherine Rush Thompson, PT, PhD, MS

Below are listed a sampling of tests used across a variety of pediatric therapy settings. Although this list is not exhaustive, it offers a range of tests that may be considered when collecting data for decision making. Learners should select the optimal measures for a given testing situation, including the situation. The situation takes into account the following:

- Demographics/characteristics of the child being assessed (eg, age, medical condition)
- Setting/specific location of testing (space for quiet test administration)
- Availability of assessment measures (available testing equipment with criteria)
- Examiner's training, familiarity with the test, and ability to perform the test reliably
- Outcomes desired from the evaluation (eg, providing information to qualify a child for services)
- Interprofessional team members (expertise, skills, concerns, and observations; keep in mind that certain tests are discipline-specific and/or require advanced training)

Consider the various cases presented throughout this book and assessments (tests and measures) that could provide the needed information to help solve the problems that these children are encountering.

1. Select a case study from one of the sections in this book.
2. Look at the following categories of tests to select appropriate assessments to provided needed information to solve problems.
3. In the selection process, ask the following:
   - Is the measure valid for the information being sought?
   - Is the measure reliable and adequately sensitive for testing and retesting a child?
   - Is the measure well designed for the population being tested?
   - Is the measure a survey or questionnaire that can be given to the parent/caregiver/teacher/child?
   - Is the measure norm referenced or criterion referenced? (Consider: Does the test need to be norm referenced to determine eligibility for services?)

Thompson CR. *Pediatric Therapy:
An Interprofessional Framework for Practice* (pp 173-180).
© 2018 SLACK Incorporated.

- Does the assessment need to be performed one-on-one with the child or does it lend itself to team administration (eg, observation of skills)?
  - Is the measure efficient for collecting needed data in a reasonable amount of time, given the child's condition?
4. In your interprofessional team, discuss your rationale for using each selected test. If the tests listed below do not provide needed information, search to see if another test exists that meets desired criteria.
5. As a team, discuss how you would inform the family about assessments selected (providing your rationale regarding how the test addresses specific concerns while avoiding jargon).

PEDIATRIC TESTS AND MEASURES

The following are examples of pediatric tests and measures listed alphabetically under their respective categories. Note that some categories overlap. Check current literature for the most recent edition of each test, as well as populations that have been successfully evaluated with each measure.[1-7]

Activities (see also Development, Fine Motor, Functional/Adaptive, Gross Motor, and Speech)

- Activities Scale for Kids (ASK)

Anthropometrics

- Observation of body dimensions, body composition, height/weight, leg length, body mass index, chest circumference, skinfold tests

Arousal (see also Behavior/Emotional Social)

- Adelaide Coma Scale
- Coma Near Coma (CNC) Scale
- Coma Recovery Scale Revised (CRSR)
- Orientation Scale
- Pediatric Glascow Coma Scale (pGCS)

Behavior/Emotional/Social (see also Cognitive/Adaptive Behavior)[8]

- Achenbach Child Behavior Checklist
- ADHD Rating Scale-IV
- Autism Behavior Checklist (ABC)
- Autism Diagnostic Observation Scale

- Behavioral and Emotional Screening System Student Self-report Form (BESS)
- Brief Infant-Toddler Social and Emotional Assessment (BITSEA)
- Carey Temperament Scales
- Childhood Autism Rating Scale (CARS)
- Devereux Early Childhood Assessment—Clinical Form (DECA-C)
- Devereux Early Childhood Assessment for Infants and Toddlers (DECA I/T)
- Disruptive Behavior Rating Scale
- Early Coping Inventory
- Evaluating Acquired Skills in Communication (EASIC)
- Functional Emotional Assessment Scale (FEAS)
- Gilliam Autism Rating Scale (GARS)
- Infant-Toddler Social and Emotional Assessment (ITSEA)
- Modified Checklist for Autism in Toddlers, Revised with Follow-Up (M-CHAT-R/F)
- NICU Network Neurobehavioral Scale (NNNS)
- Patient Health Questionnaire
- Screen for Child Anxiety Related Emotional Disorders
- Temperament & Behavior Scale (TABS)
- Vineland Social-Emotional Early Childhood Scale

Cardiopulmonary

- Blood pressure, heart rate, incentive spirometry, oxygen saturation, respiratory pattern and rate, skin color

Cognitive/Adaptive Behavior

- Bay Area Functional Performance Evaluation (BAFPE)
- Bayley Scales of Infant and Toddler Development (Third Edition)
- California Verbal Learning Test Children's Version (CVLT-C)
- Cogstate Brief Battery (CBB)
- Columbia Mental Maturity Scale (CMMS)
- Conners' Continuous Performance Test II (CPT II)
- Dynamic Occupational Therapy Cognitive Assessment for Children
- Functional Emotional Assessment Scales (FEAS)
- Kaufman Assessment Battery for Children (Second Edition) (KABC-II)
- Lowenstein Occupational Therapy Cognitive Assessment
- McCarthy Scales of Children's Abilities (MSCA)

- NEPSY: A Developmental Neuropsychological Assessment
- Peabody Individual Achievement Test-revised (PIAT-R)
- Raven Progressive Matrices (RPM)
- Rey-Osterrieth Complex Figure Test (ROCF)
- Scales of Cognitive Ability for Traumatic Brain Injury (for adolescents)
- Stanford-Binet Intelligence Scales (5th Edition) (SB-5)
- Trail Making Test (TMT)
- Vineland Adaptive Behavior Scales (VABS)
- Wechsler Individual Achievement Test (Second Edition) (WIAT-II)
- Wechsler Preschool and Primary Scale of Intelligence (Third Edition) (WPPSI-III)
- Wide Range Achievement Test 3 (WRAT-3)
- Wide Range Assessment of Memory and Learning (WRAML)
- Woodcock-Johnson III Tests of Achievement (WJ III Ach)
- Woodcock-Johnson III Tests of Cognitive Abilities (WJ-III Cog)

Communication

- Communication and Symbolic Behavior Scales: Developmental Profile
- MacArthur-Bates Communicative Development Inventories
- Peabody Picture Vocabulary Test (Third Edition) (PPVT-III)
- Preschool Language Scale-5 (PLS-5)
- Receptive Expressive Emergent Language Scale III (REEL III)
- Receptive One Word Picture Vocabulary Test
- Reynell Developmental Language Scales—American Version
- Rosetti Infant Toddler Language Scale
- Sequenced Inventory of Communication Development (SICD)
- SKI-HI Learning Development Scales (Hearing Impaired 0-3)
- Test of Early Communication and Emerging Language

Coordination

- Clinical Observation of Motor and Postural Skills (COMPS)
- Florida Apraxia Screening Test
- Gross Motor Performance Measure (GMPM)

- Lafayette Grooved Pegboard (GPT)
- Selective Control Assessment of the Lower Extremity
- Test of Ideational Praxis

Development

- Ages & Stages Questionnaires (ASQ-3)
- Alberta Infant Motor Scale
- Assessment, Evaluation, and Programming System for Infants and Toddlers (Second Edition) (AEPS)
- Batelle Developmental Inventory (Second Edition)
- Bayley Infant Neurodevelopmental Screener (BINS)
- Bayley Scale of Infant Development (Third Edition)
- Brigance Inventory of Early Development III (IED III)
- Carolina Curriculum for Infant and Toddlers with Special Needs (CCITSN)
- Carolina Curriculum for Preschoolers with Special Needs (CCPSN)
- Developmental Assessment of Young Children-2 (DAYC-2)
- Developmental Profile 3
- Early Learning Accomplishment Profile (ELAP)
- FirstSTEp Screening Test for Evaluating Preschoolers Motor Skills Acquisition in the First Year and Checklist
- Hawaii Early Learning Profile (HELP)
- Infant Toddler Developmental Assessment (IDA)
- Infant Development Inventory (IDI)
- INSITE (for visually/multi-sensory impaired)
- Merrill-Palmer–R Scales of Development (M-P-R)
- Movement Assessment Battery for Children (Movement ABC-2)
- Mullen Scales of Early Learning (MSEL)
- Peabody Developmental Motor Scales (Second Edition) (PDMS-2)

Endurance/Energy Expenditure

- Early Activity Scale for Endurance (EASE)
- Energy Expenditure Index
- 6-Minute Walk Test
- 30-Second Walk Test

Environment

- Pediatric Environmental Home Assessment[9]

Fine Motor

- Assisting Hand Assessment

- Bruininks-Oseretsky Test of Motor Proficiency (BOTP-2)
- Erhardt Developmental Prehension Assessment
- Evaluation Tool of Children's Handwriting
- Halstead–Reitan Grip Strength Test
- Harris Infant Motor Test (HINT)
- Jebsen Taylor Test of Hand Function
- Melbourne Unilateral Upper Limb Function (MUUL)
- Nine-Hole Peg Test
- Peabody Developmental Motor Scales (Second Edition) (PDMS-2)
- Shriner's Upper Extremity Assessment

Fitness

- FitnessGram
- Presidential Physical Fitness Test
- Sit and Reach Test

Functional/Adaptive Skills

- Canadian Occupational Performance Measure (COPM)
- Do-Eat Assessment Evaluation ToolKit
- Functional Independence Measure (WeeFIM)
- Goal-Oriented Assessment of Life Skills (GOAL)
- Oral-Motor/Feeding Scale
- Pediatric Evaluation of Disability Inventory (PEDI)/ PEDI-CAT
- POSNA Pediatric Musculoskeletal Functional Health Questionnaire
- Vineland Adaptive Behavior Scales

Gross Motor

- Alberta Infant Motor Scale (AIMS)
- Bruininks-Oseretsky Test of Motor Proficiency (BOTP-2)
- Dynamic Gait Index (DGI)
- Functional Mobility Assessment
- Gross Motor Function Measure (GMFM)
- Gross Motor Performance Measure
- High Level Mobility Assessment Tool (HIMAT)
- Motor Function Measure
- Observational Gait Scale (OGS)
- Peabody Developmental Motor Scales (Second Edition) (PDMS-2)
- Standardized Walking Obstacle Course
- Test of Gross Motor Development (Second Edition) (TGMD-2)

- Test of Infant Motor Performance (TIMP)
- Timed Obstacle Ambulation Test
- Timed Up and Down Stairs Test
- Timed "Up & Go" (TUG)
- Toddler and Infant Motor Evaluation (TIME)

Health Status

- Child Health and Illness Profile Adolescent Edition (CHIP-E)
- Child Health Assessment Questionnaire (CHAQ)
- Child Health Questionnaire (CHQ)
- Health Utilities Index-Mark

Hearing

- Conditioning Play Audiometry (CPA)
- Early Listening Function (ELF)
- Evoked Otoacoustic Emissions (OAE)
- Pure tone hearing test (air)
- Select Picture audiometry
- Speech Awareness Thresholds (SAT)
- Speech Discrimination Test
- Tympanometry Visual Reinforcement Audiometry (VRA)

Integumentary

- Lund Browder Chart
- Observation of skin color/skin turgor
- Pediatric Burn Assessment
- Starkid Skin Scale

Language Comprehension

- Clinical Evaluation of Language Fundamentals-4 (CELF-4)
- Comprehensive Assessment of Spoken Language (CASL)
- Fullerton Language Test for Adolescents (Second Edition)
- Functional Communication Profile
- Oral-Written Language Scale (OWLS)
- Oral-Written Language Scale-2 (OWLS-2)
- Test of Adolescent and Adult Language (Third Edition) (TOAL-3)
- Test of Language Development-Intermediate (Third Edition) (TOLD-I:3)
- Test of Language Development-Primary (Third Edition) (TOLD-P:3)

Language Development—Preschool

- Clinical Evaluation of Language Fundamentals-Preschool (CELF-pre)
- Preschool Language Assessment Instrument (PLAI)
- Preschool Language Scale-5 (PLS-5)
- Receptive-Expressive Emergent Language Test (Third Edition) (REEL-3)
- Rossetti Infant-Toddler Language Scale
- Structured Photographic Expressive Language Test-Preschool (SPELT-P)
- Test of Early Language Development (Second Edition) (TELD-2)

Language Expression

- Expressive Language Test (ELT)
- HELP Test—Elementary
- Patterned Elicitation Syntax Test (PEST)
- Structured Photographic Expressive Language Test (Third Edition) (SPELT-3)
- Test for Examining Expressive Morphology (TEEM)
- Test of Narrative Language (TNL)
- WORD Test—Adolescent
- WORD Test—Elementary

Language—Receptive

- Language Processing Test—Revised (LPT-R)
- Listening Test
- Rhode Island Test of Language Structure (RITLS)
- Test of Auditory Comprehension of Language (Third Edition) (TACL-3)
- Token Test for Children

Language—Vocabulary

- Assessing Semantic Skills through Everyday Themes (ASSET)
- Carolina Picture Vocabulary Test for Deaf and Hearing Impaired (CPVT)
- Comprehensive Receptive and Expressive Vocabulary Test (Second Edition) (CREVT-2)
- Expressive One-Word Picture Vocabulary Test (EOWPVT)
- Expressive One-Word Picture Vocabulary Test-Upper Extension (EOWPVT-UE)
- Expressive Vocabulary Test (EVT)
- Peabody Picture Vocabulary Test-III (PPVT-III)
- Receptive One-Word Picture Vocabulary Test (ROWPVT)

Mental Health/Coping

- Abuse Assessment Screening
- Bright Futures Surveillance Questions
- Depression Scale for Children (CES-DC)
- Devereux Early Childhood Assessment (DECA)
- Early Coping Inventory
- Multidimensional Scale of Social Support Parent Stress Inventory
- Revised Children's Anxiety and Depression Scale
- SAD PERSONS Scale (for suicide risk)
- Strengths and Difficulties Questionnaire

Motor Planning/Motor Processing Skills

- Assessment of Motor and Processing Skills (AMPS)
- Kaufman Speech Praxis Test for Children (KSPT)
- Motor Planning Maze Assessment
- School Assessment of Motor and Processing Skills (AMPS)

Neurological

- Quick Neurological Screening Test-II (QNST-II)

Oral Speech

- Stuttering Prediction Instrument
- Stuttering Severity Instrument (Third Edition) (SSI-3)
- Stuttering Severity Scale
- Test of Childhood Stuttering (TOCS)

Pain

- Behavioral Pain Scale
- Children's Hospital of Eastern Ontario Pain Scale (CHEOPS)
- CRIES Scale (Cries, Require Oxygen, Increased Vital Signs, Expression, Sleep)
- FACES Pain Scale
- FLACC (Faces, Legs, Activity, Crying, Consolability Behavioral Pain Scale)
- Individualized Numeric Pain Scale (INRS)
- Infant Pain Scale (IPS)
- Neonatal Pain, Agitation and Sedation Scale (NPASS)
- Numeric Scale
- Oucher Scale
- Visual Analog Scale (VAS)

Participation

- Adaptive Behavior and Participation Scales
- Adaptive Behavior Scales (VINELAND-II OR VABS)
- Assessment of Functional Living Skills (AFLS)
- Developmental Assessment for Individuals with Severe Disabilities–Third Edition (DASH-3)
- Functional Assessment and Curriculum for Teaching Everyday Routines (FACTER)
- Functional Independence Skills Handbook (FISH)
- Scales of Independent Behavior-Revised (SIB-R)
- School Function Assessment (SFA)

Personal Factors

- HABITS questionnaire[10,11]
- Pediatric Motivation Scale

Play

- Knox Preschool Play Scale
- Preschool Play Scale
- Revised Children's Assessment of Participation and Enjoyment and Preferences for Activities of Children (CAPE/PAC)
- Test of Playfulness (ToP)
- Transdisciplinary Play-Based Assessment, Second Edition (TPBA2)

Posture/Balance

- Early Clinical Assessment of Balance (ECAB)
- Movement Assessment of Infants (MAI)
- Pediatric Balance Scale (PBS)
- Pediatric Clinical Test of Sensory Interaction for Balance (P-CTSIB)
- Pediatric Reach Test (Pediatric Functional Reach Test)
- Timed Up and Down Stairs Test

Quality of Life/Participation

- Assessment of Life Habits (LIFE-H)
- Canadian Occupational Performance Measure (COPM)
- Child Occupational Self-Assessment
- Children's Assessment of Participation and Enjoyment (CAPE)
- Kidscreen
- Miller Function and Participation Scales
- Participation and Environment Measure-Children and Youth (PEM-CY)

- Pediatric Outcomes Data Collection Instrument (PODCI)
- Pediatric Quality of Life Inventory (PEDS QL)
- Preferences for Activities of Children (PAC)
- Quality of Well Being Scale (QWB)
- School Function Assessment (SFA)
- Short Child Occupational Profile
- Spinal Cord Injury—Quality of Life Anxiety
- Spinal Cord Injury—Quality of Life Psychological Trauma
- Vineland Adaptive Quality of Life: Child Health Index of Life with Disabilities

Range of Motion

- Ely's Test
- Hamstring Length Test
- Modified Ober Test
- Popliteal Angle
- Prone Hip Extension Test
- Spinal Alignment and Range of Motion Measure (SAROMM)
- Straight Leg Test
- Thomas Test

Reflexes (Developmental Reflexes: see Appendix A)

- Movement Assessment of Infants (MAI)
- Peabody Developmental Motor Scales (Second Edition) (PDMS-2)

Sensory Integrity

- Cranial nerve testing, sensory testing of superficial and combined sensations

Sensory Integration and Praxis

- Sensory Integration and Praxis Test (SIPT)

Sensory Processing

- Adolescent/Adult Sensory Profile
- Child Sensory Profile 2
- Sensory Integration and Praxis Test
- Sensory Processing Measure (SPM)
- Sensory Profile
- Test of Sensory Functioning in Infants

Spasticity

- Modified Ashworth Scale (MAS)
- Modified Tardieu Test

Speech—Articulation

- Arizona-3
- Clinical Assessment of Articulation and Phonology (CAAP)
- Contextual Probes of Articulation Competence (CPAC)
- Fisher-Logemann Test of Articulation Competence
- Goldman Fristoe Test of Articulation-2 (GFTA-2)
- Hodson Assessment of Phonological Patterns-3 (HAPP-3)
- Photo Articulation Test (Third Edition) (PAT-3)
- Weiss Comprehensive Articulation Test (WCAT)

Speech—Phonology

- Assessment Link between Phonology and Articulation (ALPHA)
- Assessment of Phonological Processes-Revised (APP-R)
- Comprehensive Test of Phonological Processing (CTOPP)
- Hodson Assessment of Phonological Patterns-Third Edition (HAPP-3)
- Khan-Lewis Phonological Analysis-2 (KLPA-2)
- Phonological Awareness Test

Strength/Muscle Power

- Dynamometry
- Manual muscle testing
- Selective Control Assessment of the Lower Extremity (SCALE)

Structural Integrity

- Adam Forward Bend Test
- Anterior/Posterior Drawer Test
- Apley's Test
- Arch Index
- Beighton Scale of Hypermobility
- Craig's Test
- Galleazi Sign
- Heel Bisector Angle
- Lachman's Test
- McMurray's Test
- Navicular Drop Test
- Ryder's Test
- Talar Tilt
- Transmaleolar Axis

Swallowing

- Endoscopic assessment
- Modified barium swallow
- Observation (posture, behavior, oral motor control)

Vision/Visual Motor/Perception

- Beery-Buktenica Developmental Test of Visual-Motor Integration (6th Edition) (Beery Vmi)
- Bender Visual Motor Gestalt Test (Bender)
- Developmental Test of Visual Motor Integration
- Developmental Test of Visual Perception (DTVP-2)
- Motor Free Visual Perception Test (4th Edition) (MVPT-4)
- Oregon Project Global Assessment Tool
- Test of Visual Motor Skills-3 (TVMS-3)

REFERENCES

The list of measures is adapted from a combination of sources listed below:

1. American Academy of Pediatrics. Mental health screening and assessment tools for primary care. https://www.aap.org/en-us/advocacy-and-policy/aap-health-initiatives/Mental-Health/Documents/MH_ScreeningChart.pdf. Accessed April 2, 2017.
2. American Physical Therapy Association, Section on Pediatrics. List of pediatric assessment tools categorized by ICF model. https://pediatricapta.org/includes/fact-sheets/pdfs/13%20Assessment&screening%20tools.pdf. Published 2012. Accessed March 30, 2017.
3. Home Speech Home. 90+ speech therapy test descriptions and report outlines. http://www.home-speech-home.com/speech-therapy-test-descriptions.html. Accessed April 2, 2017.
4. American Speech-Language-Hearing Association. Feeding and swallowing disorders (dysphagia) in children. http://www.asha.org/public/speech/swallowing/Feeding-and-Swallowing-Disorders-in-Children/. Accessed April 2, 2017.
5. East Michigan University Library. Occupational therapy – Tests, assessments, tools and measures. http://guides.emich.edu/c.php?g=259436&p=2081301. Accessed April 1, 2017.
6. Illinois Department of Human Services. arly Intervention Approved Evaluation and Assessment Instruments. http://www.dhs.state.il.us/page.aspx?item=86067. Published August 1, 2016. Accessed December 11, 2017.
7. Rehabilitation Institute of Chicago, Center for Rehabilitation Outcomes Research, Northwestern University Feinberg School of Medicine Department of Medical Social Sciences Informatics Group. Rehabilitation measures database. http://www.rehabmeasures.org/default.aspx. Accessed March 31, 2017.
8. Campbell JM, Brown RT, Cavanagh SE, Vess SF, Segall MJ. Evidence-based assessment of cognitive functioning in pediatric psychology. *J Pediatr Psychol*. 2008;33(9):999-1014.

9. National Center for Healthy Housing. Pediatric environmental home assessment. http://healthyhousingsolutions.com/wp-content/uploads/2014/12/HHAPP_Ex_2_PEHA_Survey-Nov2013.pdf. Accessed April 4, 2017.

10. Tatla SK, Jarus T, Virji-Babul N, Holsti L. The development of the Pediatric Motivation Scale for rehabilitation. *Can J Occup Ther.* 2015;82(2):93-105.

11. Wright ND, Groisman-Perelstein AE, Wylie-Rosett J, Vernon N, Diamantis PM, Isasi CR. A lifestyle assessment and intervention tool for pediatric weight management: the HABITS questionnaire. *J Hum Nutr Diet.* 2011;24(1):96-100.

Appendix C

Interprofessional Collaboration
Wheelchair and Seating Evaluation

Catherine Rush Thompson, PT, PhD, MS

The interprofessional team should work closely together with children and their families to buy needed assistive technology, including assistive, adaptive, and rehabilitative devices for mobility, communication, and engagement in daily activities. A wheelchair can be a costly piece of customized equipment, so detailed features and accessories for the wheelchair should be discussed by all team members before recommending a specific model with expensive adaptations.

The wheelchair evaluation begins with an interview of the child and family, focusing on the family's needs, their daily routines, and general lifestyle. For children who spend time outside of the home (eg, preschool, school, sports activities, community activities), others' inputs are critical for determining whether one chair is suitable to meet the child's needs and what special features are needed to meet multiple demands. Those with the greatest expertise, generally the pediatric therapists, should offer recommendations for optimal positioning and functioning in the wheelchair. Those typically involved in wheelchair and seating teams include the physical therapist, the child (if old enough to contribute ideas), family members involved in decision making, a family advocate (if needed), the occupational therapist, the speech therapist, and the rehabilitation technology supplier/durable medical equipment vendor.

Examples of questions to ask the family and others include the following:

1. What are the purposes of the wheelchair (eg, mobility, therapeutic positioning, sports, recreation, travel, classroom activities)?

2. What features are most important to the child and the family?

3. What activities will the wheelchair be used for less frequently?

4. What daily activities must be accommodated (eg, use of computer or assistive technology, carrying objects, moving through narrow spaces, use on rugged terrain)?

5. Where will the wheelchair be used the most (eg, home, school, transportation, community)?

6. How will the wheelchair be moved from place to place (eg, self-propelled, motorized, collapsible)? The team should consider distances inside the home, at the school, and in the community to determine whether

Thompson CR. *Pediatric Therapy:*
An Interprofessional Framework for Practice (pp 181-182).
© 2018 SLACK Incorporated.

the child has the ability to maneuver in a wide range of environments.

7. How much of the day will the child be spending in the wheelchair?

8. Does the wheelchair have features that will allow functional independence (eg, transfers, fine motor function, self-feeding)?

9. Does the wheelchair have features that enable safe mobility and transportation (eg, anti-tip devices, locks)?

10. What environmental features should be considered (eg, various surfaces, slopes, doorways)?

11. What is the cost, and who pays for the wheelchair?

12. How soon can the wheelchair arrive (to address possible growth between when the wheelchair is ordered and when it arrives)?

13. When is the child eligible for another new wheelchair (to take into account the need for potential growth over several years)?

The team should consider the range of options available, including the weight of the wheelchair, its portability, its versatility, and its ability to tilt in space, among others. A comprehensive summary with findings and recommendations can outline special features that the team justifies for a medical prescription. A letter of justification is typically written by a person familiar with the child/family and the product recommended, then signed by a physician. Usually it is a therapist, but, in some cases, experienced rehabilitation technology suppliers write them. This letter takes the recommendations that come out of the evaluation team and correlates them to the features of a recommended wheelchair or seating system. This letter of justification helps the third-party payer understand why certain features or characteristics of the recommended equipment are *medically necessary*. It is important to state the long-term benefits of recommended features, which can include the following:

- Bone growth and postural alignment
- Strengthening of antigravity muscles
- Development of eye-hand coordination
- Opportunity for cognitive growth
- Respiratory activity
- Development of postural control
- Social acceptance
- Improved self-esteem
- Participation in daily activities
- Mobility (potentially independent)

As a team, make recommendations for the following case studies:

1. Bobby is a 22-month-old with transverse myelitis at the C6 level (comparable to a complete C6 lesion). He needs a mobility device in his early childhood special education setting.

2. Joanie is a 6-year-old with cerebral palsy (spastic quadraparesis). She has poor head control, moderate spasticity of her extremities, and low tone in her trunk. She is nonambulatory and nonverbal, and her gross and fine motor skills are significantly impaired. She can move a lever forward 2 inches with her right hand, she can log roll from prone to supine, and she has difficulties with feeding and swallowing. Her home is full of equipment: therapy balls, mats, a stander, and a few different adapted chairs. At home, Joanie spends most of her day on the floor. The elementary school and family are seeking a wheelchair that will enable Joanie to participate in the activities throughout the school day while ensuring safety when Joanie is bused to and from school.

Appendix D

Pediatric Professional Role Play
A Case for Assistive Technology

Pamela Hart, PhD, CCC-SLP

The goal of this case is to encourage critical thinking regarding the design and use of augmentative and alternative communication (AAC) strategies for individuals with cerebral palsy or other severe speech and physical impairments.

BASIC LEARNING OBJECTIVES

The learner will:
1. Define assistive technology and AAC.
2. Describe the roles of various professionals who work with individuals who use AAC strategies.
3. Describe the communication needs of individuals with cerebral palsy.
4. Describe why AAC is often needed for individuals with cerebral palsy and how this affects the development of speech skills.
5. Define human factors and how these apply to everyday life.

6. Explain the importance of various types of human factors and how these impact the successful implementation of AAC.
7. Apply Baker's ergonomic equation to the study of human factors and AAC.

CASE DESCRIPTION

Bailey is a 7-year-old girl with cerebral palsy who is unable to walk or speak. She has limited functional use of her hands and is dependent on her caregivers for most activities of daily living, such as bathing, eating, and mobility. Due to her severe physical impairments, Bailey is unable to communicate verbally. Instead, she communicates by pointing to pictures that represent various basic needs, such as "hungry," "tired," and "pain." The picture cards are kept on her wheelchair tray and are also laminated on a communication board for times when she is not in her wheelchair. Bailey attends school in a program for children with orthopedic impairments. Her parents have also sought outside services for Bailey at a pediatric rehabilitation, where she works

Thompson CR. *Pediatric Therapy:*
An Interprofessional Framework for Practice (pp 183-187).
© 2018 SLACK Incorporated.

with a variety of professionals, including a speech-language pathologist, occupational therapist, physical therapist, and consultant special education teacher. Additionally, Bailey receives care from her pediatrician, neurologist, and orthopedic specialist on a regular basis. Bailey's health concerns include (a) mild strabismus, (b) limited fine and gross motor skills, (c) inability to communicate verbally, and (d) a mild intellectual impairment.

For the most part, Bailey understands everything that is said to her, but she is extremely limited in her ability to respond. She has a form of spastic cerebral palsy that results in hypertonic muscles, which makes volitional movement of her extremities difficult to control. Recently, Bailey's speech-language pathologist suggested the team begin to explore AAC devices to assist Bailey with her ability to make a wider range of needs known and understood. The team has decided to meet as a group and discuss Bailey's strengths, needs, and potential to benefit from AAC. Some of the dialog from this initial meeting is provided here:

Speech-language pathologist: "Thank you for taking the time to meet today. I would like to discuss Bailey's communication challenges. She is working hard in therapy to vocalize sounds, but it is difficult, and she hasn't progressed as much as I would have liked. She is doing well communicating basic wants and needs with her picture cards on her wheelchair tray. I think it is time to consider a high-tech AAC device that will allow her to have access to unlimited vocabulary to meet both her social and academic needs."

Bailey's mom: "Will using an AAC device keep Bailey from learning how to speak? I really want her to continue working on developing her speech skills."

Speech-language pathologist: "No, if anything, AAC helps to promote verbal speech development. Bailey will be able to relax and communicate for longer periods of time, which will also help her general level of language development too."

Occupational therapist: "I think it is a good idea to try AAC. My concern is whether she will be able to access the device with her hands. She is able to isolate a finger to point, but the devices require varying levels of pressure to activate the messages, and I'm not sure if she will be successful with that."

Speech-language pathologist: "Yes, I think potentially there will be several areas to problem solve as we try this. The devices can be adjusted to allow for differing levels of sensitivity, and we can also put a key guard over the screen to help with her accuracy."

Physical therapist: "I think we will need to be cautious that we do not wear her out with requiring too much motor control to access the device. I think we should start slow and maybe just use the device during certain activities to let her become familiar and see how she responds."

Speech-language pathologist: "I will be able to obtain some devices on loan through the assistive technology loan

library. We will have the devices for several weeks so we can try them out in different settings without requiring too much of her all at one time."

Occupational therapist: "Visually, she should do okay differentiating between the pictures on the communication device screen. I think the main challenge will be getting Bailey excited to use the device and finding access methods that will allow her to be as independent as possible."

BASIC KNOWLEDGE QUESTIONS

1. What is cerebral palsy? When and how does it occur?

2. What are the characteristics of spastic cerebral palsy? How do these characteristics differ from ataxic and dyskinetic cerebral palsy?

3. Describe the professional roles of speech-language pathologists, occupational therapists, and physical therapists in working with children who have severe speech and physical impairments such as cerebral palsy.

4. Why do you think is it important to use an interdisciplinary team when working to determine appropriate assistive technologies for clients with severe physical and communication impairments?

ASSISTIVE TECHNOLOGY AND AUGMENTATIVE AND ALTERNATIVE COMMUNICATION

Assistive technology includes any devices or equipment used to give individuals with special needs the ability to participate as fully as possible in their family, community, educational, and vocational needs. It includes items such as assistive listening devices, prosthetics, adapted computer access, mobility aids, environmental control aids, adapted play tools, and AAC devices. Most humans are able to meet their communication needs by verbal speech. However, for some individuals, physical and/or cognitive impairments limit the effectiveness of their verbal speech communication. AAC is one type of assistive technology designed to help individuals with severe speech impairments to communicate.

Populations who benefit from AAC include children and adults with developmental disabilities such as autism and Down syndrome, physical disabilities affecting speech production such as cerebral palsy, and acquired disabilities such as traumatic brain injury and stroke. AAC strategies range from high-tech computerized systems for voice output to low-tech picture-based systems and communication books. The goal is to help the individual to become a more competent communicator.[1] The myth that using AAC will hinder or limit verbal speech production has long been disproven. It has been found that in individuals with developmental disabilities, AAC increases verbal speech production modestly.[2,3]

APPLICATION QUESTIONS: AAC AND ASSISTIVE TECHNOLOGY

1. Why is it important to involve an interdisciplinary team in the assessment of individuals who require assistive technology?
2. Search for vendors of assistive technology equipment on the internet. Review the equipment and describe some of the assistive technologies for mobility and communication that might benefit individuals such as Bailey.
3. How might the assistive technology needs of individuals with congenital disabilities differ from those with acquired disabilities?
4. Critique the following systematic review and discuss the ideas presented by the authors that AAC promotes rather than hinders verbal speech development.[2]

HUMAN FACTORS

Human factors is a field of study that analyzes the ways that human beings interact with technology. Formally defined by the International Ergonomics Association, human factors is "the scientific discipline concerned with the understanding of the interactions among humans and other elements of a system, and the profession that applies theoretical principles, data and methods to design in order to optimize human well-being and overall system performance."[4]

This type of analysis helps technology companies develop equipment that is safe and easy to operate and has built-in error prevention strategies. In daily life, human factors has many implications. For example, in many cars, the fuel gauge is on the same side of the dashboard as the fuel tank is positioned on the outside of the car. This way, drivers know which side of the car needs to be next to the gas pump when pulling into a gas station. Don Norman's book, *The Design of Everyday Things*, explores and critiques daily life experiences with design. For example, Norman describes the experiences of a friend who became trapped between 2 sets of doors because the design of the doors made it difficult to determine whether they should be pushed or pulled, and they lacked handles or other cues. Human factors affect our lives every-day as we attempt to interact with devices and technologies that sometimes do not lend themelves to error free or obvious use.

Human factors is a critical component of any AAC device. Individuals who require AAC often experience not only communication problems but also fine motor, gross motor, vision, cognitive, and hearing difficulties. As such, considerations of the global needs of the individual must be considered when choosing an AAC device. Baker's ergonomic equation (1986) provides a way to understand how human factors impact the success or failure of assistive technologies and AAC. In this equation, the motivation of the individual to use the assistive technology must exceed the sum of the physical effort, cognitive effort, linguistic effort, and time load to operate the technology. Physical effort includes the individual's ability to produce the motor movements that result in accurate activation and use of the assistive technology. Cognitive effort consists of the level of cognitive resources required to understand and operate the technology. Specifically related to AAC, cognitive effort includes the individual's ability to remember where the messages are stored within the device, the ability to problem solve when communication breakdowns occur, and the ability to go through the multiple steps of the communication process using the device. Linguistic effort is the individual's ability to understand the mode of language representation within the AAC device. Options for representing linguistic information include written words, line drawings, colored pictures, and/or photos of real objects. The level of abstractness the individual is able to understand related to their ability to use symbols to represent language impacts their ability to understand what the pictures within the device represent. Time load is how long it takes the individual to work through the sometimes multiple steps to create and activate a message. Motivation is sometimes misunderstood in AAC. Most individuals are highly motivated to communicate, but their ability to realize this goal will be largely impacted by their team's ability to anticipate and balance the human factors of physical, cognitive, linguistic, and time load to make this possible. If a person with a communication impairment is told that she will be given a check for $1000.00 if she can say the word "eat," it could be assumed the individual is highly motivated. If, however, there is no efficient or effective means the individual is able to use to convey this message, all the motivation in the world will not enable her the ability to communicate the word "eat."

APPLICATION QUESTIONS: HUMAN FACTORS

1. Describe a time when your motivation to learn a new piece of technology was not enough to overcome the

cognitive, time, physical, and/or linguistic load factors to learn the new technology.

2. Describe a time when you were highly motivated to learn to use a piece of technology but the design of the technology made it very difficult to understand. What do you think could have been improved within the design of the technology to correct this?

3. What are ways to decrease the cognitive load for an individual learning to use an AAC device?

4. What are ways to decrease the physical load for an individual with cerebral palsy who is learning to use a high-tech AAC device?

5. What would be some ways to decrease the linguistic load factors for an individual who was struggling to learn how to use his AAC device because the symbols were too abstract?

6. How does the concept of motivation apply to individuals learning to communicate via AAC?

TEAM DECISION

After the initial meeting, Bailey's team decided to conduct an 8-week trial with a high-tech dedicated AAC device. During the evaluation, Bailey was able to use direct selection (pointing and pushing with her finger) to make selections on the AAC device as long as there are no more than 6 pictures/messages on each page. This required Bailey to access multiple levels of the device to find the relevant vocabulary for meal times. For example, Bailey chose the icon for "food" from the main page, which then took her to another screen, where she selected either breakfast, lunch, dinner, or snacks. Once she selected an item on this page, she was taken to another set of icons, where she chose the particular food item she would like to have.

1. Working in groups, visit the websites for manufacturers of high tech AAC devices such as DynaVox and Prentke Romich. Review the communication devices on the websites and discuss the pros and cons of each device for a child such as Bailey. Develop a table to compare and contrast the features of 5 devices that your group believes could provide Bailey with adequate vocabulary and a feasible access method for her current and future needs.

2. Explain how the initial setup described previously (multiple pages with a few choices on each page) would affect the physical, cognitive, linguistic, and time load factors for Bailey.

After completing a few weeks of the trial, Bailey's occupational therapist informs the team that she feels it might be easier for Bailey to have more choices on each page. With this change, however, Bailey will no longer be able to use direct selection to activate the device. Instead, she will need to use a switch and an automatic scanning option within the device so that when she pushes the switch, the device begins to highlight the messages on the screen one at a time, and when the correct message is highlighted, Bailey pushes the switch again to choose that message.

1. Explain how this change will affect the various human factors across cognitive, linguistic, physical, and time considerations.

2. Review websites for manufacturers of various switched input products such as AbleNet and Enabling Devices. Which type of switch do you think might work best for Bailey to access with a light touch of her finger?

Bailey's speech-language pathologist knows that Bailey needs access to a lot of vocabulary to be able to demonstrate her academic and personal knowledge. She also wants Bailey to communicate to meet many functions and intentions of communication. She advocates for the vocabulary of the device to include messages that help Bailey meet several language functions, including requesting, asking questions, establishing social closeness, and using her imagination when she is playing.

1. Why is it not enough for Bailey to have a means to communicate her basic wants and needs?

2. Think of all the different ways you use communication in a typical day. Make a list of all the categories of vocabulary words you need. Now, consider Bailey's needs in home, community, and school environments and make a list of additional vocabulary Bailey will need to be a successful communicator.

3. Discuss how the role of the assistive technology team in Bailey's case will change and grow now that Bailey has a communication device. What do you see as the role of each team member as Bailey moves through the next few years of school? Specifically, answer the following:

   a. Who will make sure vocabulary is updated on a regular basis?

   b. What will be the expectation for home use if Bailey is already able to use nonverbal strategies to communicate at home?

   c. Who will provide caregiver training on the features and maintenance of the device?

   d. If the device needs to be sent out for repairs, what is the backup plan to allow Bailey to communicate while waiting for repairs to be made to the device?

REFERENCES

1. Beukelman DR, Mirenda P. *AAC: Supporting Children and Adults with Complex Communication Needs*. 4th ed. Baltimore, MD: Paul H. Brookes; 2013.
2. Millar DC, Light JC, Schlosser RW. The impact of augmentative and alternative communication intervention on the speech production of individuals with developmental disabilities: A research review. *J Speech Lang Hear Res*. 2006;49:248-264.
3. Romski M. Augmentative communication and early intervention: Myths and realities. *Infants and Young Children*. 2005;18(3):174-185.
4. King TW. Assistive Technology: Essential Human Factors. Needham Heights, MA: Allyn & Bacon; 1999.

TEACHING RESOURCE

Buzolich M. Collaborative Teaming for students who require AT/AAC. Augmentative Communication & Technology Services Web site. http://www.acts-at.com/resources/AAC-PROGRAM-SUPPORT/Buzolich%20Collaborative%20Teaming.pdf. Accessed December 11, 2017.

Appendix E

Evaluating and Using Professional Websites

Catherine Rush Thompson, PT, PhD, MS

WEBSITE EVALUATION

It is important to evaluate each source of information to determine whether it is authentic, accurate, objective, and current. The following sites offer rubrics and other resources for evaluating websites:

- Cornell University Library. Evaluating Web Pages: Questions to Consider: Categories. http://guides. library.cornell.edu/evaluating_Web_pages. Accessed March 25, 2017.
- University of Maryland. University Library Guides: JOUR202 - Editing for the Mass Media - Evaluating Websites. http://lib.guides.umd.edu/c. php?g=327107&p=2195123. Published Nov 9, 2017. Accessed December 11, 2017.
- University of Southern Maine. USM Libraries. Checklist for Evaluating Web Resources. https://usm.maine.edu/ library/checklist-evaluating-web-resources. Publication 2017. Accessed December 11, 2017.

Select a relevant topic of interest, find a website featuring this topic, and review the website using evaluation criteria suggested above. Would you recommend this site as a good source of information for your interprofessional team? Would you recommend it for use by families of children with special needs? If so, provide your rationale for recommending it. If not, describe what is missing based upon your evaluation of the resource.

PROFESSIONAL WEBSITES FOR PEDIATRIC THERAPISTS

- American Physical Therapy Association: www.apta.org
- American Occupational Therapy Association: www.aota.org
- American Speech-Language-Hearing Association: www.asha.org

WEBSITES FOR FAMILIES AND PROFESSIONALS

- American Academy of Pediatrics: Healthy Children: https://www.healthychildren.org/English/Pages/default.aspx

Thompson CR. *Pediatric Therapy:*
An Interprofessional Framework for Practice (pp 189-190).
© 2018 SLACK Incorporated.

- American Association on Intellectual and Developmental Disabilities: https://aaidd.org/home
- The Arc: For People with Intellectual and Developmental Disabilities: www.thearc.org/
- Center for Disease Control and Prevention: Children Diseases: https://www.cdc.gov/parents/children/diseases_conditions.html
- Easter Seals: http://www.easterseals.com
- Family Voices: http://www.familyvoices.org/
- Federation for Children with Special Needs: http://fcsn.org/
- Friendship Circle: http://www.friendshipcircle.com/
- Goodwill Industries: http://www.goodwill.org/
- Medscape: Look for "Pediatrics" http://emedicine.medscape.com/

- National Institutes for Mental Health: Child and Adolescent Mental Health: https://www.nimh.nih.gov/health/topics/child-and-adolescent-mental-health/index.shtml
- National Association of Councils on Developmental Disabilities: http://nacdd.org/
- Parents Helping Parents: http://www.php.com/
- Pathways: Information on Typical and Atypical Child Development: www.pathways.org
- Pediatric Therapy Network: http://www.pediatrictherapynetwork.org/
- Special Needs Alliance: http://www.specialneedsalliance.org/
- Special Olympics: http://www.specialolympics.org/
- United Cerebral Palsy: http://ucp.org/

Appendix F

Educational Resources
Videos and Books Related to Pediatric Therapy

Catherine Rush Thompson, PT, PhD, MS

RECOMMENDED BOOKS RELATED TO PEDIATRIC THERAPY

Interprofessional Reference Books

- *1001 Pediatric Treatment Activities: Creative Ideas for Therapy Sessions* by Ayelet H. Danto
- *Early Childhood* by Barbara Chandler
- *Imaging in Pediatrics (First Edition)* by Arnold Carlson Merrow and Selena L Hariharan
- *Neonatal and Pediatric Pharmacology: Therapeutic Principles in Practice* by Jacob V. Aranda, MD, PhD, FRCP(C) and Sumner J. Yaffe, MD
- *Pediatric Rehabilitation: Principles and Practice (Fifth Edition)* by Michael A. Alexander, MD and Dennis J. Matthews, MD
- *Pediatrics (Series: Rehabilitation Medicine Quick Reference)* by Maureen R. Nelson, MD

Occupational Therapy

- *Best Practices for Occupational Therapy in Schools* by Gloria Frolek Clark and Barbara Chandler
- *Collaborating for Student Success: A Guide for School-Based Occupational Therapy (Second Edition)* by Barbara Hanft and Jayne Shepherd
- *Kids Can be Kids: A Childhood Occupations Approach* by Shelly J. Lane and Anita C. Bundy
- *Occupational Therapy Evaluation for Children: A Pocket Guide (Second Edition)* by Shelley E. Mulligan, PhD, OTR
- *Occupational Therapy for Children and Adolescents (Seventh Edition)* by Jane Case-Smith EdD, OTR/L, FAOTA and Jane Clifford O'Brien, PhD, OTR/L
- *Pediatric Occupational Therapy and Early Intervention* by Jane Case-Smith, EdD, OTR/L, FAOTA
- *Pediatric Occupational Therapy Handbook: A Guide to Diagnoses and Evidence-Based Interventions* by Patricia Bowyer, EdD, OTR/L, BCN and Susan M. Cahill, MAEA, OTR/L

Thompson CR. *Pediatric Therapy:*
An Interprofessional Framework for Practice (pp 191-193).
© 2018 SLACK Incorporated.

Physical Therapy

- *Campbell's Physical Therapy for Children Expert Consult (Fifth Edition)* by Robert J. Palisano, Margo Orlin, and Joseph Schreiber
- *Pediatric Physical Therapy (Fifth Edition)* by Jan Tecklin
- Peds Rehab Notes: Evaluation and Intervention Pocket Guide by Robin L. Dole
- *Physical Therapy for Children (Fourth Edition)* by Suzann K. Campbell, Robert J. Palisano, and Margo Orlin

Speech-Language Pathology

- *Communication Assessment and Intervention with Infants and Toddlers* by Barbara Weitzner-Lin
- *Helping Children to Improve Their Communication Skills: Therapeutic Activities for Teachers, Parents and Therapists* by Deborah Plummer
- *Intervention in Child Language Disorders* by Ronald B. Hoodin
- *Language and Communication Disorders in Children (Sixth Edition)* by Deena K. Bernstein

VIDEOS RELATED TO PEDIATRIC THERAPY

These following videos are posted on YouTube and provide audiovisual information that may help in demonstrating key concepts addressed in the various practice settings. Note that these videos were produced and posed with voluntary permission by those who appear in the video and are publicly available. These videos may be used, unaltered, for professional development (with appropriate citation).

Neonatal Intensive Care

- "Days in the Life: NICU" (https://www.youtube.com/watch?v=Zt7R-4LmusY)
- "How do Neonatal Therapists work with OT/PT/SLP in NICU?" (https://www.youtube.com/watch?v=ovDJeuoN7Us)
- "Neonatal Intensive Care for Premature Baby" (https://www.youtube.com/watch?v=AFGkNAeE4Wo&list=PLotU4X0mUnSXwscLg7NIBk6RcH0uAvX8C&index=7)

Early Intervention

- "10 Early Signs of Autism" (https://www.youtube.com/watch?v=r1CqboCzxSc)

- CONNECT Modules: Instructor Supports: http://community.fpg.unc.edu/connect-modules/instructor-supports. CONNECT (The Center to Mobilize Early Childhood Knowledge) provides videos and activities for an evidence-based practice approach to professional development.
- CONNECT Videos: https://www.youtube.com/playlist?list=PLBB64DAC64304E785. The Center to Mobilize Early Childhood Knowledge (CONNECT) created a series of 139 web-based modules for national educational use by early childhood instructors and learners, including Foundations of Inclusion Birth to Five and Early Intervention: A Routines-Based Approach—Part 1: Traditional vs Routines.
- "Early Intervention: Helping babies with visual impairments" (https://www.youtube.com/watch?v=6rbHOAtBNew)
- "Early Intervention Home Visits" (https://www.youtube.com/watch?v=8fOJGmIdj0c)

Early Childhood Special Education

- "Challenging Behavior in Young Children" (https://www.youtube.com/watch?v=8eCfnrGu5xo)
- "Peek into early childhood education: Meet Billy" (https://www.youtube.com/watch?v=a0NAptuWZz4)
- "Lee Ann Britain Infant Development Center"(https://www.youtube.com/watch?v=CKeByRhRGxE) The Lee Ann Britain Infant Development Center is dedicated to serving children with developmental disabilities from birth to 6 years of age. The Lee Ann Britain Infant Development Center uses a unique program that gets siblings and parents involved in the process of therapeutic treatment and education.
- "Go Baby Go! - Mobility for kids with disabilities" (https://www.youtube.com/watch?v=kW_gzM3iGlM)

Elementary School

- "ABA Autism Classroom Case Study 2008" (https://www.youtube.com/watch?v=w9N0_7D_Re8)
- "Engaging Families and Creating Trusting Partnerships to Improve Child and Family Outcomes" (https://www.youtube.com/watch?v=fvwVOi_8Xd0)

High School

- "My Transition Story" (https://www.youtube.com/watch?v=WXqkuZkJ5Xo)
- "Popular Special Education Videos" (https://www.youtube.com/playlist?list=PLIXtN8GZ_10ypqBORZLMfz_p-fp_J6h2F)

Medical Care (Inpatient, Outpatient, Rehabilitation, and Clinic Care)

- "Brachial Plexus Center/Cincinnati Children's" (https://www.youtube.com/watch?v=q_kzRJVZ4S8)
- "Burn Care Splinting" (PT/OT splinting for burn patients) (https://www.youtube.com/watch?v=2VMlvntxSco)
- "Child Pain Management" (https://www.youtube.com/watch?v=wBpPwGpkiIY)
- "Pediatric Occupational and Speech Therapy" (https://www.youtube.com/watch?v=PGb3hFFXwfw)
- "Physical Therapy and Occupational Therapy" (https://www.youtube.com/watch?v=iXu0ntBTEXg)
- "What is Feeding Therapy? Sample Session from JCFS' Integrated Pediatric Interventions" (https://www.youtube.com/watch?v=X2nGk2DoOt8)

Accommodations and Modifications

- "Accommodations and Modifications for Students with Disabilities" (https://www.youtube.com/watch?v=O0xdaCEqrU0)
- "iPads for Special Needs" (https://www.youtube.com/watch?v=So2eDnKosJc)
- "iPads & Autism at Manhattan Childrens Center by Andrew J Parsons 2010" (https://www.youtube.com/watch?v=OZmpQj7WhBc)
- "Kids Like Me (with disabilities)—I believe!" (https://www.youtube.com/watch?v=wJQQtM6240s)

Index